Applied Ethics in Mental Health

Basic Bioethics
Arthur Caplan, editor

A complete list of the books in the Basic Bioethics series appears at the back of this book.

Applied Ethics in Mental Health Care
An Interdisciplinary Reader

edited by Dominic A. Sisti, Arthur L. Caplan, and
Hila Rimon-Greenspan

The MIT Press
Cambridge, Massachusetts
London, England

MIT Press books may be purchased at special quantity discounts for business or sales promotional use. For information, please email special_sales@mitpress.mit.edu or write to Special Sales Department, The MIT Press, 55 Hayward Street, Cambridge, MA 02142.

This book was set in Sabon by Toppan Best-set Premedia Limited, Hong Kong. Printed and bound in the United States of America.

Library of Congress Cataloging-in-Publication Data

Applied ethics in mental health care : an interdisciplinary reader / edited by Dominic A. Sisti, Arthur L. Caplan, and Hila Rimon-Greenspan.
    p. ; cm. — (Basic bioethics)
Includes bibliographical references and index.
ISBN 978-0-262-01968-2 (hardcover : alk. paper)—ISBN 978-0-262-52501-5 (pbk. : alk. paper)
I. Sisti, Dominic A. II. Caplan, Arthur L. III. Rimon-Greenspan, Hila. IV. Series: Basic bioethics.
[DNLM: 1. Psychiatry—ethics. 2. Patient Rights—ethics. 3. Professional-Patient Relations—ethics. 4. Psychotherapy—ethics. 5. Substance-Related Disorders—therapy. WM   21]
RC455.2.E8   2013
174.2'9689—dc23
2013011580

10   9   8   7   6   5   4   3   2   1

Contents

Series Foreword

I am pleased to present the thirty-eighth book in the Basic Bioethics series. The series makes innovative works in bioethics available to a broad audience and introduces seminal scholarly manuscripts, state-of-the-art reference works, and textbooks. Topics engaged include the philosophy of medicine, advancing genetics and biotechnology, end-of-life care, health and social policy, and the empirical study of biomedical life. Interdisciplinary work is encouraged.

Arthur Caplan

Basic Bioethics Series Editorial Board
Joseph J. Fins
Rosamond Rhodes
Nadia N. Sawicki
Jan Helge Solbakk

Foreword

For mental health professionals, there is no scarcity of ethical challenges. Some of the conundra that arise in everyday mental health work derive from the nature of the disorders and conditions that mental health professionals evaluate and treat. A second set of ethical issues originates in the treatments we use. Additional layers of moral complexity are contributed by the settings in which mental health professionals work. Taken together, it can safely be said that ethical challenges inhere in every aspect of mental health practice.

Mental disorders themselves create a variety of dilemmas. Severe conditions such as schizophrenia or bipolar disorder, and to a lesser extent depression, can impair decision-making capacity, at the extreme rendering patients unable to make competent decisions for themselves. Determining when the line has been crossed from impairment to incapacity involves the application of normative conclusions about the necessary preconditions for decisional autonomy to complicated factual situations. Who determines incapacity, with what degree of protection for the rights of the patient, and who then decides on the patient's behalf are questions freighted with value judgments, and after four decades of argument and litigation, these are still closely debated.

Along with vulnerability to impaired decision making, a second characteristic of mental disorders—their putative association with violence—has led the state to endow mental health professionals with the power to use coercive means to detain and treat some proportion of persons with serious mental illnesses. This stands in marked contrast to practices regarding general medical disorders, which are usually treated on a voluntary basis and rarely over a patient's objections. The power to abrogate a person's liberty and impose treatments that are clearly unwanted is so potent as to suggest that it be used only with the greatest care. To be sure, the courts as agents of a broader society are often involved in these decisions, though not always at the inception. In any event, mental health professionals routinely need to determine when and on what basis to deprive a person with mental illness of the freedom that the rest of us take for granted.

If these issues have existed for scores and even hundreds of years, and they have, their newer permutations present dilemmas of their own. Where once deprivation of liberty meant confinement in a mental hospital, today outpatient commitment, mental health courts, and specialty mental health probation services extend the reach of the state into the community. With these mechanisms, the lives of people with mental disorders, including substance abuse, may be shaped in more subtle ways, blurring even further the line between treating and coercing. Even such widely acclaimed approaches as assertive community treatment (ACT) teams have engendered concerns regarding their intrusive and coercive potential. Moreover, new populations have been targeted for coercive treatment as well, with nearly half the states in the United States enacting laws allowing civil commitment of dangerous sex offenders. Insofar as these statutes appear to be punitive and preventive rather than rehabilitative in intent and practice, the ethics of mental health professional participation in these programs is at best unclear.

By their very nature, treatments used in mental health practice often raise ethical concerns as well. Psychotherapy, especially in its more traditional, psychodynamic form, takes place within a framework in which patients are encouraged to speak frankly about their most intimate fears and fantasies, with some assurance—implicit or otherwise—that the information will remain closely held and secure. As in so many other contemporary venues, however, the privacy of the consulting room is much less secure than it may seem. Conflicting desiderata, each supported by its own set of ethical arguments, impinge on the isolation of the therapist-patient relationship, from protecting third parties from harm to reporting abuse of children, the elderly, or disabled persons. Even harder are the decisions that must be made about revealing information in what are presumed to be the patient's interests, albeit without the patient's consent, for example, disclosing suicidal ideation to family members who may thereby be induced to watch the person more closely to prevent self-harm.

Creation of an intimate space within which the revelations necessary for psychotherapy can take place depends on the maintenance of clear boundaries between psychotherapists and patients. Proscriptions of sexual contact with patients have become widely accepted over the past quarter-century, and there is some reason to believe that violations of this principle have become less frequent over time. However, difficult line-drawing challenges remain. To what extent should therapists disclose their own stories, becoming "real people" for their patients? How should self-disclosure be managed online? For example, should a therapist have a Facebook page and if so, what should (and should not) be on it? If sexual relationships are off-limits, what about platonic friendships, business relationships, and other involvements in patients' lives? Answering these questions requires negotiating a twisting path that runs between avoiding conditions that may lead to exploitation of the patient and respecting the patient as an autonomous person capable of responsible choice.

At the same time that technology has made it harder for therapists to present themselves as a blank slate, it has multiplied the channels through which mental health treatment can take place. Telepsychiatry, once dependent on expensive equipment and dedicated land lines, has given way to therapy by means of online videoconferencing. Mental health professionals and patients communicate by e-mail or text messages. In addition to concerns about the confidentiality of these communications, what it means for patients to be able to reach their therapists at any time of day and for therapists always to be accessible remains to be explored. Nor are advances in technology limited to means of communication. Treatments unimagined a short time ago, such as the insertion of electrodes into the brain (i.e., deep brain stimulation) for the treatment of depression and perhaps other mental disorders, evoke questions about when highly intrusive treatments, with more substantial risks than are common in mental health practice, should be used, and how desperate patients can be helped to make decisions without falling prey to unreasonable expectations of a miracle cure, often stoked by media hyperbole.

Solo practitioners working in private offices once dominated the world of mental health, but that is no longer the case. Mental health professionals now typically find themselves working in organized systems of care—hospitals, clinics, health maintenance organizations, schools, and prisons—where the interests of their patients may be in conflict with organizational imperatives. A patient's need for a few more days of hospital care may be compromised by the facility's desire to hold down length of stay and the charge of the managed care company that is overseeing the patient's insurance benefit to reduce the costs of care. Patients' desires to keep potentially compromising information about mental health treatment out of the hands of their other caregivers become less viable when an organization adopts an integrated medical record aimed at sharing data to improve the quality of care. Clinicians find themselves caught between the entity paying their salaries and the people whose interests they feel obliged to protect.

Even more pointed examples of the dilemmas created by the context in which care is rendered arise in the military and in correctional facilities. Military regulations may require mental health professionals to disclose information regarding violations of rules, including drug use and the commission of adultery, even when they do not directly compromise the military mission, although there is reason to believe that clinicians may not always abide by the regulations. Diagnostic labels that are commonplace in civilian treatment settings must be used with care in the military, where they could lead to the end of a service member's career. Prisons and jails, with the primacy they give to security considerations, often make similar demands of mental health staff regarding information on contraband, including drugs, threats toward personnel and other prisoners, and other serious violations of rules. Mental health professionals in these settings face difficult choices between preserving their patients' confidences, which may be essential for meaningful treatment, and conforming to the demands of the institution, which is serving an important societal role of its own.

Mental health evaluation has long had particular salience for the courts, including assessment of the mental state of criminal defendants at the time of the crime and prior to court proceedings. In addition, issues of mental impairment are frequently material to civil litigation as well. Participation in the justice system, though, takes the mental health professional to new ethical terrain where familiar rules may no longer apply. Rather than seeking the best interests of a patient, the forensic evaluator is there to assist the administration of justice, even when that is to the disadvantage of the person being evaluated. Moreover, persons subject to evaluations are not always willing participants, turning the consent process into something closer to mere disclosure, with emphasis on the assessor's role and the very real limits on confidentiality. Mental health professionals who lose sight of the differences between clinical and forensic settings threaten to compromise their own integrity and the interests of the people whom they assess.

The ubiquity of ethical issues that mental health professionals confront is motivation enough for inquiry into the underlying principles and values of alternative courses of action. But it is worth noting one additional benefit of education about the ethical challenges facing mental health professionals. As this very partial catalog of the area makes clear, many of the challenges derive from outside the mental health professions, from law, institutional rules, and economic forces. Who better to help shape policy at both the macro and micro levels than informed mental health professionals who know firsthand the competing values at stake? This compendium of notable articles addressing some of the most critical ethical dilemmas in mental health today is an excellent place to begin acquiring the knowledge that can make informed involvement possible.

Paul S. Appelbaum, MD
Columbia University and New York State Psychiatric Institute
New York, New York

Acknowledgments

We thank the Thomas Scattergood Behavioral Health Foundation for its ongoing and generous support of our work. In particular, we thank Joe Pyle, the foundation's president, for his advice, patience, and encouragement. We thank current and former members of the ScattergoodEthics Advisory Board: Paul Appelbaum, Marna Barrett, Cindy Baum-Baicker, Donna Chen, Gail Edelsohn, Dwight Evans, Barry Fabius, Marc Forman, Renée Fox, Gregg Gorton, John Maher, Frederick Reamer, Anthony Rostain, Ilina Singh, and Paul Root Wolpe.

Katherine Buckley deserves distinct recognition and credit for her substantial editorial assistance in the preparation of the final manuscript and her support of the ScattergoodEthics Program.

Several others provided support, resources, advice and encouragement in completing this project, including Ezekiel Emanuel, chair of the Department of Medical Ethics and Health Policy at the University of Pennsylvania, and Clay Morgan of MIT Press. We thank also Rebecca Johnson, Allison Rosenbloom, Jason Schwartz, Daniel Reid, Anna Barnwell, and Ceara O'Brien for their assistance.

Finally, we thank our spouses—Corinne Sebesta Sisti, Margaret Caplan, and Itay Greenspan—for their patience and support of all our work.

I

Foundational Questions

Unlike other areas of medicine, psychiatry and the behavioral sciences involved in the diagnosis and treatment of mental illness are the subjects of great contention about the reality of what it is that they diagnose and treat. Practitioners do not always agree on how to draw the boundaries between illness and health. Nor do members of the general public agree with the determinations that those expert in mental health offer. Many core public policy questions hinge on how these foundational questions are answered from simple issues such as the number of persons who have a mental illness, which determines how much money is allotted for diagnosis and treatment, to what sort of training is deemed appropriate for a mental health practitioner, to vexing problems such as whether to hold a person suffering from a mental illness legally culpable and responsible for any antisocial act he or she might commit.

Charles Rosenberg, a distinguished historian of medicine, leads us into this challenging set of problems with a review of how the relationships among disease concepts and painful or socially problematic behaviors have been and continue to be contested and recontested across time and place. This is in part because many behaviors—substance abuse, sexual conduct, political dissent, violence—are tied to beliefs about morality as much as they are to beliefs about pathology.

Rosenberg notes that in trying to shift deviant or disliked conduct from sin to illness, mental health practitioners have placed great weight on the discoverability of somatic pathology in the brain as underlying mental illnesses. The discovery of germs and genes helped clarify the nature of physical ailments and permitted specificity in diagnosis. Nineteenth-century mental health pioneers were quick to try to fit mental illness into this somatic-pathology framework. They repeatedly referred to the brain as the organ of mind and mental illness as a product of brain disorder. The social and moral sides of mental illness were downplayed in favor of abnormal brain physiology.

This biological reductionism is being challenged on many fronts today. Some would argue that there is no single study of brains or behavior that could determine whether children exhibiting problematic restlessness in school suffer from disease or are at one end of the spectrum of normal human diversity, which may not serve them well in a classroom. Biology may count, but what constitutes disease is a function of what particular societies at particular times value in terms of character and behavior.

We include here a historical curiosity by Ralph Little and Edward Strecker, who in 1956 offered a peek back at a different foundational question: "How ought a psychiatrist negotiate a conflict between the rights of an individual patient and the greater good?" They illustrate this conflict by asking their colleagues about cases involving the limits of doctor-patient confidence, such as this anachronistic query: "What is your ethical responsibility when one of your unmarried patients becomes pregnant during treatment and informs you that she has arranged to have a criminal abortion?"

After reporting the results of their survey, Little and Strecker argue not for hard-and-fast rules but for judgment and reflection when challenges to boundaries and confidentiality arise between psychiatrists and their patients. They might have been surprised to learn how thinking in this area has evolved with respect to both the widely recognized duty to break confidentiality and warn others if a therapist believes one's patient ready to harm another and in the use of ethics committees to face some of the most challenging issues of research and therapy. The rise of concerns about privacy and the presence of a more diverse range of practitioners in terms of gender and sexual orientation has been accompanied by a tightening of limits over what a practitioner may and may not do in interacting with a patient.

Toksoz Karasu, and then Jennifer Radden and John Sadler, struggle with the challenge of how to deal with the ineradicable presence of values in the practice of psychological therapy. Karasu notes that a shift had taken place from paternalism, where the benevolent doctor led the way in therapy, toward a contract, where patient and therapist together negotiate the outcome sought from therapy. The rise of autonomy as a core value in medical ethics generally, particularly in the United States, United Kingdom, Canada, the Netherlands, and Australia, has continued to shape the respect accorded patients, even those with fairly significant mental illness, to determine whether they will seek care and, if so, what that care will have as its goal or goals.

Radden and Sadler see the resolution of these challenges—the goals of treatment and the nature of the therapist-patient relationship—through the inculcation of virtue among care providers. Rather than setting out bright lines to guide practice, they argue that the best outcomes for diagnosis and treatment are to be obtained by those armed with good character and virtue. They go on to describe how they think these can best be instilled in novice practitioners in the mental health field.

1

Contested Boundaries: Psychiatry, Disease, and Diagnosis

Charles E. Rosenberg

Some years ago, the *New York Times* front page reported the outcome of a much-discussed courtroom drama, the Andrew Goldstein murder trial. Previously diagnosed and treated—or more often not treated—as a chronic schizophrenic, Goldstein had killed a random young woman by pushing her in front of a subway train. Despite his unchallenged diagnosis, the jury convicted Goldstein of second-degree murder. "He seemed to know what he was doing," one juror said after the trial. "He picked her up and threw her. That was not a psychotic jerk, an involuntary movement." Another juror explained that they had thought the defendant was "in control and acted with intent to kill." "It was staged and executed," he said of the lethal attack. "There was forethought and exquisite timing" (Barnes 2000).

This is a story of intellectual and institutional conflict, of inconsistent conceptions of disease and impulse control, and of a chronically ill-starred relationship between law and medicine. It is also a story that might have been written in 1901 as well as in 2001; and, of course, the formal categories of the cognitively defined right-and-wrong test for criminal responsibility still lingers in most American courtrooms. Not too long ago, our media retailed the story of Houston mother Andrea Yates, who drowned her five children. The local prosecutor argued that there was no question concerning her responsibility. She knew right from wrong, he was quoted as saying: "You will also hear evidence that she knew it was an illegal thing, that it was a sin, that it was wrong" (*New York Times* 2002).

But such highly publicized forensic dramas represent just one—in some ways far from typical—example of a much larger and more pervasive phenomenon: the negotiation of disease in public and the particularly ambiguous status of hypothetical ailments whose presenting symptoms are behavioral or emotional. Most of us would agree that there is some somatic mechanism or mechanisms (whatever their nature or origin) associated with grave and incapacitating psychoses, but as the dilemma of criminal responsibility illustrates, even in such cases we remain far from agreement about management and precise disease boundaries. But there is a much larger group of individuals who represent a more elusive and ambiguous picture. They are men and women who experience incapacitating emotional pain, who have difficulties in impulse control—or who, even if they have not violated a criminal statute, behave in ways that seem socially or morally unacceptable to many of their generational peers.

Sociologists and social critics have, for more than a quarter-century, spoken of the medicalization of deviance, of the tendency to recategorize sin(s) as pathology(ies) and to consign the management of such conditions to appropriately certified practitioners.[1] But this is only one subset of a larger phenomenon that is in a literal sense coterminous with the history of medicine as a specialized calling. I refer to the assignment of certain aspects of human pain and incapacity to the realm of medicine and to the physician's care and explanatory authority. "Medicalization" might perhaps be better understood as a long-term trend in Western society toward reductionist, somatic, and—increasingly—disease-specific explanations of human feelings and behavior as well as unambiguously physical ills.

Nevertheless, the phenomenon remains complex, inconsistent, and contingent, even if expansive and increasingly pervasive. The relationships among disease concepts and painful or socially problematic behaviors have been and are being contested and recontested, not only in melodramatic courtroom situations, but in countless clinical, bureaucratic, and administrative contexts. Moreover, deviance is hardly a discrete and objective thing: it is time-, place-, and even class-specific. Think of now casually accepted sexual behaviors that a century ago would have been seen as certainly deviant and possibly pathognomonic—ranging from masturbation to "excessive" female sexuality. A bright line between disease and willed misbehavior or culpable self-indulgence—or idiosyncratic emotional discomfort—will not easily be agreed upon, while the cultural and bureaucratic need to create such boundaries will hardly disappear. Meanwhile individual men and women, lay and professional, act out complex and not always consistent agendas shaped by personal, familial, generational, and social locational realities.

Criminal responsibility and the vexed relationship between law and medicine constitute only one such area of recurring negotiation. The media provide countless instances of such public controversy, only a very small minority of which are acted out in criminal courts. I need only refer to a number of problematic categories, entities such as gender identity disorder, attention deficit hyperactivity disorder, social anxiety disorder, or chronic fatigue syndrome, not to mention road rage and premenstrual syndrome or putatively—and thus potentially exculpatory—pathological addictions to gambling and sex. A local outpatient psychiatric facility has recently offered treatment for "computer addiction"—an inability to refrain from the Internet (McLean Hospital n.d.). Readers are informed that the hospital offers a full range of "specialized clinical programs in addition to those for computer addiction . . . [including] . . . those dealing with anxiety, depression, alcohol and drug abuse, Alzheimer's, dementia, personality disorders, bipolar and psychotic illnesses, dissociative disorders, trauma, sleep disorders, human sexuality, and women's and men's issues."

Public policy in regard to drug and alcohol use represents another tenaciously contested occasion for debating the applicability and legitimacy of disease concepts.

Billions of dollars and many thousands of lives have been altered by deeply felt and widely disseminated assumptions concerning what has come to be called substance abuse. Are such behaviors the symptoms of a chronic disease (with a biochemical and perhaps genetic substrate) that demands treatment? Or are they crimes to be punished? "Addiction is a chronic disease that demands a medical and public health response," one advocate of the disease model contended in a typical letter to the editor. "It is not a moral lapse" (*Boston Globe* 2001). Such conflicts surrounding the ontological status—and thus social legitimacy—of behavioral and emotional ills have been endemic since their widespread articulation well over a century ago. Patterns of cultural and clinical visibility change, but that ambiguity remains; today, for example, problems of mood constitute a particularly pervasive and diagnostically tendentious category. Is depression a thing? Or a dimension of human diversity and the human condition? And—or—an appropriate response to situational realities? These questions have become all too familiar in the past generation.

Perhaps the most embarrassingly public of such debates over the epistemological legitimacy of a disease category took place more than a generation ago and was occasioned by a planned revision of the American Psychiatric Association's *Diagnostic and Statistical Manual*. In retrospect, the most egregious aspect of this conflict was the series of votes surrounding a reconsideration of the problematic category "homosexuality."

Was this a disease? Or a choice? And how could a legitimate disease—in most physicians' minds a biological phenomenon with a characteristic mechanism and predictable course—be decided by a vote? A vote, moreover, influenced by feverish lobbying and public demonstrations (Bayer 1987). Though it has become routine, many Americans still find it unseemly that diagnoses can be shaped in part by advocacy groups and Web sites, or that disease-targeted research funding can be determined in part by lobbyists, lay advocates, and journalists, and not by the seemingly objective and inexorable logic of laboratory findings. (Although lobbying for federal support of cancer research and treatment has come to seem normal politics, a similar worldly judgment seems not so easily accepted when applied to ailments of mood and behavior.) And in the private sector, we have seen in the past half-century how pharmaceutical industry research and marketing decisions have helped reshape both medical and lay notions of emotional illness and its treatment. But we have also witnessed the articulation of a vigorous critique of such trends, a criticism not only of specific corporate tactics, but also of the social role of business, its relationship to government, and the problematic nature of psychiatry's diagnostic categories.[2]

What I should like to do in the following pages is to outline the key characteristics of an era of expanding nosological boundaries—beginning in roughly the last third of the nineteenth century and extending into the present—and then specify some of the reasons that controversy often continues to surround disease categories that promise to explain behavior and emotional pain.[3] Much of what I will be discussing falls into psychiatry's domain of clinical responsibility. For more than a century, the psychiatrist has been the designated trustee of those social and emotional dilemmas that can plausibly—and thus usefully—be framed as the product of disease. We contest the precise definitions and appropriate clinical and social responses to somatic ills as well, but behavioral and emotional ailments constitute a particularly sensitive and contingent subset of problems. Since its origins as a specialty in the nineteenth century, psychiatry has been a definer of boundaries, a delineator and designated manager of the normal and abnormal, and thus unavoidably a key participant in this never-ending debate. At the same time it has suffered from a recurrent status anxiety—one might call it procedure envy, or organic inferiority. Psychiatry has been chronically sensitive to its inability to call upon a repertoire of tightly bounded, seemingly objective, and generally agreed-upon diagnostic categories based firmly on biopathological mechanisms (Grob 1998). Ailments such as pellagra and paresis, which had been the psychiatrist's responsibility when their cause and treatment was obscure, left the specialty's domain when their mechanisms were understood and their treatment established. Psychiatry remains the legatee of the emotional, the behavioral, and the imperfectly understood. In this sense it has been a poor relation of its specialist peers in surgery and internal medicine. And one need hardly speak of psychiatry's history of uncritical flirtations with seemingly effective somatic interventions.[4] Think, for example, of insulin shock and lobotomy.

The Specificity Trap

Though diverse, the examples of contested ills I have cited exhibit a number of core similarities. All illustrate the social and intellectual centrality of specific disease entities and the assumption that a legitimate disease is discrete and that it has a characteristic clinical course; perhaps equally important, behavioral and emotional symptoms are presumed to reflect an underlying mechanism. In other words, what some sociologists and social critics have for decades called "medicalization" is in practice the use of time- and place-specific vocabularies of disease entities as a tool for at once conceptualizing and managing behavior and feelings. And these disease models have ultimately to be specific and somatic if they are to find wide acceptance.

A somatic identity is perhaps most fundamental. It is no accident that today's advocates for the mentally ill state again and again that "it" is a physical ailment no different from diabetes or cancer—and no more deserving of censure or less-than-equal insurance coverage. "The brain is an organ," as a *New York Times* (1999) editorialist put it in formulaic language, "and diseases related to this organ should be treated like any other medical illness." It was no wonder that President Clinton should have described it as "morally right" for insurance companies to set the same annual and lifetime coverage limits for mental as for physical ills. Like the rules of criminal responsibility, insurance coverage presents a continuing occasion for debating the nature and treatment of emotional and behavioral ills. It is also not surprising that such claims inevitably generate not only novel entities, but also—and equally important— somatic rationalizations for the existence of such ailments. As I edited this article, for example, my morning newspaper reported that "a national study . . . reported that at some point in their lives, about 5 per cent of people have such frequent, serious blow-ups that they qualify as suffering from Intermittent Explosive Disorder, a full-fledged psychiatric diagnosis."

The reporter also cited the comments of an authority on anger: "It's not simply bad behavior," the expert explained: "There's a biology and a psychology and a genetics and a neuroscience behind this, and you can come up with strategies for intervention just like for anything else, like diabetes or hypertension or depression" (Goldberg 2005). All such examples—and one could cite hundreds of others from contemporary print and electronic sources—reflect the underlying historical reality I have already discussed: the cultural pervasiveness of somatic, mechanism-based ideas of disease specificity, and the problems associated with using such concepts to manage deviance, rationalize idiosyncrasy, and explain emotional pain.

I have been interested for many years in the history of such putative disease categories (Rosenberg 2002, 2003). One theme that seems to me particularly fundamental is the idea of disease specificity itself—the notion that diseases can and should be thought of as entities existing outside their unique manifestations in particular men and women. These ideas did not become culturally pervasive until the last third of the nineteenth century. And, not so coincidentally, it was only in this period that such hypothetical disease entities began to be used widely and routinely to explain an increasing variety of socially stigmatized or self-destructive behaviors. Of course, there are earlier examples of similar phenomena: even nonhistorians have come across such conditions as hypochondriasis, hysteria, and melancholy, and references in literature to a variety of painful moods explained in terms of a speculative but materialist pathophysiology. Humoral explanations of temperamental peculiarity are as old as Western medicine itself, but the disease concepts they rationalized were fundamentally different from those most of us take for granted today. Conditions such as melancholy or hysteria were as much flexible descriptions of individual life-course outcomes as diseases conceived of in terms of modern notions of specificity.

The late nineteenth century was an era of expanding clinical boundaries—a period in which hypothetical ailments such as homosexuality, kleptomania, neurasthenia, railroad spine, and anorexia were delineated—one might say put into cultural play—as disease entities. Some of these terms persist, while others have an archaic ring or altered meanings, yet all were described as novel clinical phenomena by enthusiastic late-nineteenth century physicians. The timing is no accident. The first three-quarters of the century had provided a series of intellectual building blocks, cumulatively suggesting a new emphasis on disease as discrete entity. Earlier interest in clinical description and postmortem pathology had articulated and disseminated a lesion-based notion of disease, but the late nineteenth century saw a hardening in this way of thinking, reflecting the assimilation of germ theories of infectious disease as well as a variety of findings from the laboratories of physiologists and biochemists. The gradual assimilation of the notion that specific micro-organisms constituted the indispensable and determining cause of par-ticular clinical entities seemed to endorse the specificity of infectious disease—and thus, by a kind of intellectual contagion, the notion of specific disease itself. Also supportive of such views was the growing prestige of what we have come to call the biomedical sciences: histology, biochemistry, physiology, and pharmacology. Collectively they spoke a reductionist, mechanism-oriented, and antivitalist language, providing a compelling and seemingly objective store of tools, procedures, models, and data that promised to delineate disease in newly precise, measurable—and thus portable—terms. The late-nineteenth-century vogue for heredity and evolution constituted another significant factor, linking biology and behavior, mind and body, past and present. And many of the putative behavioral ills described in the late nineteenth century were in fact seen as constitutional.[5] Alcoholism and homosexuality were prominent cases in point. Heredity seemed increasingly a determining—inexorable—force, rather than one among a variety of factors interacting to deter-mine health and disease. Like the germ theory, heredity provided many late-nineteenth-century physicians a reassuringly somatic mechanism with which to explain a variety of unsettling emotions and problematic behaviors.

Expanding Boundaries and the Reductionist Project, 1870–1900

Such explanations increasingly took the form of hypothetical disease entities, and neurasthenia was particularly prominent among such con-cepts (Gijswijt-Hofstra and Porter 2001; Rosenberg 1962; Sicherman 1977). Coined in the late 1860s by George M. Beard, a New York neu-rologist, the term *neurasthenia* incorporated an eclectic mixture of symp-toms: depression, anxiety, compulsions and obsessions, sexual dysfunction and deviance, and fleeting aches and pains both physical and mental. Although the concept might be thought in retrospect a forerunner of the twentieth-century idea of neurosis—itself a catchall description for mal-adaptive individual adjustments in Freudian and post-Freudian models of personality and pathogenesis—Beard rationalized his discovery in relentlessly material terms. He had no choice if it were to be taken seriously by his peers: social legitimacy presumed somatic identity. In Beard's view, the elusive and ever-shifting symptoms that characterized neurasthenia were reflections of an underlying weakness in the individual sufferer's constitutional allotment of nervous energy. "Physiology," Beard (1884) explained, "is the physics of living things; pathology is the physics of disease" (p. 15). Although neurasthenia was characterized by feelings and behavior alone, Beard was confident that it rested on a firm if still obscure somatic basis. "I feel assured," he wrote in 1869, "that it [neurasthenia] will in time be substantially confirmed by microscopical and chemical examinations of those patients who die in a neurasthenic condition" (p. 218). The postmortem pathology that had so impressively delineated, for example, the lesions of tuberculosis and Bright's disease in the first half of the nineteenth century would soon illuminate this even more elusive but ultimately somatic condition.

This speculative somaticization of behavioral ills by physicians was, as we have seen, a medical tactic far older than Beard's Gilded Age "discovery" of neurasthenia. Hypochondria, for example, was as much the result of somatic causes as any physical ailment. Half a century earlier, Benjamin Rush (1812) had sought to combat the judgmental and widespread view that such ills were "imaginary," mere self-indulgence. Hypochondria, he explained, "has unfortunately been supposed to be an imaginary disease only, and when given to the disease in question is always offensive to patients who are affected with it. It is true, it is seated in the mind; but it is as much the effect of corporeal causes as a pleurisy, or a bilious fever" (p. 75).

Nineteenth-century physicians repetitively and formulaically referred to the brain as the organ of mind and mental illness as a product of brain disorder.[6] What might be called the assumption of an ultimately somatic pathology had never been questioned in regard to the etiology of grave and incapacitating mental ills, but it had been broadened in scope by the late nineteenth century to include a variety of putative disease pictures that Rush and his generational peers would hardly have regarded as appropriate objects for clinical attention. In Beard's era of self-referred outpatient neurology, a variety of compulsions and obsessions, emotional pain (often termed mood disorders today), and what might be called problems of identity (as in homosexuality) began to populate that novel urban space, the consulting neurologist's waiting room.

It is not surprising that would-be ailments as diverse as homosexuality and railroad spine, anorexia and neurasthenia were all articulated in roughly the same period, the 1860s and 1870s. All were presumed to have some somatic if not constitutional basis, yet all explained behavior that seemed individually painful and dysfunctional, or socially problematic. Let me elaborate this argument with another example: the mid-nineteenth-century ailment called "railroad spine" or "spinal concussion," diagnoses even less familiar today than neurasthenia. These novel diagnoses were associated with a growing mid-nineteenth-century anxiety—and lawsuits—following the era's frequent railroad accidents. It reflected as well a widespread disquietude in confronting the seemingly unnatural and feverish pace of railroad travel. The pathological concept was associated with John Erichsen, a London surgeon, just as neurasthenia was associated with George Beard. Erichsen's *On Railway and Other Injuries of the Nervous System* (1866), originally a series of lectures given to students at University College Hospital, soon became a standard reference. And like Beard's formulation, Erichsen's diagnostic neologism reflected a more widespread sense of cultural uncertainty. Even before Erichsen's work, the *Lancet* had editorialized about the neurological sequalea of railroad trauma.

These symptoms are manifested through the nervous system chiefly, or through those physical conditions which depend upon the perfect physiological balance of the nerve-forces for their exact fulfillment. They vary . . . from simple irritability, restlessness and malaise after long journeys up to a condition of gradually supervening paralysis, which tells of the insidious disease of the brain or spinal cord, such as . . . follows on violent shocks or injuries to the nervous centres. These latter are the symptoms which frequently ensue from the vehement jolts and buffetings endured during a railroad collision. (Harrington 2001, p. 42)

One can discern a rough filiation among neurasthenia, spinal concussion, soldier's heart, and shellshock, in a clinical tradition that linked particular clusters of emotional and behavioral symptoms with a parallel dependence on a legitimating (if, in retrospect, hypothetical) physical mechanism. And all served in some measure as occasion and vehicle for social comment. It is no accident that George Beard wrote a much-cited book called *American Nervousness* (1881) and another, *Sexual Neurasthenia* (1884); both addressed widespread cultural anxieties about self and society.

Many novel late-nineteenth-century entities such as sexual inversion and neurasthenia were soon adopted and widely cited but nevertheless remained controversial—to some clinicians and intellectuals real diseases, but to others mere self-indulgence or symptoms of a larger cultural decay. Diseases were deployed as rhetorical weapons in recurrent battles over cultural values and social practices. "Overstress," for example, was a condition noticed in late-nineteenth-century secondary schools and attributed to the urban middle class's relentless competitiveness, while sterility and hysteria could be seen as the inevitable cost incurred by higher education for women. An urban, technology-dependent—and thus unnatural—life could be stigmatized as psychically as well as physically pathogenic.

This all seems neat and tidy, with disease concepts mirroring and mediating both cultural angst and a widespread faith in the explanatory power of disease models. The dots are nicely connected. But the story on the ground is rather more complicated. These pathologizing tactics were neither universal nor consistently accepted in late-nineteenth- and early-twentieth-century America. While many were attracted by the certainties of somatic and reductionist styles of explaining sickness and health, others found this approach less than congenial. Christian Science, consistently enough, like Spiritualism, Seventh Day Adventism, and the Emmanuel movement, all developed in their several ways in tension with this polarizing development: at one pole a way of thinking about behavior reducible to somatic mechanisms (with an implied deterministic understanding of behavior), at the other pole a holistic, spiritual framework emphasizing faith and agency in their impact on health outcomes. One might think of them as two rather different styles of reductionism. Of course, many Americans—and not only lawyers—who shared a general faith in the progress of scientific understanding remained skeptical of the legitimacy and exculpatory implications of such would-be ills as alcoholism, kleptomania, anorexia, and nervous exhaustion; a parallel aura of ambiguity and disdain surrounded the older but still current diagnosis of hysteria. These behavioral and emotional ills and their presumed social causes echoed morally resonant controversies over class, appropriate gender behavior, and a variety of other issues—clashes in an endless cultural war in which we still struggle over the legitimacy of ills such as chronic fatigue syndrome, anorexia, fetal alcohol syndrome, alcoholism, and homosexuality, without arriving at a stable consensus.

The More Things Change

Some aspects of medicine's social history have changed dramatically in the past century; others comparatively little. One that has changed little is the mediating role of psychiatry. Medicine in general and psychiatry in particular remain boundary managers: border police examining and certifying transit documents in an unceasing battle over depression and anxiety, sexuality and addiction. Psychiatry remains the peculiar legatee of such problems, an obligate participant in every generation's particular cultural negotiations—a kind of canary at the pitface of cultural strife. It is by no means the only player. Civil and criminal courts, welfare officers, media commentators, a variety of other specialists—not to mention patients and families—all play a role.

The search for somatic mechanisms with which to legitimate behavioral ills seems in retrospect a parallel and logically related continuity. The twentieth-century psychodynamic tradition with its emphasis on family setting and individual psychological development and associated talk therapies seems almost a kind of byway in relation to mainstream medicine, an oppositional—if culturally significant—counterpoint to a consistently dominant reductionism. Even at the height of its influence (from the 1940s through the 1970s), psychodynamic explanations of behavior and emotions remained in an uneasy and even marginal relationship to much of mainstream medicine, despite the widespread influence of such ideas outside the profession. That very marginality helps explain the recurrent attraction of intrusive therapies in twentieth-century psychiatry (Braslow 1997; Pressman 1998; Scull 2005; Valenstein 1986, 1998).

The dominance of reductionist styles has a long history in the explanation of human behavior, but it has an extraordinarily salient place today. We have never been more infatuated with visions of molecular and neurochemical—ultimately genetic—truth. "We're now at the point where we can begin articulating the physical basis of some of the mysterious brain functions that exist . . . learning, memory, and emotion. . . . We're at a point where we can move miraculously from molecule to mind" (Wade 2001). In the not-too-distant past we have seen claims for the discovery of genetic bases for dyslexia, obesity, risk taking, homosexuality, even aggression. Many of us can remember the widespread discussion of chromosomal explanations for criminality. Today's fashionable evolutionary psychology adds a metahistorical style of biological reductionism to our culturally available store of mechanism-oriented and determinist explanations for behavioral and emotional pathologies (as well, of course, as the "normal").

But there remains a historical irony. We are in a moment of peculiar and revealing paradox, a complex and structured mix of reductionist hopes and widespread criticism of such sanguine assumptions. As a culture we are relentlessly reductionist in presuming somatic (and ultimately genetic) causation for behavior, yet at the same time we are reflexive, critical, and relativist in our approach to existing disease classifications and therapeutic modalities. We have never been more aware of the arbitrary and constructed quality of psychiatric diagnoses, yet in an era characterized by the increasingly bureaucratic management of health care and an increasingly pervasive reductionism in the explanation of normal as well as pathological behavior, we have never been more dependent on them. I need only underline the way in which the DSM has evolved from its originally modest format—a hundred-page spiral-bound, soft-covered form in 1952 and 1968—to today's ponderous octavo (with its numerous epitomes, visual aids, and commentaries), while wry commentators lay and professional scoff at the seemingly transparent arbitrariness of its categories (Kirk and Kutchins 1992; Kutchins and Kirk 1997).

This inconsistency struck me, for example, with particular force in reading *Girl, Interrupted*, Susanna Kaysen's 1993 memoir of her late 1960s inpatient stay in McLean Hospital. The book includes a revealing section in which the author is seated in her "corner Cambridge bookstore" reading DSM III and deconstructing the substance and language of the borderline personality disorder diagnosis that had justified her treatment almost thirty years before (Kaysen 1993). She underlines the arbitrariness, the gender stereotypes, and the social control built into the seemingly objective language of clinical description. Kaysen's agnostic point of view reflects and incorporates three decades of political, epistemological, and feminist criticism of psychiatric nosology; there has never been a more skeptical and reflexive period. Explicit and fundamental criticism of psychiatric nosology has in fact been widespread for a half-century; one need only cite the works of Thomas Szasz, R. D. Laing, and a variety of feminist and sociological critiques of psychiatric authority and the epistemology that justified it.

The paradoxical reality of such fundamental skepticism coexisting with a triumphalist reductionism is exemplified as well in the current debate over the use of psychoactive drugs. In the past half-century, the widespread prescribing of such drugs implies and has helped legitimate the specific entity idea: bipolar disease is what responded to lithium; depression is legitimated ontologically by the drugs that treat it. But as current controversies over Ritalin and a variety of antidepressants and antipsychotic drugs, for example, suggest, these relationships have simply constituted a new site and designated players for the contestation of social values. Who would have guessed a generation ago that an American president would choose the pediatric use of psychoactive drugs as a public issue, as Clinton did during his presidency? And that we would accept with barely a second thought such public contestation of a seemingly clinical problem?[7] Just as attention deficit was, for example, being widely discussed and accepted, it stimulated—through a kind of cultural dialectic—a variety of forceful rejections of such categories as arbitrary social constructions. It was not just that children and increasingly adults "are too casually offered stimulants like Ritalin," as a letter to the *New York Times* charged almost a decade ago, "but that biological reductionism lies behind the tendency to ignore the deeper social, psychological and cultural issues . . . in favor of assuming there is a disease located within their heads" (Kohn and Armstrong 1997). Such critical sentiments may be in the minority, but they have been widely and articulately voiced in the past decade—with little effect (DeGrandpre 2000).

It is, of course, not simply a technical (pharmacological) problem, or a problem of diagnostic precision, or of pharmaceutical industry marketing strategies. No quantity of well-conceived epidemiological studies will bring consensus with regard to children exhibiting a problematic restlessness; it is at some level a problem of human diversity, of social class, of gender, and of bureaucratic practice. Clinical epidemiological studies play a role, but as only one voice in a complicated and discordant discourse. Concepts such as hyperactivity are meaningful only in specific contexts. Even if the most extreme and intractable behaviors are ultimately products of still-undeciphered but ultimately specifiable genetic and neurochemical mechanisms, their social evaluation remains contingent and a subject of inevitable contestation. What are appropriate levels of attention? Of hyperactivity? What is normal and what is, in fact, being measured? When does therapeutics stop and enhancement begin? (Elliot 2003) The terms *hyperactive* or *attention deficit* are context dependent by definition, reflections of specific institutional realities and cultural needs. And one of those needs, as I have suggested, is the recourse to medical personnel, authority, and conceptual categories as at once legitimation and framework for the institutional management and cultural framing of awkward social realities.

Similar judgments could be made in regard to a variety of such multicausal and nonspecific ills. A phenomenon such as fetal alcohol syndrome—like attention deficit hyperactivity disorder—might be thought of as a statistically configured point on a spectrum of behaviors and seemingly linked physical characteristics, perhaps reflecting an underlying biological substrate even if we can define and defend such a core as constituting a usefully predictive entity, fetal alcohol syndrome, a presumably gestational phenomenon, would still serve as only one element in a more complex and multidimensional social reality. A disease entity so defined would incorporate not only the ideal-typical core of presumed victims of fetal alcohol syndrome, but also all the effects surrounding it. Like a stone dropped into a body of water, the ripples are real indeed, ranging from labels on alcoholic beverages, to individual guilt and anxiety, to pleas for reduced responsibility in criminal justice contexts—or, as we have seen, expanded responsibility placed on ethanol-addicted mothers (Armstrong 2003; Golden 2005). Depression constitutes a parallel and even more pervasive phenomenon. What we call "major depression" may have a biochemical substrate, but the relationship between etiology and individual clinical outcome remains obscure. How do we balance the determined and the contingent, the genetically given and the situationally negotiated? And what is the relationship between such disabling ills and the spectrum of emotional states we casually term "depression"? What is the gradient of that slippery slope from temperament and situational reaction to something rather different and categorically pathological? Laypeople today often put that functional distinction in linguistic terms when they say a person has a "clinical depression"—presumably an extreme point on the necessary spectrum of human pain and varieties of mood.

Despite such indeterminacy, our repertoire of specific entities constitutes a powerful reality, providing a resource for individuals in thinking about themselves and for society in conceptualizing behaviors, as can be indicated in the varied histories of such current and obsolete entities as hysteria, hypochondria, hypoglycemia, chronic fatigue syndrome, Gulf War syndrome, or gender identity disorder. There are scores of such problematic ills, and the very social utility of these categories implies their contestation. There are always winners and losers in the negotiations surrounding the attribution of such diagnoses, as the social legitimacy—and often social resources—associated with the sickness role constitutes a prize worth contesting. Advocacy groups and the Internet have only exacerbated such debates, as some individuals claim the sick role's legitimacy offered by certain controversial disease entities—chronic Lyme disease, for example, or chronic fatigue syndrome—while others scorn them as mere excuses for self-indulgence.

Conflict and Continuity

I have tried to describe a phenomenon that is always in process, always contested, and never completed. Sociologists and historians have described the linked phenomena of medicalization and bureaucracy as having mounted a powerful campaign for cultural and institutional authority over problematic behaviors and suspect emotions. And, in fact, the boundaries of presumed disease have in general expanded relentlessly in the past century and a half. But these boundaries remain contested even as they move outward. At least some medical and lay hearts and minds remain only partially converted to these new and expansive models of pathology.

This is only to have been expected. There are a number of continuities that guarantee both the continued centrality and contestation of behavioral and emotional ills. One such controversy turns on the paradox of using reductionist means for holistic—cultural—ends. As disease definitions have become more and more dependent on seemingly objective signs (first physical diagnosis, then laboratory findings and imaging results), ailments that cannot easily be associated with such findings were naturally segregated into a lesser status. Behavioral ills thus fall into a lowly position in a status hierarchy that is at once social, moral, medical, and epistemological. When allied with the fear, punitiveness, hostility, stigmatization, personal guilts, and pain often associated with such contested behaviors, it is hardly surprising that individuals exhibiting emotional and behavioral "symptoms" would not be consistently well served by the mechanism-oriented specific-entity style of legitimating and conceptualizing disease.

And when there is no cultural consensus—as in regard to homosexuality or substance abuse—there is no basis for a nosological consensus. But it is equally, if ironically, inevitable that the powerful concept of disease specificity has been—and will continue to be—employed as a tool for the ideological management of problematic emotions and behaviors. It is a tool, moreover, available to laypeople as well as clinicians and administrators. There is always an eager market for disease labels, whether found on a Web site, in a magazine, or in a nosological table. Insofar as our ideal-typical conception of disease is specific and mechanism based, this reductionist model will remain to a degree inconsistent with the cultural—and, as I shall argue, bureaucratic—work performed through the articulation and deployment of such disease categories.[8]

A second factor is a never-ending negotiation over agency and responsibility.

Post-nineteenth-century models of disease bear with them an aura of determinism and can thus have a potentially significant role in shaping the social role allotted the sick. We want moral meaning in the narratives we impose on ourselves and others, and it is hard to find it in the random nemesis of genetics and neurochemistry. It is not only in the courtroom, but in society more generally that we seek to preserve responsibility for individual decisions (and thus meaning in misfortune). Contemporary debates over "obesity" represent an example of such ambiguity. Is it a disease or a failure of character? Does "it" represent the working out of genetic destiny, or does a predisposition toward weight gain constitute just one aspect of a complex and poorly understood biological and psychosocial identity? When does idiosyncrasy become pathology?

A third factor both nurturing the use of lexicons of disease categories and, at the same time, guaranteeing conflict about their definition and legitimacy are the linkages that structure medicine into a bureaucratized and highly institutionalized society. Each diagnosis links an individual to a network of bureaucratic relationships and often specialty practice. If it can't be coded, as the saying goes, it doesn't exist. But those coding decisions are potential sites of social contestation in which the legitimacy of individual diagnoses can become structured points of conflict and contestation. Linkage means connections, but differing institutional interests and practices breed conflict over policy, authority, and jurisdiction, as in the case of debates over workman's compensation or product liability, as well as the more obvious questions relating to disability or criminal responsibility. And, of course, individuals do not track neatly on to generalized disease categories and related practice guidelines. The potential arbitrariness of such clinical realities is often apparent to both physician and patient.

We may consign certain feelings and behaviors to the sphere of medicine, but medicine itself is not clearly bounded. Government policies on health care reimbursement, for example, or Food and Drug Administration regulatory procedures—like the (often not unrelated) corporate decisions of pharmaceutical companies in the private sector—have in their various ways shaped disease definitions, accepted therapeutics, and thus individual experience. Powerful stakeholders are involved in all these decisions, and all relate ultimately to the clinical practices and legitimating concepts of contemporary medicine—and nowhere more markedly than in psychiatry. Consumer advertising as well as randomized clinical trials figure in the creation and diffusion of hypothetical disease entities, but the process is complex and elusive. Despite the expenditure of millions of advertising dollars, it is not clear, for example, that erectile dysfunction has been accepted as a legitimate, value-free, disease entity; it is still surrounded by a penumbra of stigma, whimsy, and self-conscious cultural irony.

Fourth, psychiatry and its concepts bleed constantly and unavoidably into the larger culture. This is a phenomenon by no means limited to the past century. I need only refer to the linguistic archeology of once technical terms adapted into everyday discourse: *nostalgia, hypochondria, sanguine, hysterical, paranoid, narcissism, degenerate, nymphomaniac, psychopath, inferiority complex, obsessive-compulsive.*

Usages have changed, but the process by which ordinary men and women appropriate once-technical medical language and explanatory frameworks to think about human behavior and its social management remains straightforward. Behavioral and emotional ills seem more accessible than "somatic" ills to laypeople, who often question such categories as depression or attention deficit but rarely interrogate and are generally unaware of the indeterminacy built into the diagnosis or staging of a somatic ill such as cancer.

Thirty years ago, I wrote an essay on what I called "The Crisis in Psychiatric Legitimacy" (Rosenberg 1975), in which I emphasized the difficult role played by psychiatrists and suggested that it would continue to be ambiguous, no matter what technical progress might take place: "Unless all psychiatry should thaw, melt, and resolve itself into applied pharmacology there seems little possibility of these difficulties redefining themselves" (p. 147). Perhaps psychiatry *has* in good measure resolved itself into applied pharmacology in the past three decades. But the range of human dilemmas that we ask medicine to address has if anything expanded, from depression to anxiety, from bereavement to dysfunctional marriage. So long as medicine in general and psychiatry in particular remains our designated manager of such problems, specific disease categories will always be an indispensable tool in the performance of that social role. So long as we ask medicine to help in doing the cultural work of defining the normal and providing a context and meaning for emotional pain, we will continue to fight a guerrilla war on the permanently contested if ever-shifting boundary dividing disease and deviance, feeling and symptom, the random and the determined, the stigmatized and the deserving of sympathy.

Notes

1. For a recent sociological overview of the state of play, see Clarke et al. 2003; Conrad 2005; and Horwitz 2002. This is not an essay about the idea of medicalization and its history, but I do want to express a word of caution about the tendency to conceptualize medicalization as a reified, monolithic, and inexorable

thing—a point of view that obscures the complex, multidimensional, and inconsistent nature of the way in which medical concepts and practices have laid claim to larger realms of social action and authority. Conrad (2005), for example, refers to the role of pharmaceutical companies and managed care as "engines that are driving . . . [the] medicalization train . . . into the twenty-first century" (p. 12). Trains are material things that move forward in one direction only—along predetermined tracks. For Conrad's earlier formulations, see Conrad 1976 and Conrad and Schneider 1992.

2. David Healy (1997) has been particularly influential in his linkage of pharmaceutical company strategies with a shift in psychiatric nosology and clinical practice.

3. Many of these generalizations might be seen as applying to chronic disease as well, in which the stigmatization of cultural deviance is transformed into the seemingly neutral language of risk, and in which agency and the discussion of behavior in the form of lifestyle management becomes central (Rosenberg 1995).

4. As one advocate for the specialty put it in 1902: "The work done by the alienist cannot remain long in the condition in which it is at present and still be considered worthy of respect by members of other branches of the medical profession" (Paton 1902, p. 434). Not surprisingly, he called not only for a parity in the treatment of mental illness with that available for typhoid fever or pneumonia sufferers, but also for investment in high-status physical chemistry and a sharpening of the alienist's embarrassingly vague diagnostic categories. After all, psychiatry was presented with problems "involving . . . all questions for the preservation and continuance of the normal mental activities in a community" (p. 442).

5. This instance implies a complex relationship between the notion of specific disease and that of patterned deviant behavior as a determined outcome of a general constitutional makeup. Fashionable degeneration theory provided a general framework for explaining such phenomena (Pick 1989).

6. This is not to obscure the early-nineteenth-century physician's assumption that moral—emotional—causes could over time bring about somatic change. Mind and body were continuously and necessarily interactive.

7. Of course, psychoactive drugs are not alone in attracting public debate. One thinks of the public debates over screening mammography or hormone replacement therapy—not to mention stem cell research—in the even more recent past, complete with newspaper editorials, op-ed battles, full-page ads, and television coverage.

8. It is, of course, no easy matter to fit moods and behaviors into neat, defensible, and differentiable boxes, a point underlined in many critiques of the DSM. Moreover, the power of the specific entity ironically focuses clinical attention on any related states that might be construed as early stages of slippery slopes along the way to a full-blown disease. Anxieties and minor depressions are thus reshaped by their presumed relationship to well-marked conditions that they may signal (and possibly constitute), like hypertension or elevated cholesterol levels in cardiovascular disease.

References

Armstrong, E. M. (2003). *Conceiving risk, bearing responsibility: Fetal alcohol syndrome and the diagnosis of moral disorder.* Baltimore: Johns Hopkins Univ. Press.

Barnes, J. (2000). Insanity defense fails for man who threw woman on to track. *New York Times,* March 23.

Bayer, R. (1987). *Homosexuality and American psychiatry: The politics of diagnosis.* New Jersey: Princeton Univ. Press.

Beard, G. [M.]. (1869). Neurasthenia or nervous exhaustion. *Boston Medical and Surgical Journal, 80,* 217–221.

Beard, G. M. 1881. *American nervousness: Its causes and consequences. A supplement to nervous exhaustion (neurasthenia).* New York: G. P. Putnam's.

Beard, G. M. 1884. *Sexual neurasthenia [nervous exhaustion]: Its hygiene, causes, symptoms and treatment.* New York: E. B. Treat.

Boston Globe. (2001). Letter to the editor, February 20.

Braslow, J. T. (1997). *Mental ills and bodily cures: Psychiatric treatment in the first half of the twentieth century.* Berkeley: Univ. of California Press.

Clarke, A. E., et al. (2003). Biomedicalization: Technoscientific transformations of health, illness, and U.S. biomedicine. *American Sociological Review, 68,* 161–194.

Conrad, P. (1976). *Identifying hyperactive children: The medicalization of deviant behavior.* Lexington, MA: Lexington Books.

Conrad, P. (2005). The shifting engines of medicalization. *Journal of Health and Social Behavior, 46,* 3–14.

Conrad, P., & Schneider, J. W. (1992). *Deviance and medicalization: From badness to sickness.* Philadelphia: Temple Univ. Press.

DeGrandpre, R. J. (2000). *Ritalin nation: Rapid-fire culture and the transformation of human consciousness.* New York: Norton.

Elliot, C. (2003). *Better than well: American medicine meets the American dream.* New York: Norton.

Erichsen, J. E. (1866). *On railway and other injuries of the nervous system.* London: Walton and Mabry.

Gijswijt-Hofstra, M., & Porter, R. (Eds.). (2001). *Cultures of neurasthenia: From Beard to the First World War.* Amsterdam, NY: Rodopi.

Goldberg, C. (2005). Out of control anger. *Boston Globe,* August 9.

Golden, J. (2005). *Message in a bottle: The making of fetal alcohol syndrome.* Cambridge: Harvard Univ. Press.

Grob, G. N. (1998). Psychiatry's holy grail: The search for the mechanisms of mental illness. *Bulletin of the History of Medicine, 72,* 189–219.

Harrington, R. (2001). The railway accident: Trains, trauma, and technological crises in nineteenth-century Britain. In M. S. Micale & P. Lerner (Eds.), *Traumatic pasts: History, psychiatry, and trauma in the modern age, 1870–1930* (pp. 31–56). Cambridge: Cambridge Univ. Press.

Healy, D. (1997). *The anti-depressant era.* Cambridge: Harvard Univ. Press.

Horwitz, A. V. (2002). *Creating mental illness.* Chicago: Univ. of Chicago Press.

Kaysen, S. (1993). *Girl, interrupted.* New York: Random House.

Kirk, S. A., & Kutchins, H. (1992). *The selling of DSM: The rhetoric of science in psychiatry.* New York: Aldine DeGruyter.

Kohn, A., & Armstrong, T. (1997). Letter to the editor. *New York Times,* September 7.

Kutchins, H., & Kirk, S. A. (1997). *Making us crazy: DSM, the psychiatric bible and the creation of mental disorders.* New York: Free Press.

McLean Hospital. (N.d.). *The computer addiction service at McLean Hospital.* Brochure. Belmont, MA.

New York Times. (1999). Equitable coverage for mental illness. June 10.

New York Times. (2002). Trial in case of drowned children opens. February 2.

Paton, S. (1902). Recent advances in psychiatry and their relation to internal medicine. *American Journal of Insanity, 58,* 433–442.

Pick, D. (1989). *Faces of degeneration: A European disorder, circa 1848–circa 1918.* Cambridge: Cambridge Univ. Press.

Pressman, J. D. (1998). *Last resort: Psychosurgery and the limits of medicine.* Cambridge: Cambridge Univ. Press.

Rosenberg, C. E. (1962). The place of George M. Beard in nineteenth-century psychiatry. *Bulletin of the History of Medicine, 36,* 245–259.

Rosenberg, C. E. (1975). The crisis in psychiatric legitimacy: Reflections on psychiatry, medicine, and public policy. In G. Kriegman, R. D. Gardner, & D. W. Abse (Eds.), *American psychiatry, past, present, and future: Papers presented on the occasion of the 200th anniversary of the establishment of the first state-supported mental hospital in America* (pp. 135–148). Charlottesville: Univ. Press of Virginia.

Rosenberg, C. E. (1995). Banishing risk: Or the more things change the more they remain the same. *Perspectives in Biology and Medicine, 39,* 28–42.

Rosenberg, C. E. (2002). The tyranny of diagnosis: Specific entities and individual experience. *Milbank Quarterly, 80,* 237–260.

Rosenberg, C. E. (2003). What is disease? In memory of Owsei Temkin. *Bulletin of the History of Medicine, 77,* 491–505.

Rush, B. (1812). *Medical inquiries and observations, upon the diseases of the mind.* Philadelphia: Kimber & Richardson.

Sicherman, B. (1977). The uses of diagnosis: Doctors, patients, and neurasthenia. *J. Hist Med, 32,* 33–54.

Scull, A. (2005). *Madhouse: A tragic tale of megalomania and modern medicine.* New Haven, CT: Yale Univ. Press.

Valenstein, E. S. (1986). *Great and desperate cures: The rise and decline of psychosurgery and other radical treatments for mental illness.* New York: Basic Books.

Valenstein, E. S. (1998). *Blaming the brain: The truth about drugs and mental health.* New York: Free Press.

Wade, N. (2001). The other secrets of the genome. *New York Times.* February 18.

2

Moot Questions in Psychiatric Ethics

Ralph B. Little and Edward A. Strecker

Medicine is a science blessed with the magnificent heritage of many great men. Men such as Pasteur, Osler, and Harvey are known to laypeople as well as to doctors.

Medicine is the concern of everyone. It is our opinion that of all the men who have contributed to medicine, no one has been more intimately reflected in its actual practice than Hippocrates.

Hippocrates, who lived over 2,000 years ago, is considered the Father of Medicine. He initiated many fine principles, including the scientific method,[1] but none has surpassed his ethical values recorded in his well-known oath, which from its inception has been the basis for medical ethics. The basic principles have remained relatively unchanged. When one considers that there is no procedure in medicine that can be performed without ethics being involved, one can understand the prominent place that this oath has attained. Dr. Robert I. Lee, in an address before the World Medical Association, stated:

The Hippocratic Oath is entirely unselfish and altruistic. It relates to the behavior of doctors for the benefit, not of doctors, but for the benefit of patients. It has been a touch of idealism in a selfish world.[2]

In America, the American Medical Association has restudied, revised, and enlarged upon the ethical principles of the profession four times since 1902. In general, it outlines ethical considerations of the character of the physician, his duties and responsibilities to his patients, to his profession, to his colleagues, and to the general public.

The first sentence of the preamble states:

These principles are intended to serve the physician as a guide to ethical conduct as he strives to accomplish his prime purpose of serving the common good and improving the health of mankind.[3]

In considering the application of ethical principles to the practice of medicine, it should be pointed out that there are many situations where ethical behavior is clear and definite. The physician is either ethical or he is not. For example, if a psychiatrist commits a patient to a mental hospital when he knows the patient is not committable, but does so for financial gain, it is obvious that he is practicing unethical medicine. When, however, as Sperry points out, you have two principles, two forces that are both valid and right but cannot exist simultaneously, and "the claim of each is equally justified, but the right of each is pushed into a wrong because it ignores the right of the other," you have a dilemma demanding ethical action.[4] Thus, if the rights of an individual patient are in opposition to the rights of society, the doctor or the psychiatrist is confronted with the necessity of making a difficult decision which intimately involves his ethical approach to the practice of medicine. In this area, there are considerations about which there is a good deal of uncertainty and divergence of opinion. It is the purpose of this presentation to attempt to obtain better understanding about these doubtful points. To learn more about ethical considerations, we sent the following questionnaire to sixty-seven of our colleagues in Philadelphia, most of them our associates at the Institute of the Pennsylvania Hospital:

Dear Doctor:
Doctor Ralph Little and I are interested in learning more about the less commonly recognized aspects of medical ethics, and have listed some situations that we feel many of us have faced. We would like to have your answers to the questions we have proposed in any way you care to answer them. You might feel that these questions should be answered by a lawyer, but in our experience in this area, psychiatric thinking is more advanced. Thus, we would like the answers to come directly from you. It is important to remember that your opinions, more than anything, determine what are our medical ethics, and that is why we feel your opinions are so important. We will not quote you in any way. Thank you.
EDWARD A. STRECKER, M. D.

(1) What is the ethical responsibility when you have definite proof that a colleague of yours, who is practicing psychiatry is: (a) a narcotic addict; (b) psychotic; (c) indulging in sexual activities with his patients; or (d) prescribing narcotics to addicts for self-administration, which is illegal in that state?

(2) What is your ethical responsibility to a minor whom you are treating, when you definitely believe this patient is homicidal and/or suicidal, and the responsible parent or guardian will not attempt to take measures to protect your patient or society?

(3) What is your ethical responsibility when a patient relates to you he has committed murder, and then forbids you to notify the police on the basis his communications to you are secret?

(4) What is your ethical responsibility when a patient tells you her husband is ill and is planning to kill her, and you have reason to believe this is true, but she will not permit commitment or help from the police, and forbids you to interfere?

(5) What is your ethical responsibility when one of your unmarried patients becomes pregnant during treatment and informs you that she has arranged to have a criminal abortion? There are no indications for a therapeutic abortion, and she forbids you to divulge her professional confidence.

(6) What is your ethical responsibility when a patient whom you are treating for narcotic addiction is securing the drug from illegal sources?

(7) What is your ethical responsibility when you know one of your patients is embezzling, and he refuses to do anything about it?

(8) What is your ethical responsibility when one of your patients takes out a large insurance policy, and plans to commit suicide as soon as the suicide clause is fulfilled, and he does not accept your recommendations for treatment?

(9) What is your ethical responsibility when a patient whom you have had in treatment for some time reveals acts of disloyalty and sabotage against the United States, and demands that you keep such information secret by his right of privileged communication?

We received forty-two responses, but, in tabulating them, could use only thirty-eight as four were too general.

It should be emphasized that the above questions were not a product of our own imaginations, but had occurred in our practice and in those of our colleagues. In tabulating the replies, whenever a psychiatrist gave more than one choice, we recorded his first choice.

To question 1a, "What is your ethical responsibility when you have definite proof that a colleague of yours, who is practicing psychiatry, is a drug addict," there was almost unanimous opinion: thirty-six felt that some action seemed indicated in this situation. Two psychiatrists felt they would take no action unless there was definite proof that the addiction caused the doctor to be negligent in his duties. However, there was a difference of opinion as to what measures should be taken. Sixteen of the thirty-six who felt they should do something about it thought they would try to help the physician by consulting with him directly. Sixteen indicated their first action would be to consult a committee on ethical procedures of their organized group, so that it might take the responsibility. One would notify his family, and three would consult with a senior psychiatrist.

In part b of the first question, "What is your ethical responsibility when one of your colleagues is psychotic?" there was a unanimous feeling that action should be taken, but again there was divergence about what should be done. Eighteen recommended consultation with an appropriate committee or authorities, fourteen would consult the doctor personally. Of the remainder, three recommended consultation with a senior colleague, two physicians would notify his family first, and one would take whatever steps necessary to achieve a solution.

To question 1c, "What is your ethical responsibility when one of your colleagues is indulging in sexual activities with his patients?" thirty-two doctors indicated they would do something and eighteen of these would recommend consulting with a committee, while nine would talk with the doctor personally. Two would consult with a colleague, and three would try to help the doctor get treatment. Of the six who indicated they felt the ethical responsibility did not require action, one said he would do something if the individual doctor was psychotic.

To the fourth part of the first question, "What is your ethical responsibility when a colleague of yours is prescribing narcotics to addicts for their own self-administration which is illegal in that state?" all but four felt definite action was indicated, and twenty-three of the 34 would seek help from an appropriate committee or authorities. Only seven would consult directly with the doctor, three would take whatever steps necessary to solve the problem, and one would consult with a senior colleague.

Question 2.—"What is your ethical responsibility to a minor whom you are treating, when you definitely believe this patient is homicidal and/or suicidal, and the responsible parent or guardian refuses to take measures to protect your patient or society?" In response to this, twenty-nine indicated they would like some definite action and would inform the proper authorities such as the police, district attorney, courts, school authorities, or the appropriate social organization. Of the nine who would not inform outside authorities, four felt they would stop treatment of the minor after informing the family, two would seek consultations, and three would continue treatment.

Question 3.—"What is your ethical responsibility when a patient relates to you that he has committed murder, and then forbids you to notify the police on the basis that his communications to you are secret?" Thirty felt they would deny the patient's request for privileged communication, and do something. Of this group, eighteen would report this action to proper authorities such as the police or district attorney. Five of the thirty indicated they would use their own judgment about informing the authorities, and this would depend on the nature of the murder and how long ago it had been committed. The remaining seven would either consult with the local society, a relative, colleague, lawyer, or stop treatment if the patient would not turn himself in.

Of eight who felt no action was necessary, one stated very definitely that there was no legal responsibility, and seven felt that they should continue treatment, the responsibility of reporting the crime being up to the patient.

Question 4.—"What is your ethical responsibility when a patient tells you her husband is mentally ill and is planning to kill her, and you have reason to believe this is true, but she will not permit commitment or help from the police, and forbids you to interfere?" Twenty-five individuals expressed responsibility for taking some action. Of these, twelve would report to legal authorities; seven would attempt to force commitment of either the husband or the wife, some feeling that the wife might be suicidal. Five would consult with a colleague, and one would refuse treatment if the patient would not accept help. Thirteen indicated they felt their only responsibility would be to continue to treat the patient, trying to point out the meaning of the patient's behavior to her.

Question 5.—"What is your ethical responsibility when one of your unmarried patients becomes pregnant during treatment and informs you that she has arranged to have a criminal abortion?" There are no indications for a therapeutic abortion, and she forbids you to divulge her professional confidence. In this question of ethical responsibility, twenty-nine indicated they would take no definite action, and most of these stated they would try to help the patient understand its psychological significance. (Four did not feel ethical responsibility was involved, and one felt there were too many variables to answer this question.) The opinions of the nine who felt their ethical responsibility demanded some action varied greatly. One would try to commit the patient if she were committable. One would try to find the name of the abortionist and report him anonymously; two would stop treatment if the patient insisted on the abortion. Of those who would report this, one would report to the district attorney, one to a public health officer, one to the parents, and one to the medical society. One felt that there were too many variables to answer the question.

Question 6.—"What is your ethical responsibility when a patient whom you are treating for narcotic addiction is securing the drug from illegal sources?" In reply to this, twenty-two felt they would do something in this situation. Thirteen would report this to the proper law enforcement authorities. Of this group, three would report and refuse treatment, three would try to hospitalize the patient and then report, and seven would just report it. The remainder who would take action indicated that three would only stop treatment, and two would report it to the appropriate committee. Four would take whatever means necessary to hospitalize the patient. Of the sixteen who would not report this, thirteen indicated they would continue treatment, and three stated they felt they had no ethical responsibility.

Question 7.—"What is your ethical responsibility when you know one of your patients is embezzling, and he refuses to do anything about it?" Responses revealed that twenty-two would not feel it their ethical responsibility to report this patient. One would, however, report only if the patient were paying his fees from the embezzled money. Two made the definite statement that no responsibility was present, and three were noncommittal. Sixteen would continue treatment. Of the sixteen who would "do something," six would stop treatment if the patient refused to report himself. Six more would only report him, to either his family, his employer, or the medical society. Two felt that the amount of money would be the determining factor of whether they would report him. One would try to commit him to a hospital, and one would report him to the local medical society.

Question 8.—"What is your ethical responsibility when one of your patients takes out a large insurance policy, and plans to commit suicide as soon as the suicide clause is fulfilled, and he does not accept your recommendations for treatment?" In this question of responsibility, eighteen felt there was no responsibility to do any more than to treat the patient without breaking his confidence, and five of this group specified they would urge hospitalization. Twenty also felt that their responsibility demanded more than to continue treatment; ten would continue treatment, but inform the family; two would insist on commitment; two would report it; one would call in a consultant; another would consult with the medical society. Three would inform the insurance company, one only if he committed suicide. One would stop treatment.

Question 9.—"What is your ethical responsibility when a patient whom you have had in treatment for some time reveals acts of disloyalty and sabotage against the United States, and demands that you keep such information secret by his right of privileged communication?" In response to this question, all but three indicated they felt there was ethical responsibility to report such information. Of these thirty-four (one wished his response would not be used), twenty-seven would report to the proper authorities, and of these, thirteen indicated that they would have to evaluate personally the seriousness of the acts before they would report them. Two would consult their lawyers, two would refuse treatment and seek medical consultation, and two would report to the medical society. One was undecided what he would do.

We would like to discuss our observations from this questionnaire with the following considerations:

We felt that the responses pointed out certain doubtful areas in the concept of privileged communication, by which we mean that the patient expects what he tells his doctor to be held in confidence. This is primarily, but not exclusively, an ethical consideration, for the right of privileged communication means that the doctor has the privilege of deciding whether he will reveal to others what is said to him in confidence. We understand that there are seventeen states that retain the common law rule under which no privilege is recognized covering communications between patient and physician. Other states respect the privileged communication, and consider the doctor liable when he reveals such information to a third party.[5]

Of all the specialties, psychiatry has to depend more than others on the idea of secrecy to be effective therapeutically. We do not see how psychiatrists could successfully treat patients with emotional problems if they cannot say to them, in effect, "Tell me about all your thoughts and feelings—no matter what they are. You don't have to worry about my telling anyone about them." This concept must be part of the very basic structure of the doctor-patient relationship. Hippocrates thought so, and so wrote in his famous oath:

Whatsoever in the course of practice I see or hear (or even outside my practice in social intercourse) that ought never to be published abroad, I will not divulge, but consider such things to be holy secrets.

The American Medical Association enlarged upon this in Chapter II, section 2, of the *Principles of Medical Ethics* of the AMA:

Confidences concerning individual or domestic life entrusted by patients to a physician and defects in the disposition or character of patients observed during medical attendance should never be revealed unless their revelation is required by the laws of the state. Sometimes, however, a physician must determine whether his duty to society requires him to employ knowledge, obtained through confidences entrusted to him as a physician, to protect a healthy person against a communicable disease to which he is about to be exposed. In such instance, the physician should act as he would desire another to act toward one of his own family in like circumstances.

Before he determines his course, the physician should know the civil law of his commonwealth concerning privileged communications.[3]

Thus, both Hippocrates and the American Medical Association seal the lips of the physician unless there is something he feels he "ought" to reveal. Therefore, when the psychiatrist learns something that, if not revealed, might cause innocent people to suffer, he may be forced into a role for which he has not had proper training. The psychiatrist may have to assume the role of a judge, without the wisdom and experience of a judge, in trying to carry out his ethical responsibilities. He may be placed in the tragic situation of trying to serve two loyalties that appear to be in conflict with each other, namely, his loyalty to the practice of psychiatry, with its allegiance to the secrecy inherent in the doctor-patient relationship, and his loyalty as an American citizen to his country and its laws. We have no way of determining how frequently this dilemma may occur in psychiatric practice, but we feel the chances are good that many psychiatrists may be faced with such problems some time during their psychiatric experience.

In making his decision, the psychiatrist will have to decide for himself what information he considers he should or should not reveal. He may differ with a patient who feels that certain information should be regarded as privileged, and may feel that the patient has no right to expect him to conceal certain information that, if kept secret, would result in harm to others. He may feel that by withholding such information, he may indirectly be giving sanction to harmful behavior. His decision about his ethical responsibility will depend on his own personality and experience. There may be times when his ego, that part of his personality that deals mainly with the realistic aspect of the entire problem, will predominantly determine his actions. At other times, his superego, that facet of the mind that is closely allied to his conscience, may take the leading role in arriving at his ethical actions. In coming to a decision, we feel it is important to remember what John W. Reed, of the University of Michigan, wrote to a doctor about this consideration:

It appears that a psychiatrist is under no legal duty to report to law enforcement officials a confession of crime made by a patient in the course of professional treatment. If he does report, he runs the clear risk of a lawsuit at the instance of the patient, there being in the few decisions on the subject a continuing assumption by the courts that there is a civil liability for *unwarranted* breach of confidence. Should such a lawsuit occur, the psychiatrist could apparently prevail over the patient by showing that the disclosure was for the purpose of guarding the community against the possibility of further harm at the hands of the patient.

We would like to discuss the divergence of opinions we received to this questionnaire. We have felt that all the men who received it had the highest ethical responsibility, and for anyone who might question this, the burden of proof would most decidedly be on him. It might be felt that we did not have a fair cross section of psychiatric opinion, for we had responses of men primarily from a certain area of Philadelphia. This may be true, but we are proud of our psychiatry in Philadelphia and of our five medical schools (we had representatives of each in our responses), and we do not feel that we are out of touch with the best psychiatric opinion in the country. Certainly, we do not know of any registered complaints against our ethics. Another objection could possibly be that we might have had different responses if our study had demanded that the responses be anonymous. We can point out that some did send in anonymous replies.

We did not feel that because some of our colleagues believed it their ethical responsibility to do something about some of these matters, while others felt they had no responsibility, that some were ethical and others were not—just as one is not right and the other is not wrong.

These responses did indicate that there are moot questions in psychiatric ethics. The reason for the diversity of opinion seemed to indicate to us a commonly understood fact that each one's own ethical activity is determined by his personality and experience.

There are, of course, advantages and disadvantages in this, and it is our hope that by further discussion of the uncertain areas of ethical conduct, a greater understanding of our responsibility will ensue.

The advantages are, we feel, centered around the idea of freedom. Medicine continues to make rapid advances, the benefits of which will most likely have some effect directly or indirectly on all of us. Progress in the lessening of human suffering has been accomplished in an atmosphere of freedom, which the physician respects and feels he needs for his work. Because a physician works in an area of freedom, his ethical behavior will reflect this, and it would seem deplorable if any attempt were to be made that would legislate his activities, for he is very jealous of his freedom and has certainly put it to good use.

The disadvantages of divergences of ethical responsibilities in psychiatry are that some individual will possibly suffer because of this. We can only hope that this suffering is minimal. We want to repeat that no procedure in medicine can be carried out without ethics being involved, and this emphasizes the importance of further enlightenment on the subject.

We would like to be so bold as to make some recommendations from the observations we have drawn from this study. There seemed to be a feeling that it would be helpful if there were an active committee on ethics in the local medical societies to whom doctors could go with their problems. Such a committee would be available to psychiatrists, promoting discussions and increasing our understanding of our ethical responsibilities.

We want to point out that we have not in any way indicated that we have the answers to these moot questions in psychiatric ethics. We only point out their existence. We also hope that additional discussion between ourselves and our colleagues in the law profession might ensue. Any attempt to further our understanding of our ethical responsibilities can help us, for as Hippocrates stated, if his oath is adhered to by doctors, then "may I enjoy honor in my life, and art among all men for all time: but if I transgress and forswear myself, may the opposite befall me." And, as Gladstone has written, "It is not men who ennoble medicine, but medicine that ennobles men."[6]

If this article has in any way brought about a wish for individual reflection on this subject, and for further discussion and clarification, we shall consider that it has been worthwhile.

References

1. Humphries, S. V. J. (1951). *J. Internat. Coll. Surg.*, 15, 506.

2. Lee, I. R. (1952). *World Medical Association Bulletin*, 4: 148.

3. *Principles of Medical Ethics* of the American Medical Association.

4. Sperry, Willard L. (1948). *New Engl. J. Med.*, 239 (December 23).

5. Guttmacher, M. S., & Weihofen, H. (1952). *Psychiatry and the Law* (p. 271). New York: Norton.

6. Galdston, I. (1948). *On the Psychology of Medical Ethics. Victor Robinson Memorial Volume: Essays on Historical Medicine.* New York: Froben Press.

3

The Ethics of Psychotherapy

Toksoz B. Karasu

In 1978 Spiegel (1) suggested that we have evolved from an Age of Anxiety to an Age of Ethical Crises. Progressive loss of faith in traditional institutions and the erosion of authority are now being met with the increasing challenge of existing standards and widespread concern for safeguarding human values and rights. Today's growing climate of anti-establishment, antiprofessional, and antirational sentiment has direct implications for the roles and responsibilities of the psychotherapist. Growing skepticism about the sanctity of science, medicine, and psychiatry means that these fields are no longer above rebuke or exempt from active moral review by their recipients, professional peers, and others outside their practice, such as third-party payers. The psychotherapist, once left relatively undisturbed in the private confines of his or her office, has now been besieged from within (2) and without (3). The siege from within reflects psychiatry's own members and critics, who extol widely different models and criteria of mental illness and its treatment, which are confusing and divisive to the field and its future. The siege from without reflects the public voice and confusion regarding the functions, procedures, and powers of the psychotherapist. There is an increasing expectation and demand for accountability, that is, that the patient be granted, indeed is owed, health as a right and greater participation in determining and assessing the goals and activities as well as the outcome of treatment. Simultaneously, social, political, and personal pressures oblige the psychotherapist (under the prospect of national health insurance) to assess and review his or her practices. Michels (4) attributed the failure of the profession itself to stave off this challenge and criticism to four factors: (a) a fundamental disappointment with the limitations of science and reason in answering the problems of mankind, (b) an antielitism that aims to mitigate the power of professionals as symbolic representations of the inequitable distribution of resources in society, (c) the compounding of the antiprofessional stance by members of the profession who have failed and then have turned against it in response to exclusion from membership, and, most relevant for the morality issue in psychotherapy, (d) the fear of overgeneralization of the authority of the professional from scientific to ethical arenas.

The Interface between Science and Ethics in Psychotherapy

The issue of the relationship of science to ethics in psychotherapy may be considered the conceptual heart of the matter. *Webster's New World Dictionary* defines *ethics* as "the system or code of morality of a particular person, religion, group or profession; *morals* as "relating to, dealing with, or capable of making the distinction between right and wrong in conduct"; and *science,* which psychotherapy presumes to be, as "a branch of knowledge or study concerned with establishing or systemizing facts." Theoretically, science and ethics have been viewed as two distinct and separate entities, almost antithetical: science as descriptive, ethics as prescriptive; science as resting on validation, ethics as relying on judgment; and science as concerned solely with "what is," ethics as addressing "what ought to be" (5). The lines become less sharply drawn, however, when the complexities of social reality are brought into the picture, when the psychotherapist is obliged to act as a "double agent" (6) to accommodate conflicts of interest posed between patient and therapist and by third parties to whom the therapist holds allegiance, such as family members and school, hospital, and military authorities (7). The lines become even less clear as the therapist confronts the ambiguity between the science and the art of psychotherapy, dual attitudes of the psychotherapist's identity that differ in degree and quality (8). In fact, there is still a question of whether psychotherapy is a science at all, in that it deals with hermeneutics rather than explanation, is humanistic rather than mechanistic, seeks private rather than public knowledge—in all, in that it is not a science but a body of knowledge with a special status, which frees it from obligations that other sciences share (9).

In addition, although the distinction between the principles of science and those of ethics may more readily hold for the researcher inside his or her laboratory, it is simply less applicable to the clinician in daily practice (10). Lifton (6) highlighted this point in describing his work with Vietnam veterans, which required him to combine sufficient detachment to make psychological evaluations with involvement that expressed his own personal commitments and moral passions. (He had taken an active antiwar advocacy position during the Vietnam conflict and expressed profound interest and concern for Hiroshima survivors.) Lifton aptly concluded, "I believe that we [therapists] always function within this *dialectic between ethical involvement and intellectual rigour.*" He went even further to recommend that "bringing our advocacy 'out front' and articulating it makes us more, rather than less, scientific. Indeed, our scientific accuracy is likely to suffer when we hide our ethical beliefs behind the claims of neutrality and that we are nothing but 'neutral screens.'"

With the above in mind, we may say that it is inevitable for the boundaries between science and ethics to become blurred. To the extent that the therapist implicitly, if not explicitly, cares about "what ought to be" as well as "what is," ethical issues will inhere in virtually all of his or her work. In the broadest terms, then, there has been a growing recognition that subjective commitment (unconscious as well as conscious) places inevitable constraints on the presumed purity and verity of objective treatment. More specifically, the idyllic notion of psychotherapy (and the psychotherapist) as value free is now widely accepted as a fallacy (11). This is supported by current research demonstrating many contradictions in expressed belief versus reported practices in psychotherapy (12). Buckley and associates (12) hypothesized the presence of a "two-tier" system: one, the ideal or correct (i.e., value-free, nonsuggestive); the other, the practical or applied view (i.e., direct suggestions, encouragement of specific goals), which loosens the adherence to a value-free frame of reference. In brief, when actually applied, psychotherapy represents neither pure science nor pure ethics but a branch of the healing profession that resides somewhere in between. Therefore, Erikson (13) concluded that psychotherapy can find its ethical place only by locating a legitimate and unique area between the two ideological extremes of being an objectively applied true science and representing an ideology of healthy conduct.

Concern with the interface of science and ethics or healthy conduct and with the place of values in treatment is certainly not new to the field of psychotherapy. A major controversy has long pivoted on the degree to which psychoanalysis inherently propounds any particular value system. Some believe it does not do so (14). Others imply that it is political and repressive by definition (15, 16), that it favors particular cultural values, especially biases toward certain social classes over others (17), and that its basic tenets are inherently biased against women (18). Still others, although they accept that psychotherapy cannot be value free and even believe that in its overall goals it should not be (19), see the fundamental issue as whether the imposition of such values is "deliberate and avowed" or "unrecognized and unavowed" (13).

On a more concrete level, Freud can be credited with the discovery and longtime recognition of the unique power and intensity of the transferential relationship (both to cure and to be resisted) and the inevitable influence of the therapist and his or her values in treatment. This has been classically dealt with in great depth in analytic attempts to maintain the purity of the therapeutic relationship (transference) through the technical neutrality of the therapist, and, when inadvertently violated, the full exploration and understanding of the therapist's countertransference. Freud certainly held an ethical ideal about the conduct of psychotherapy when he wrote, "One must not forget that the relationship between analyst and patient is based on a love of truth, that is, on the acknowledgment of reality, and that it precludes any kind of sham or deceit" (20, p. 248).

The Goals of Psychotherapy

The Principles of Medical Ethics of the American Medical Association (21), first adopted in 1847, set down the standards of practice for physicians. Although psychiatrists are assumed to have the same goals as all physicians, APA added to the *Principles with Annotations Especially Applicable to Psychiatry* (22). The rationale for these annotations was that "there are special ethical problems in psychiatric practice that differ in coloring and degree from ethical problems in other branches of medical practice" (22). These annotations made no alterations whatever in the original AMA standards.

Section 3 of the AMA *Principles* was the only one not annotated for psychiatry. It states that a physician (and therefore a psychiatrist) "should practice a method of healing founded on a scientific basis; and he should not voluntarily associate professionally with anyone who violates this principle." In the annotation to section 6 of the *Principles,* the psychiatrist is advised that "he/she should neither lend the endorsement of the psychiatric specialty nor refer patients to persons, groups, or treatment programs with which he/she is not familiar, especially if their work is based only on dogma and authority and not on scientific validation and replication."

Fisher and Greenberg (23) suggested that the question of the scientific credibility of Freud's theory and therapy, despite extensive exploration, has not been decisively settled in the minds of psychiatrists themselves, although their hearts may tell them otherwise. Moreover, the proliferation of well over 100 supposed schools of psychotherapy,[1] each with its own, albeit overlapping, theory of mental illness and health, therapeutic agents, overall goals, and specific practices (24), reflects the massive nature of investigating therapeutic efficacy and the complexity of establishing scientific guidelines. Given the stunning diversity of therapeutic forms now being offered to potential patients, how does one ethically equate the goals encompassed in a screaming cure (Janov's primal therapy), a reasoning cure (Ellis's rational therapy), a realism cure (Glasser's reality therapy), a decision cure (Greenwald's direct decision therapy), an orgasm cure (Reich's orgone therapy), a meaning cure (Frankl's logotherapy), and even a profound-rest cure (transcendental meditation)? For example, Leo (25) quoted Slavson's assessment of "feeling therapy, nude therapy, marathon therapy, and other new remedies of the ailing psyche." Slavson concluded that "these activities [are] untested, theoretically weak, and potentially very dangerous." More specifically, he asserted that "latent or borderline psychotics with tenuous ego controls and defenses may, under the stress of such groups and the complete giving up of defenses, jump the barrier between sanity and insanity." However, the data on the efficacy of these practices are not yet in. Does the psychotherapist have an ethical responsibility to force closure on these events, especially if his or her judgments are premature?

Such tremendous confusion in the state of the art has led to a virtual identity crisis for psychiatry and the psychotherapist (26–28), highlighted negatively (29) in the recent growth of the antipsychiatry movement, which makes it possible for a psychiatrist to be a psychiatrist by training, accreditation, affiliation, and status but at the same time an antipsychiatrist in ideology and action. (All this under one ethical psychiatric roof.) Indeed, the goals and responsibilities of the psychotherapist are now so broadly and vaguely defined that Raskin (30) said ours is a profession without a "role-specific function" and Vispo (31) said our practices run the gamut from "science to social revolution." Redlich and Mollica (7) described the quandary of whether the practical purpose of psychiatry and the psychotherapist as its agent is "to diagnose, treat, and prevent a relatively defined number of psychoses? To perform this task on a number of neurotics? to make unhappy and incompetent persons happy and competent? or to tackle poverty and civil and international strife?" Although these are not beyond the legitimate concern of psychotherapists in their quest to improve the psychological welfare of their patients, there is a question as to whether these goals are beyond their legitimate competence. Where does one draw the line?

Although broadly recognized goals can include Freud's love and work and variants of growth and maturation, self-realization, self-sufficiency, and security and freedom from anxiety—all of which may be noble aspirations—ethical issues inhere in the practices that are conducted in their name. Across a spectrum of possibilities have been posed questions of freedom to change or not to change versus coercion, helping and healing versus shaping and imposing the therapist's influence, and issues of "cure" of illness versus positive growth. Szasz (32), probably the most prolific and vocal propounder of an antipsychiatry position, views conventional therapy by definition as "social action, not healing" and as "a series of religious, rhetorical, and repressive acts." The basis of the controversy is the medical model's designation of "patient," which presupposes restrictive conceptualizations of normality and health.

One of the most fundamental ethical dilemmas directly related to the goal of therapy is whether to encourage the patient to rebel against a repressive environment or to adjust to his or her condition (33). This issue is illustrated by psychiatry's standard definition and traditional treatment of homosexuals. "Homosexuality" as a "sexual deviation" (*DSM-II*) and its implications have been ardently challenged by advocates for gay rights, and sufficient pressure was brought to bear on APA that the official designation was changed to "sexual orientation disturbance." A review of the psychotherapy and behavior therapy literature indicates that therapists generally regard homosexuality as undesirable, if not pathological (34). On the less theoretical plane of actual treatment goals, the therapist may be obliged to take a position, implicitly if not explicitly, as to whether a heterosexual orientation is a valid ultimate goal for the patient or the patient should maximize the quality of his or her life adjustment as a homosexual. The latter stance, often unpopular, was subject to debate when a behavior therapist treating a man who was sexually attracted to boys provided the patient with methods to transfer that attraction to men, not women (11, 35, 36). Obviously, definitions of goals not only vary between therapists but change with the times as definitions of normality evolve.

Another ethical dilemma in establishing therapeutic goals pertains to the dual allegiance of the therapist to the patient and to society's representatives. This was placed in bold relief in the role of psychiatrists who were treating soldiers in Vietnam (6). Lifton stated that in such instances the therapist is forced to tread the thin line between advocacy and corruption. With adjustment to the military as the goal of therapy, the psychiatrist most likely "helped" the troubled soldier to remain on military duty. This meant that the soldier had to continue the commission of war crimes, which is what he was expected to do in Vietnam. Thus psychiatry served unsuspectingly "to erode whatever capacity [the soldiers] retained for moral revulsion and animating guilt" (6), and the goals of psychotherapists became inseparable from those of military authority.

Aside from conflictual goals in psychotherapy posed by the individual versus the larger society, Hadley and Strupp (37) found that a major area of negative effects of psychotherapy according to a survey of practitioners and researchers in the field was "undertaking unrealistic tasks or goals." These authors listed false assumptions concerning the scope and potency of therapy's purported goals first among tendencies in the conduct of treatment that have profound ethical implications. Misleading impressions may be imbued by therapists when their need to instill hope in the patient and the omniscience endowed them (by themselves and/or the patient) become intertwined. Although some degree of positive expectation or hope is regarded as requisite for producing therapeutic effects in all psychotherapies (38), the patient may get the erroneous impression that therapy and the therapist can solve everything. This can perpetuate unrealistic expectations and goals that are ultimately deleterious to the patient. Such tendencies are often compounded by the failure to discuss, describe, or even acknowledge the reality of goals during treatment or when the stated goals are too broad or obscure.

Special technical problems with ethical implications also arise when goals explicitly or implicitly exceed the patient's capabilities, which fosters false hopes of speedy progress that cannot be realized if the patient actually requires longer treatment. Another problem occurs when the patient has accomplished certain goals but the therapist alters the goals to prolong treatment because he or she is unwilling to terminate it. Greenson (39) aptly warned that any form or aspect of therapy that makes the patient an addict to therapy and to the therapist is undesirable.

Therapists are obliged to ask themselves, How ethical is it to have limited goals when the needs of the patient may change or evolve as the therapy progresses, or when the patient is in need of long-term treatment but either financial or administrative expediencies will not permit it? Can superficial interpretations, made in the interests of time, shortchange patients? Where does one draw the line in serving long-term goals? For example, psychotherapists tend not to prescribe medication for moderate insomnia, anxiety, or depression, the presumed justification being the potentially motivating aspect of discomfort and suffering for psychological work. If this is the case, has the patient been informed of the means and ends of the therapist?

In summary, the issue of the goals of psychotherapy is complex and subtle, including professional versus personal, long versus short term, nonspecific versus specific, and overt versus covert goals. It is the last that is ethically the most problematic and the one most under the therapist's and the patient's control.

The Therapeutic Relationship

The therapeutic relationship or special power relationship that exists between doctor and patient constitutes psychotherapy's strength as well as its weakness. The duality inheres in the concept of authority, which may be defined in many ways (40). In its purist sense, it refers to an individual who is a specialist in his or her field and is entitled to credit or acceptance on this basis; in another sense, it refers to power that requires submission. Different types of therapeutic relationships have been formed with different therapies (24) or at different times in the process of the same therapy (41). A common ethical problem for psychotherapy pivots on the degree to which the therapeutic relationship is authoritarian versus egalitarian or, more specifically, to what extent the pervasive power of the therapeutic transference relationship, which offers the therapist a unique vehicle for exercising enormous influence over another human being, is balanced by a true "therapeutic alliance" (39) or "therapeutic partnership" (42). Redlich and Mollica (7) pointed out that in general psychiatry, "the fiduciary system, in which a patient puts his trust in the physician's ability and willingness to make crucial decisions, is being replaced by a contractual system." This trend applies as well to the current psychotherapies.

An egalitarian therapeutic relationship is gaining in prominence and is considered more humanitarian and facilitative of free exchange between patient and therapist than the traditional medical model (i.e., doctor-to-patient) or the behavioral model (i.e., teacher-to-student) (24). Might some aspects of this model, however, have negative implications for the therapeutic endeavor in general? Parsons (43), in his analysis of social structure and the dynamic process, identified certain requirements of the doctor-patient relationship necessary for successful treatment. One of the most essential was the "social distance" between practitioner and client. In their study of human organization Burling and associates (44) concluded, "We are coming to understand that faith in the doctor is a necessary element in cure, [and] that he will not be able to exercise therapeutic leverage if we, as patients, regard him in too prosaic a light" (p. 71). These authors suggested that the therapist's power to claim the patient's confidence and the therapist's effectiveness will be impaired by growing familiarity. Where, then, does one draw the line between the good use of power in the traditional model and its abuse? Where do the new boundaries of partnership end and those of "real" familiarity and friendship begin? More important for the times, will there be new ethical dilemmas in the egalitarian relationship between therapeutic partners?

Goldberg's exposition of the equitable "therapeutic partnership" (42) suggests that it is not only the nature of the therapeutic alliance (i.e., its power distribution) that is critical but the degree to which it is made explicit. Often within its nonexplicit nature lies the ethical rub of psychotherapy. Goldberg recommended that a therapeutic contract establish a mutually agreed on and explicitly articulated working plan (comparable to the medical model's treatment plan), the essence of which is how each agent will ultimately use or restrict his or her use of power. This should consist not only of agreed-on goals but established means, evaluation of therapeutic work during its course, and methods of addressing dissatisfactions in the working alliance. Articulating in practice what one intends in theory, however, is an admirable but not easily accomplished task. In addition to goal ambiguity, noted earlier, the distinction between theory and practice has also been a criticism of newer modalities like encounter group therapy (45, 46). Despite appearances of therapeutic virtues like openness, autonomy, and mutuality, encounter group therapy often gives little attention to the specificity of individual participants' psychological needs (45), and treatment is often started without defining what the patient wants or expects to be the result of the encounter (46).

How the therapeutic relationship is manifested also relates to one of the most prominent negative effects of the traditional therapeutic relationship, according to a 1976 survey (37): its insufficient regard for the patient's intentionality or will. This can be exacerbated in many ways. For example, in the analyst's fervent search for unconscious determinants, the therapy may soon become an end in itself and the therapist may assume priority over all other people in the patient's life. This can occur in an even more extreme form in the newer, "spiritual" therapies, which encourage pious belief in the therapist that overrides the realities of life itself (witness the tragedy of Guyana). In either event, the therapist's power is greatly exaggerated for reasons that may have more to do with the therapist's needs than those of the patient.

Dependency, nonetheless, is one of the most common characteristics of all patients and allows for the early establishment of the helper-helpee relationship. Other relationships (e.g., transference and a working alliance) that help to play out that dependence and ultimately aid the therapist in encouraging independence in the patient develop in the process of treatment. Some patients, however, need lifelong supervision of their lives even after much of the psychotherapy work is done; often they may take action themselves and terminate treatment. It is also possible that a therapist, because of lack of experience or for less benign reasons (e.g., financial or pathological needs), perpetuates the dependency and unresolved transference of the patient. Although most often viewed within the arena of a technical problem of treatment, the question remains, When does this technical problem in therapy become an ethical issue as well?

Confidentiality

The issues of confidentiality and privileged communication in psychotherapy have had national implications in the last decade, exemplified by the Watergate scandal and the attempt to steal Daniel Ellsberg's records from his psychiatrist's office, but these issues are generally more subtle in everyday psychotherapeutic practice. Although psychotherapists need be concerned here with the ethical rather than the legal aspects of confidentiality, the subject is often complicated by the specter of legal sanction.

The sanctity of confidentiality for the psychotherapeutic endeavor is crucial because of the inherently personal nature of its communications, which plumb the depths of the patient's innermost thoughts, fantasies, and feelings. A number of states, in fact, have statutes that grant the relationship between psychiatrist and patient the same absolute protections from public policy as are accorded to the relationship between husband and wife and attorney and client, to grand jurors, and to secrets of state (47). Indeed, the most elaborate clause of APA's *Annotations* to *The Principles of Medical Ethics* (section 9) (22) relates to this subject. It calls for extreme care in matters of both written and verbal communications, especially in instances of consultation with other professionals, with clinical notes and records, and in case presentations and other use or dissemination of confidential teaching materials. In addition, Redlich and Mollica (7) warned against the more insidious dangers of "gossip" between therapists that might inadvertently prove detrimental to the patient and the therapeutic relationship.

Having to meet current demands for detailed record keeping in anticipation of the requirements and wishes of third-party payers and peer review organizations means that the confidential boundaries of the traditional dyadic relationship between therapist and patient have greatly enlarged and eroded. Both the domain for potential communication (i.e., who is privy to confidential information) and the risk of violation of confidentiality have geometrically increased. Plaut (48) has said that an escalating conflict exists between the right to secrecy and the right to information because of (a) increasing government involvement in areas that were previously considered private affairs; (b) the electronic revolution in data collection, storage, and retrieval; and (c) the prevailing atmosphere of high suspiciousness between individuals and government authorities, for whom knowledge has always meant power.

In view of these new outside pressures, the major questions of confidentiality in psychotherapy are, Whose agent is the psychotherapist (the patient's? the family's? society's? the law's?)? What are the goals of divulging confidential material (better treatment? evaluation? consensual validation? support?)? What are the risks? (Will the therapeutic relationship be jeopardized? Will the patient terminate treatment?) Conversely, will rigid adherence to a rule of confidentiality between therapist and patient blind the therapist to worse fates for the patient—the risk of danger to self or others?

Sometimes the confusion of the therapist's allegiance inheres in the nature of the psychotherapy he or she is conducting—individual, family, or society oriented. Although individual-oriented psychotherapy may limit itself to the more orthodox dyadic goals within the private framework of the patient's inner thoughts and feelings, other goals may be more society oriented and may use the information communicated between therapist and patient to influence the patient's social milieu. A serious question that often arises is the therapist's role and responsibility to the family of the patient. In general, the less healthy the patient, the more important this issue can become. With relatively stable and independent individuals, there is usually no need to contact family members, nor would the therapist encourage any communication from them. Should the latter occur, it is usually in the patient's best interests that he or she be promptly informed of the family contact and that the contact become material for the sessions themselves, grist for the mill of the psychotherapeutic treatment. However, more disturbed patients may not only need the support of the family; they may involve family members with the therapist as an extension of their disturbance. In such circumstances, each communication with the family not only complicates the treatment but also raises serious ethical questions about breaches of confidentiality and whose interests the therapist is serving. In family therapy, whose purported goal is "to treat the family as the patient" (49), the situation may be reversed in that an individual's confidences may be subverted in the therapeutic service of the marital unit or family.

Thus whether a therapist adheres to an individual or a family orientation may determine not only the goals of treatment but also the nature of its treatment of the individual within each mode. How does the therapist determine whether it is in the individual patient's best interests to be seen alone or within the context of the family unit? How ethical is it to impose a systems approach in treatment (e.g., husband and wife, parents and children) because one views the problem as stemming from the family or marriage? On the other side of the coin are instances in which dynamic psychotherapists so strongly believe in utmost confidentiality and individual privacy of the dyadic relationship that they fail to divulge confidences or share information with family members that may prove vital to the welfare of the patient.

Indeed, the only exception to the overall rule of confidentiality between therapist and patient is that of "dangerousness" to others. This concept was legally stipulated by the famous *Tarasoff* decision (50), which enunciated the maxim that "protective privilege ends where public peril begins." According to this decision, therapists must warn authorities specified by law as well as potential victims of possible dangerous actions of their patients. (The legal case involved a young man's confidential announcement to his therapist that he intended to kill his girlfriend. After the therapist had consulted with two psychiatrists and notified the police that the man was dangerous, the young man was detained. However, he was released when he denied such violent intentions. Simultaneously, in response to his therapist's breach of confidence, he broke off treatment. Two months later he murdered his girlfriend. The therapist and his psychiatrist-supervisor were then sued by the woman's parents for failing to warn them of her peril.)

The case, while highly unusual, places in bold relief the dilemmas of therapists in balancing the rights to confidentiality of individuals with the protection of society from danger. Several psychotherapists (51, 52) have been antagonistic to the decision because of its conceptual and practical flaws and its negative implications for psychiatry. Roth and Meisel (51), for example, stated that the decision assumes a degree of expertise in predicting violence or danger that the psychiatrist simply does not possess; that the result will be a confusion and lowering of the threshold of dangerousness for issuing warnings to intended victims, which can compromise the patient's right to confidentiality and possibly his or her treatment; that the psychiatrist is liable not only if he or she fails to warn but also for invasion of privacy or defamation of the patient if the threat of harm does not materialize; and, finally, as actually happened in the *Tarasoff* case, the patient's dangerousness was probably increased because of his sense of betrayal at the therapist's commitment attempt and the patient's premature termination of the very treatment he needed. On a more conceptual level, Gurevitz (52) stated that the *Tarasoff* decision erroneously "defines and reenforces a social control function for psychiatry" by allying the psychotherapist "more with the goal of protecting society than with that of healing patients." It is not, Gurevitz pointed out, that psychiatrists reject the need to balance these functions; in fact, most psychiatrists attempt to fulfill both responsibilities. However, they have done so with procedures that have not mandated them to routinely perform a duty that is "counter to their power of prescience."

Despite the *Tarasoff* decision, and no doubt because of it, alternative courses of action that can be taken by psychotherapists short of actual warning have been recommended. For example, due to their very strong convictions about the importance of confidentiality in the doctor-patient relationship, in no instance have Roth and Meisel (51) directly warned a potential victim without first obtaining the patient's permission. Since actual violence is relatively rare, they stated that it is prudent to "rely on odds and not warn." In addition, they suggested that therapists should inform the patient of the boundaries and limits of confidentiality. Even when danger seems imminent, the therapist should consider a number of social or environmental manipulations to reduce dangerousness before he or she makes the decision to compromise confidentiality. When confronted with a potentially violent patient, the therapist has options that include (a) continued therapeutic management of the patient, (b) involuntary hospitalization, (c) notifying the police, and (d) notifying the potential victims. Each of these choices of action places a differing weight on the competing values of confidentiality versus protection of the social order (or protection from "public peril").

There is also the question of the more private peril of the patient's danger to himself or herself. The following questions remain: Is the therapist able to predict danger to self any better than he or she can predict danger to others? If not, at what point does the duty to warn enter? Where does one draw the confidentiality line when the patient is a threat to himself or herself? Here issues of suicide and its active prevention may also ethically relate to the therapist's ideological position. Recently publicized cases of so-called rational suicide, especially under the psychological and physical specter of terminal illness, along with the call for increased options for dealing with dying, suggest that the psychotherapist may be increasingly faced with the need to respect such choices by patients as part of his or her ethical responsibilities. In each such instance, the therapist and patient alike are obliged to confront and resolve their ethical dilemmas together.

Therapist-Patient Sex and Sexism

The Hippocratic Oath pledges that "with purity and holiness I will practice my art. . . . Into whatever houses I enter I will go into them for the benefit of the sick and will abstain from every voluntary act of mischief and corruption, and further from the seduction of females or males, of freemen and slaves" (53). The *Annotations Especially Applicable to Psychiatry* of *The Principles of Medical Ethics* (22) less eloquently but no less unequivocally upholds this moral tradition by stating simply, "Sexual activity with a patient is unethical." Indeed, it is the only specific activity deemed unethical between doctor and patient that is presented in so unambiguous a fashion. As part of the requirement that the physician "conduct himself with propriety in his profession and in all the actions of his life" (22), the dictum regarding sexual activity is especially important in the case of the psychiatrist because the patient tends to model his or her behavior after that of the therapist by identification. Further, the intensity of the therapeutic relationship may activate sexual feelings and fantasies on the part of both patient and therapist, while weakening the objectivity required for treatment. Insofar as it has earned a position of such priority, therapist-patient sex may be considered the ultimate expression of the overt misuse and exploitation of the transference relationship.

Nonetheless, sexual activities (including sexual intercourse and various forms of erotic contact between therapist and patient) have been increasingly reported in the literature; they have involved clinicians at all levels of training, from psychiatric resident to training analyst (54–61). Despite appearances, this is hardly a new problem for psychotherapists, who have reported erotic transferences and their vicissitudes since the dawn of psychoanalysis. Mesmer, Breuer, Janet, and Charcot, as well as Freud, have amply described the emergence of strong sexual feelings in treatment and the inevitable problems wrought by their presence. Although affairs between therapist and patient were never sanctioned by Freud or his followers, they did occur. However, therapists were often saved from moral indictment, as they still are, by marriage to the patient (and, of course, the termination of treatment by the spouse-therapist). Such a "shotgun" resolution between therapist and patient may be a rather extreme and limited option for dealing with sexual acting out deriving from the therapeutic relationship. The question still remains, What are the ethical options if the therapist does not marry the patient?

In a current assessment of the legal and professional alternatives in deterring, disciplining, or punishing sexual activity between therapist and patient, Stone (62) cited four possible avenues of approach: (a) criminal law (e.g., charges of rape by fraud or coercion), (b) civil law (e.g., malpractice suits), (c) medical boards (e.g., revoked licensure), and (d) professional associations (e.g., pressure to limit referrals and threatened career opportunities). Each in its turn has been virtually ineffectual thus far in providing an effective system of control. In the instance of criminal law, rape charges, which were strongly recommended by Masters and Johnson (63), are rarely brought and rarely stick; most cases involve psychological coercion, not physical coercion. Both force and fraud appear to be required, and the prevailing judicial view is that if the patient consents and the therapist never claimed that sexual activity was treatment, there has been neither force nor fraud. In the instance of civil law damages or malpractice cases, again no legal course may be available if the therapist has not misidentified the sexual activity as treatment. In one recent publicized incident, two factors were held in the therapist's favor: the patient pressed charges a year and a half after the sexual relationship began, and the patient presumably did not have a normal transference. (Legally the therapist was found "negligent," and he continued to practice without his medical license.) Medical licensing boards are not consistent from state to state and often do not have a close relationship with members who are psychiatrists. Finally, professional associations generally have no subpoena power and little expertise in evidentiary investigation, either to protect the due process rights of the therapist charged or if the therapist sues them. Davidson (34) pointed out that going into treatment may be another way for the seductive psychiatrist to escape censure; treatment thus serves to sabotage efforts at discipline. Given the above failings of sanctions from without, Stone (62) was forced to conclude that in the end "patients must depend on the decent moral character of those entrusted to treat them."

What constitutes "decent moral character," however, may be changing with the times, at least according to the findings of some psychotherapists. We have not only Masters and Johnson's extreme stance on the matter (i.e., therapists who have sex with their patients should be charged criminally with rape, no matter who initiated the seduction) (63) but also attitudes on the other side of the scale. Evidence suggests that the sexual value system of psychiatric clinicians has evolved in the direction of increased sexual permissiveness in terms of what is acceptable for themselves and what is acceptable for others (64). In addition, there is the current overt endorsement of touching and so-called nonerotic physical behaviors, especially by advocates of the human potential movement (65, 66). Such activities, far from being regarded as unethical or harmful, are viewed as promoting personal growth and enhancing the therapeutic relationship.

The range of opinions and/or activities on the matter appears to reflect not only individual predilection but also theoretical orientation (67) and major medical specialty (57). Kardener and associates' survey of physicians' erotic and nonerotic physical contact with patients (57) may be relatively heartening in that it found psychiatrists among the lesser offenders in comparison with other medical specialists. Psychiatrists' reported rates of erotic contact—10 percent—and sexual intercourse with patients—5 percent—were lower than those of general practitioners, surgeons, and obstetrician/gynecologists. Moreover, substantial differences regarding therapist-patient sex were found between psychiatrists with "psychodynamic" and those with other theoretical orientations. For example, although 86 percent of the therapists with a psychodynamic orientation felt that erotic contact with the therapist would never benefit the opposite-sex patient, this figure was substantially lower for humanistic and behavioral therapists (71 percent and 61 percent, respectively). That there is widespread ambivalence on the subject even after the fact is reflected in Taylor and Wagner's review of cases of therapists who had actually had intercourse with their patients (68). Less than half (47 percent) reported that the experience had had negative effects on either patient or therapist, 32 percent reported that it had mixed effects, and 21 percent that it had positive effects. (The authors did not survey the patients.) Butler (58), however, found that 95 percent of therapists who had sex with their patients reported conflict, fear, and guilt, yet only 40 percent sought consultation for their problems.

In brief, available evidence suggests that erotic practices with patients do not conform, nor have they ever conformed, to medicine's ethical dictates; neither are any real risks taken by those who engage in them. Those therapists who may not themselves engage in sexual activity with patients have lent subtle support to the practice by protecting their errant colleagues with silence or with treatment (34). Several questions remain: Is such behavior unequivocally unethical regardless of outcome? If erotic contact is decidedly unethical, how ethical is the "nonerotic" kissing, hugging, and touching that more than 50 percent of a sample of psychiatrists said they engaged in with patients (57)? When, if ever, are these appropriate?

Others raise a more subtle issue: Are sexual relations with a patient (nearly always a female patient) simply the tip of the iceberg of the more pervasive practice of sexism in psychotherapy (69, 70)? The ethics of psychotherapy in relation to patient gender has implications not only for its specific abuses (e.g., sex between the male therapist and the female patient) but for other forms of sexual exploitation and discrimination. They may be manifested in psychotherapy's underlying theory, training practices, and doctor-patient relationship. Although it may well be difficult (even unethical) to do otherwise because of subtle and pervasive social pressures, therapeutic theories have more often supported than questioned stereotypical assumptions about sex roles. Broverman and associates (71) noted different standards of mental health for women and men, including tacit assumptions that dependency and passivity are normal for women whereas assertiveness and independence are normal for men. Women who are unhappy in their traditional role have often been considered psychopathological (69).

In addition to the unfortunate legacy of an "antifeminine Freudian position" (69), women may also be harmed by a "blame-the-mother" tradition, especially by therapists positing their potential as "schizophrenogenic" to their children (70). Such sex role biases are then often compounded during the therapist's professional training, in which androcentrism (i.e., male chauvinism) is not likely to be corrected by a male supervisor (70). Indeed, female therapists are much less likely to have had supervisors of their own sex as role models during training: some even have had none (72). By far the most insidious issue of sexism in the practice of psychotherapy has been a function of the predominance of male therapists and the resultant tendency in psychotherapy to replicate within the dyadic relationship the "one-down" position in which women are typically placed. This may encourage the fantasy that an idealized relationship with a powerful other is a more desirable solution to life's problems than taking autonomous action (56, 70). Such a posture, in fact, may set the stage for the kind of sexual exploitation that occurs in instances of therapist-patient sex.

In the final analysis, ethical recommendations for dealing with both sex and sexism in psychotherapy would approximate the constellation of factors found in the new feminist therapies: a greater egalitarianism between therapist and patient in an active attempt to balance the therapist and patient's social power in the therapeutic endeavor and a conscious recognition of the necessity at all times to provide an ethical role model for the patient.

Conclusions

While ethical concerns have no doubt been with the field of psychiatry since its inception, *The Principles of Medical Ethics with Annotations Especially Applicable to Psychiatry* (22) provides a rather modest addendum of suggested standards for the profession. Unfortunately, some therapists feel that, however unprecedented its appearance and despite its noble aspirations, it has serious limitations in assisting them to make ethical decisions in their daily practice. It is understandably disappointing to those who confuse codes with covenants or who expect to magically produce morally scrupulous psychiatrists.

Aside from the merits or failings of a code of ethics itself, Zitrin and Klein (73) insisted that the more pressing problem is not the establishment of guidelines but their enforcement. The sentiment here is that a document can always be revised to better meet the psychiatrist's needs, but there are major problems in self or peer review processes and procedures. These problems include the voluntary nature of complaint investigations, the conflicting roles in which professional committees are required to act (as investigator, prosecutor, judge, and jury), inaccessibility and bureaucratic barriers to the system, inaccurate (and insufficient) case reporting, fear of liability by the professional reviewer, and overconcern with confidentiality, which often takes precedence over other ethical considerations and can be used as a rationalization to resist investigation (74). In actuality, however, it is exceedingly difficult to know what really occurs within the therapeutic relationship. Psychotherapists, like other professionals, are naturally reluctant to judge their colleagues, nor may they feel morally or technically equipped to do so. For example, Sullivan (75) reported that of more than 200 known charges of unethical conduct brought against psychiatrists within a twenty-six-year period (1950–1976), only eight psychiatrists were more than reprimanded.

The ethics not only of the profession but of peer review is also of concern (75). Here a major criticism is that the patient has been excluded from the design process and has been poorly informed about current procedures. Consequently, a prevailing view suggests that psychiatry at this time is simply unable to police itself (73) and that peer review, as currently constructed, is "bound to fail" (76). Nonetheless, we have made and continue to make positive headway in the peer review process (77).

The expectations held for a code of ethics and for peer review may be overendowed, especially by practitioners not directly involved in their development and implementation. For example, in his examination of the true roles and functions of a code of ethics, Moore (74) defined two major purposes as "structuring" and "sensitizing." The first has a basically preventive value and aims to hold back impulsive or unethical behavior; the latter has an essentially educative value and aims to raise one's ethical consciousness. However, a code of ethics can be misused by the moralist or therapist with personal motives that are essentially punitive, not educative or preventive. Moore made the point that a code of ethics should not be viewed as a vehicle for revenge, vindication, or private gain. Comparably, Newman and Luft (78) considered the primary purpose of the peer review process to be education, not control.

These authors suggested that an educational peer review system promoting cooperation among professionals would be of greater utility and more acceptable to clinicians than a bureaucratic system of control, which might tend to foster manipulation. Since the question remains as to how much authority should be vested in peer review committees, using such systems involves very powerful and delicate processes. Ultimately the need for continuing and remedial education for the practicing psychotherapist must be addressed, both for the clinician and for the selection, training, and evaluation of reviewers. More active development of codes of ethics as basic guidelines, not disciplinary instruments, can be used to help elucidate ethical conflicts and the part they play in the life of every psychotherapist.

In conclusion, as I have suggested throughout this paper, the problem of ethics in the practice of psychotherapy is not entirely soluble in that there is no single answer to the varied and complex dilemmas psychotherapists face in relation to the patient and to society. Thus at this time we cannot completely rely on codified instruments—nor should we. Ideally, with the guidance of our professional peers, we must seek individual answers to the ethical problems that inevitably arise. I think the following suggestions would maximize the exercise of ethical choices by the psychotherapist:

1. Greater exploration of the philosophical foundations of therapeutic practice and the ethical assumptions on which psychotherapy is predicated.

2. Awareness of one's own self and personal commitments, for example, by constant examination and analysis of attitudes and behaviors within and outside of the therapeutic relationship.

3. Active development within the treatment endeavor of a "therapeutic alliance" or partnership in which there is equal power and participation by both parties toward mutual goals and responsibilities.

4. Greater allegiance to a code of ethics and its development to better sort out one's ethical choices and their implications for both patient and therapist.

5. Greater responsibility by the clinician for the maintenance of professional competence for himself or herself and others of the profession.

6. Openness to consultation with others and receptivity to outside opinions in making the best ethical decisions in treatment.

7. Greater understanding of human nature and morality from which timely and productive ethical alternatives can be derived.

As Bernal y del Rio (79) aptly put it, "By definition, ethical problems remain unresolved. By their unresolved quality, they provoke a continuous anxiety in the practicing psychiatrist and concomitantly a desire to search, to oppose, to think, and to research."

Note

1. M. Parloff, "Twenty-five years of research in psychiatry." Department of Psychiatry. Albert Einstein College of Medicine. New York, NY, Oct. 17, 1975.

References

1. Spiegel, R. (1978). Editorial: On psychoanalysis, values, and ethics. *Journal of the American Academy of Psychoanalysis*, 6, 271–273.

2. Osmond, H. (1973). Psychiatry under siege: The crisis within. *Psychiatric Annals*, 3(11), 59–81.

3. Freedman, D. X., & Gordon, R. P. (1973). Psychiatry under siege: attacks from without. *Psychiatric Annals, 3*(11), 10–34.

4. Michels, R. (1976). Professional ethics and social values. *International Review of Psycho-Analysis, 3,* 377–384.

5. Fletcher, J. (1971). Ethical aspects of genetic control. *New England Journal of Medicine, 285,* 776–783.

6. Lifton, R. J. (1976). Advocacy and corruption in the healing professions. *International Review of Psycho-Analysis, 3,* 385–398.

7. Redlich, F., & Mollica, R. (1976). Overview: Ethical issues in contemporary psychiatry. *American Journal of Psychiatry, 133,* 125–136.

8. Jasnow, A. (1978). The psychotherapist—artist and/or scientist? *Psychotherapy (Chicago, IL), 15,* 318–322.

9. Edelson, M. (1977). Psychoanalysis as science: Its boundary problems, special status, relations to other sciences, and formalization. *Journal of Nervous and Mental Disease, 165,* 1–28.

10. London, P. (1964). *The Modes and Morals of Psychotherapy.* New York: Holt, Rinehart and Winston.

11. Strupp, H. (1974). Some observations on the fallacy of value-free psychotherapy and the empty organism: Comments on a case study. *Journal of Abnormal Psychology, 83,* 199–201.

12. Buckley, P., Karasu, T. B., Charles, E., et al. (1979). Theory and practice in psychotherapy: Some contradictions in expressed belief and reported practice. *Journal of Nervous and Mental Disease, 167,* 218–223.

13. Erikson, E. (1976). Psychoanalysis and ethics—avowed and unavowed. *International Review of Psycho-Analysis, 3,* 409–415.

14. Marcuse, H. (1955). *Eros and Civilization.* Boston: Beacon Press.

15. Szasz T. (1961). *The Myth of Mental Illness.* New York: Hoeber-Harper.

16. Torrey, E. F. (1974). *The Death of Psychiatry.* Radnor, PA: Chilton.

17. Hollingshead, A., & Redlich, F. (1958). *Social Class and Mental Illness: A Community Study.* New York: Wiley.

18. Horney, K. (1939). *New Ways in Psychoanalysis.* New York: Norton.

19. Fromm-Reichmann, F. (1959). *Psychoanalysis and Psychotherapy.* Chicago: University of Chicago Press.

20. Freud, S. (1964). Analysis terminable and interminable (1937–1939). In J. Strachey (Trans., Ed.) *Complete Psychological Works* (Vol. 23). London: Hogarth Press.

21. American Medical Association. (1971). *Opinions and Reports of the Judicial Council.* Chicago: AMA.

22. *The Principles of Medical Ethics with Annotations Especially Applicable to Psychiatry.* (1968). Washington, DC: APA.

23. Fisher, S., & Greenberg, R. P. (1977). *The Scientific Credibility of Freud's Theories and Therapy.* New York: Basic Books.

24. Karasu, T. B. (1977). Psychotherapies: An overview. *American Journal of Psychiatry, 134,* 851–863.

25. Leo, J. (1969). Danger is found in some remedies: Group psychotherapy body urges thorough study. *New York Times,* February 9, 92.

26. Brill, N. (1973). Future of psychiatry in a changing world. *Psychosomatics, 14,* 19–26.

27. Kety, S. (1974). From rationalization to reason. *American Journal of Psychiatry, 131,* 957–963.

28. Yager, J. (1974). A survival guide for psychiatric residents. *Archives of General Psychiatry, 30,* 494–499.

29. Cerrolaza, M. (1973). The nebulous scope of current psychiatry. *Comprehensive Psychiatry, 14,* 299–309.

30. Raskin, D. (1972). Psychiatric training in the 70s—toward a shift in emphasis. *American Journal of Psychiatry, 128,* 119–120.

31. Vispo, R. (1972). Psychiatry—paradigm of our times. *Psychiatric Quarterly, 46,* 208–219.

32. Szasz T. (1978). *The Myth of Psychotherapy.* New York: Anchor/Doubleday.

33. Blatte, H. (1973). Evaluating psychotherapies. *Hastings Center Report* (Sept.): 4–6.

34. Davidson, V. (1977). Psychiatry's problem with no name: Therapist-patient sex. *American Journal of Psychoanalysis, 37,* 43–50.

35. Garfield, S. (1974). Values: An issue in psychotherapy. Comments on a case study. *Journal of Abnormal Psychology, 83,* 202–203.

36. Davison, G. C., & Wilson, G. T. (1974). Goals and strategies in behavioral treatment of homosexual pedophilia: Comments on a case study. *Journal of Abnormal Psychology, 83,* 196–198.

37. Hadley, S. W., & Strupp, H. H. (1976). Contemporary views of negative effects in psychotherapy: An integrated account. *Archives of General Psychiatry, 33,* 1291–1302.

38. Frank, J. (1961). *Persuasion and Healing: A Comparative Study of Psychotherapy.* Baltimore: Johns Hopkins University Press.

39. Greenson, R. (1967). *The Technique and Practice of Psychoanalysis* (Vol. 1). New York: International Universities Press.

40. Miller, D. (1977). The ethics of practice in adolescent psychiatry. *American Journal of Psychiatry, 134,* 420–424.

41. Karasu, T. B. (1980). General principles of psychotherapy. In T. B. Karasu & L. Bellak (Eds.), *Specialized Techniques in Individual Psychotherapy.* New York: Brunner/Mazel.

42. Goldberg, C. (1977). *Therapeutic Partnership: Ethical Concerns in Psychotherapy.* New York: Springer Publishing Co.

43. Parsons, T. (1951). *The Social System.* Glencoe, IL: Free Press.

44. Burling, T., Lentz, E. M., & Wilson, R. N. (1956). *Give and Take in Hospitals: A Study of Human Organization.* New York: Putnam.

45. American Psychiatric Association. (1970). *Encounter Groups and Psychiatry. Task Force Report 1.* Washington, DC: APA.

46. Goldberg, C. (1970). *Encounter: Group Sensitivity Training Experience.* New York: Science House.

47. Dubey, J. (1974). Confidentiality as a requirement of the therapist: Technical necessities for absolute privilege in psychotherapy. *American Journal of Psychiatry, 131,* 1093–1096.

48. Plaut, E. A. (1974). A perspective on confidentiality. *American Journal of Psychiatry, 131,* 1021–1024.

49. Bloch, D. A. (1976). Family therapy, group therapy. *International Journal of Group Psychotherapy, 26,* 289–299.

50. Tarasoff v. Regents of the University of California. (1974). 118 Calif. Rep. 129, 529 P.2d 553.

51. Roth, L. H., & Meisel, A. (1977). Dangerousness, confidentiality, and the duty to warn. *American Journal of Psychiatry, 134,* 508–511.

52. Gurevitz, H. (1977). *Tarasoff:* Protective privilege versus public peril. *American Journal of Psychiatry, 134,* 289–292.

53. Braceland, F. J. (1969). Historical perspectives of the ethical practice of psychiatry. *American Journal of Psychiatry, 126,* 230–237.

54. Dahlberg, C. (1970). Sexual contact between patient and therapist. *Contemporary Psychoanalysis, 6,* 107–124.

55. Truax, C. B., & Mitchell, K. M. (1971). Research on certain therapist interpersonal skills in relation to process and outcome. In A. E. Bergin & S. L. Garfield (Eds.), *Handbook of Psychotherapy and Behavior Change: An Empirical Analysis.* New York: Wiley.

56. Chesler, P. (1972). *Women and Madness.* Garden City, NY: Doubleday.

57. Kardener, S., Fuller, M., & Mensh, I. (1973). A survey of physicians' attitudes and practices regarding erotic and nonerotic contact with patients. *American Journal of Psychiatry, 130,* 1077–1081.

58. Butler, S. (1975). *Sexual contact between therapists and patients* (doctoral dissertation, California School of Professional Psychology).

59. Robertiello, R. (1975). Iatrogenic psychiatric illness. *Journal of Contemporary Psychotherapy, 7,* 3–8.

60. Stone, M. (1975). Management of unethical behavior in a psychiatric hospital staff. *American Journal of Psychotherapy, 29,* 391–401.

61. Marmor, J. (1976). *Some psychodynamic aspects of the seduction of patients in psychotherapy.* Presented at the 129th annual meeting of the American Psychiatric Association. Miami Beach, FL, May 10–14.

62. Stone, A. A. (1976). The legal implications of sexual activity between psychiatrist and patient. *American Journal of Psychiatry, 133,* 1138–1141.

63. Masters, W. H., & Johnson, V. E. (1976). Principles of the new sex therapy. *American Journal of Psychiatry, 133*, 548–554.

64. Roman, M., Charles, E., & Karasu, T. B. (1978). The value system of psychotherapists and changing mores. *Psychotherapy (Chicago, IL), 15*, 409–415.

65. Levy, R. B. (1973). *I Can Only Touch You Now.* Englewood Cliffs, NJ: Prentice-Hall.

66. Pattison, J. E. (1973). Effects of touch on self-exploration and the therapeutic relationship. *Journal of Consulting and Clinical Psychology, 40*, 170–175.

67. Holroyd, J. C., & Brodsky, A. M. (1977). Psychologists' attitudes and practices regarding erotic and nonerotic physical contact with patients. *American Psychologist, 32*, 843–849.

68. Taylor, B. J., & Wagner, N. N. (1976). Sex between therapists and clients: A review and analysis. *Professional Psychology, 7*, 593–601.

69. Rice, J. K., & Rice, D. G. (1973). Implications of the women's liberation movement for psychotherapy. *American Journal of Psychiatry, 130*, 191–196.

70. Seiden, A. M. (1976). Overview: Research on the psychology of women, II. Women in families, work, and psychotherapy. *American Journal of Psychiatry, 133*, 1111–1123.

71. Broverman, I. K., Broverman, D. M., Clarkson, F. E., et al. (1970). Sex-role stereotypes and clinical judgments of mental health. *Journal of Consulting and Clinical Psychology, 34*, 1–7.

72. Seiden, A., Benedek, E., Wolman, C., et al. (1974). *Survey of women's status in psychiatric education: report of the APA Task Force on Women.* Presented at the 127th annual meeting of the American Psychiatric Association, Detroit, MI, May 6–10.

73. Zitrin, A., & Klein, H. (1976). Can psychiatry police itself effectively? The experience of one district branch. *American Journal of Psychiatry, 133*, 653–656.

74. Moore, R. A. (1978). Ethics in the practice of psychiatry: Origins, functions, models, and enforcement. *American Journal of Psychiatry, 135*, 157–163.

75. Sullivan, F. W. (1977). Peer review and professional ethics. *American Journal of Psychiatry, 134*, 186–188.

76. Klein, H. (1975). Current peer review system bound to fail. *Psychiatric News*, July 16, 21.

77. Chodoff, P., & Santora, P. (1977). Psychiatric peer review: The DC experience, 1972–1975. *American Journal of Psychiatry, 134*, 121–125.

78. Newman, D. E., & Luft, L. L. (1974). The peer review process: Education versus control. *American Journal of Psychiatry, 131*, 1363–1366.

79. Bernal y del Rio V. (1975). Psychiatric ethics. In A. M. Freedman, H. I. Kaplan, & B. J. Sadock (Eds.), *Comprehensive Textbook of Psychiatry* (2nd ed., Vol. 2, p. 2546). Baltimore, MD: Williams & Wilkins Co.

4

Character Virtues in Psychiatric Practice

Jennifer Radden and John Z. Sadler

The character-focused approach known as *virtue ethics* is especially well suited, we believe, for understanding and promoting ethical psychiatric practice. Virtues are the personal qualities, such as integrity, honesty, and compassion, that we attribute to character.[1-3] They are traits—stable dispositions and responses rather than more passing and temporary states. For this reason, they are often used in describing people. "She is a courageous person," we say, or, "He is compassionate." A virtue-based ethics, then, is one in which people's selves or characters, rather than their actions or the consequences that flow from those actions, are at the center of moral assessment.[4-11] Because virtue ethics emphasizes everyday conduct, behaving virtuously implies that everyday conduct is laden with moral value. Likewise, as we shall indicate later, everyday clinical practices and strategies can be understood as imbued with virtues (and hence with morality, too).

A virtue focus can be contrasted with other approaches to ethics, yet pluralistic forms of virtue ethics are also possible—ones in which virtues provide some strong moral reasons, but not the only moral reasons, for acting and living.[7] Moreover, only a misreading, it has been argued, could present either Kantian (emphasizing rights and duties) or utilitarian traditions (directed toward maximizing happiness) as indifferent to the importance of character virtues in the moral life.[12] Similarly, an ethical position defined by particular values or principles, such as Beauchamp and Childress's principlism, could be construed as a set of character traits:[13] the principle of beneficence resides in the benevolent character, autonomy in the character that is self-determining and respectful of others, and so on. An ethics of care (where caring and caregiving are central to the moral life) accommodates a focus on the character of the carer.[14] Even a pragmatist approach that emphasizes the need for flexibility and contextualized moral responses can be depicted in terms of virtues such as the flexibility, sensitivity to context, and open-mindedness that we associate with the pragmatic frame of mind. Thus, only differences of emphasis and framing need distinguish virtue ethics from these other approaches. Also, rather than a single group of tenets shared among virtue theorists, virtue ethics forms a family of related assumptions and emphases, not all of which are equally pertinent to the settings where psychiatry is practiced (i.e., in relation to those suffering from severe mental disorders).

In the first section of this discussion ("Habituation"), case scenarios illustrate some of the reasons that virtue ethics is applicable to psychiatric practice. These scenarios are presented unconventionally for three reasons: to avoid some of the artificiality and limitations associated with standard case material in biomedical ethics;[15] to emphasize that virtues are identifiable through the person's inner, mental life, as much as through any outward actions; and to show that behaving virtuously is a *task* requiring rehearsal, planning, focus, effort, and discipline. Using these cases, we illustrate some of the following key aspects emphasized in virtue-focused discussions: virtues are acquired through habituation; they are habits of mind as much as behavior; they are heterogeneous as a group, and individually composite; they involve affective responses; they are not impartial; they are compatible with the "role morality" required of professionals; they are responses to particular temptations and weaknesses; and they include, in the capacity for practical judgment known as *phronesis*, a means for resolving conflicts and dilemmas that arise in practice.

The approach to ethics involving virtues will likely be most useful, we believe, in the educational setting, where practitioners are learning clinical skills and being shown the broad ethos of practice. In the second part of our discussion ("Questions About Teaching the Virtues Required in Psychiatric Practice"), aspects of this educational effort are briefly reviewed, including whether it ought to be undertaken at all, whether it is possible to teach virtues, and, if so, how it is to be achieved.

For purposes other than educational ones, a virtue-based approach may be insufficient, we readily grant, and other approaches will be more useful. The purposes of professional censure, for example, along with the codification of minimal standards of professional practice, require us to identify actions as *obligatory* (as in the physician providing the best standard of care), *forbidden* (as in the case of sexual relationships with patients), or *permitted* (as in the [limited] flexibility associated with clinician self-disclosures). For the purpose of establishing these minimal standards, virtues may be insufficient; the focus on deeds and on clear rules (as found in Kantian or utilitarian frameworks) will be more helpful here even if, as most virtue theorists believe, those rules must ultimately have been derived from virtues. Nonetheless, the importance of virtues cannot be overestimated, and as we believe our cases illustrate, virtues have been too often neglected or overlooked.

As we consider various ramifications of the virtue aspects of psychiatric ethics, our cases will appear as dramatic exchanges, with the clinician's thoughts, or inner monologue, set apart in italics. The intention is to convey both the inner workings of the virtuous character as well as the behavioral enactments of virtue.[16] The cases were selected to represent ordinary and common clinical situations in order to illustrate the ubiquity of virtue concerns. Our cases are a combination of fictitious and composite clinical situations.

Part 1: Habituation

Virtues are traits that may be acquired and strengthened through habituation—which is, at least, the way that virtues have been understood, following Aristotle. The process resembles that by which we acquire and strengthen any habits; it calls for attention, conscientiousness, and repetition, together with the close observation of exemplary models. Like later philosophers—who emphasized that virtues stem from natural human tendencies, both affective and social, appropriately shaped in childhood—Aristotle recognized the importance of feelings as antecedents and preconditions, as well as ingredients, of moral virtues. But the educational setting where, as young adults, practitioners are taught professional rules of conduct presupposes that such basic moral education has been achieved.

The following brief exchange between a third-year medical student and his "attending" supervisor illustrates a student's burgeoning awareness of the need for habituation:

Dr. Chang: John, did you put Mrs. Millikan's fMRI report on the chart?
Student John: Oh, no! I left it in my backpack in the car. I should have put it on the chart right away. No, I forgot.
Dr. Chang (annoyed): So where is it?
Student John (anxious): I left it in my pack in the car last night.
Dr. Chang: I'm going to have to have a talk with this kid in private. This could have compromised the patient's care. How about going down to your car and getting it right away? Our next management decision depends on that report. Remember, "Be meticulous!"

Student John: Okay. *How many times have people told me to get organized? I should get a day planner or something.*

Student John's casual approach to the fMRI report is judged by Dr. Chang a serious failure. Orderly record keeping, careful attention to detail, and consistent follow-through are habits essential for effective and ethical practice. Indeed, to learn rules of conduct such as those embodied in the slogan "Be meticulous!" will be to acquire some virtuous habits.

Habits of Mind as Much as Behavior

Virtues are habits of mind as much as of outward behavior. Rather than the action-oriented focus of rules of conduct, "*Do* thus and so," the virtue-focused admonition is often something closer to "Strive to *be* thus and so." Of course, what a person does is also important, as are the consequences of that conduct. Nonetheless, possessing a virtue might affect not actions, but felt responses that find no immediate expression in action—habits of deliberation, concentration, imagination, and attention; or it might involve the difference between an action motivated in one way rather than another.

The following exchange occurred during a narcissistic patient's second psychotherapy session with a psychiatry resident:

Mr. Stevens: All my prior therapists have come out to the car to see my cats. It's a sign that the therapist cares about me, so when you didn't do it, it made me angry and made me wonder about whether you really care. Do you?
Dr. Fox: *It's pretty clear that I'm going to need to focus on this guy's underlying vulnerability in order to stay empathic with him. It's easy to understand why his prior resident therapists complained about his sense of entitlement and avoidance of responsibility. He's managed to annoy me already.* Of course, I care about you. I overlooked the significance of your cats. This incident, though, reminds me of what you said earlier about feeling slighted and ignored by people in the past—so this must have generated some old and unpleasant feelings for you.

The emphasis on inner states that comes with a focus on virtues fits the healing medium of psychiatric practice. The "action" or conduct involved in that practice is often imperceptible to the observer, as with Dr. Fox's insight about his patient's underlying vulnerability. Exercising judgment, applying knowledge, concentrating, recalling, imagining— these take place within the mind of the person. Even when overt, what the practitioner does is often subtle, conveying warmth and understanding through words, demeanor, and body language, rather than through grosser motor action. Dr. Fox listens and speaks only briefly during this exchange. Yet his response to Mr. Stevens will likely be effective. He allows himself to explore what lies beneath Mr. Stevens's annoying attitude. Recognizing the underlying vulnerability of this patient, Dr. Fox is able to foster the alliance and to convey regard, warmth, and a sympathetic appreciation of the effect of past painful experiences, while at the same time raising matters for further discussion and exploration.

Heterogeneous as a Group, and Individually Composite

Virtues are heterogeneous and composite. Rather than natural kinds, they are, when considered together, a loose group of qualities varying in their makeup, in their perceived value, and in the extent to which their status as moral virtues reflects agreed, stable norms. Even regarded individually, virtues are not unitary traits. Each particular quality (compassion, kindness, and so on) is a composite, made up of feelings, impulses, attitudes, capabilities, and motivations.

The following conversation took place during a meeting between the psychiatry resident from the previous example (Dr. Fox) and his psychotherapy supervisor:

Dr. Fox: Mr. Stevens spent most of his session complaining about the disappointments he has had with others. He was offended when I didn't want to go out to the parking lot and see his pet cats in his car. I know he's struggling with shame and a sense of inadequacy, but I'm having trouble crafting supportive responses to him while also getting him to acknowledge his own feelings.

Dr. Elder: This was just the second session, and there are good reasons why therapy with narcissistic patients takes a long time. Your initial focus with this man is to develop the alliance by reflecting back and contextualizing his feelings. It's hard to be patient with patients like this.

Dr. Fox: Sometimes I feel that by being empathic with him, I'm approving of his maladaptive behavior.

Dr. Elder: What's your role—being the judge, or the person who understands? Cultivate your curiosity about him.

Dr. Fox's description of his patient shows some of the mix of cognitive understanding (e.g., about Mr. Stevens's sense of inadequacy), compassionate feeling (prompted by Mr. Stevens's underlying shame), and goal-oriented perception (when he tries to get Mr. Stevens to acknowledge his sense of inadequacy and when he strives to convey empathy to further the alliance). Even curiosity, Dr. Elder points out, might be part of this mix—and a useful trait for clinical effectiveness. A number of different virtues will be required in working with this patient. Moreover, the curiosity that Dr. Fox is encouraged to cultivate illustrates the composite nature typical of each individual virtue. Curiosity comprises several subcapabilities: sensitivity, but also careful attention, empathic listening, imagination, and a kind of eagerness for discovery.

Affective

Virtues involve emotional responses: as clusters of attributes and capabilities, they usually comprise affective, cognitive, and motivational elements. This emphasis fits psychiatric practice, where affective traits are especially important. In addition to the knowledge, skill, and attention to detail with which Dr. Fox must approach Mr. Stevens (see the previous case example), compassion, empathy, and concern are required. Only with the addition of these elements, as Dr. Elder points out, will Dr. Fox achieve the alliance that is the sine qua non of effective practice. And with awareness of the vulnerability beneath Mr. Stevens's outward, narcissistic show, Dr. Fox is able to alter and soften his own attitudes and to feel compassion for his patient.

Partiality

Most accounts of virtue ethics emphasize that it avoids the kind of universalizing "impartialism" that demands that we treat other people in the same way regardless of the relationship they may have to us. The impartialism associated with ethical systems such as the Kantian and utilitarian ones has come to be regarded as an impoverished and perhaps wrongful picture of the moral life and moral deliberation.[17,18] Some central human roles and activities call for a partial, not an impartial, response toward others; for example, a parent will—and *should*—prefer her own children's welfare and safety to that of other children. Similarly, the practitioner's commitment to the interests and well-being of his own patients is a mainstay of the professional role. The practitioner-patient relationship at the center of any type of medical practice calls for such partial responses from the practitioner.

The following conversation takes place between a consultation-liaison psychiatrist and an internist who wishes to discharge a patient:

Dr. Markowitz (the psychiatrist):   *I can't believe this. Irwin is going to discharge this patient without looking at her thyroid function test results.* Dr. Irwin, all I'm asking is that we wait for the TFTs to come back before you discharge this patient. We believe her delirium is classic myxedema: note her boggy pretibial edema.

Dr. Irwin: Look, it's not my fault that psych doesn't have the beds to accept this patient, but there are three more sick patients in the ER waiting for this patient's bed. I can't justify keeping her here with only psychosis as a diagnosis. All the other labs have been negative.

Dr. Markowitz: *This patient belongs on medicine and the patient should come first.* Look, we both want what's best for the patient. Is it the bed availability? Because if that's it, we [the psychiatry consultation service] can manage the patient on another service's bed, at least until myxedema is ruled in or out.

In the face of what he sees as a too ready willingness on the part of Dr. Irwin to discharge his patient, Dr. Markowitz's concern for this patient becomes intense. It allows him to respond with vehemence, persistence, and (as is apparent with regard to finding a bed) flexibility. It has long been recognized that doctors have role-specific duties and that those duties pertain to "my patients, persons who occupy a special, especially vulnerable position and with whom I have enacted special ties and bonds."[19] These ties, moreover, involve a partiality to which virtue ethics can well be applied, in both the psychiatric and broader medical setting.

Compatible with Role Morality

The ethical codes of professions such as medicine, which involve treating one's own patients or clients with special partiality, exemplify "role morality"—that is, the obligations or constraints attaching to, and generated by, a particular social role. In this form, role morality imposes on anyone undertaking particular roles a set of moral demands exceeding those imposed on other persons.

The context for the following conversation is an end-of-the-day, follow-up medication visit between a psychiatrist and one of his patients, a professional model being treated with antidepressants:

Dr. Roma: *I'm finding it difficult to keep my mind on my work when this woman dresses this provocatively.* Ms. Veronica, you're having, in my view, an excellent response to this particular medication. I don't think you need to see me again for a couple of months. Do you have any questions for me before we finish?
Ms. Veronica: Yeah. It's really hard to get a taxi at this time of day. Any chance I could catch a ride with you uptown?
Dr. Roma (mustering composure):   Hmm. *How to say no (when I want to say yes)?* I really can't do that, but I'd be happy to get the clinic secretary to make some calls to see if she can find a taxi for you.

Because the demands imposed by medical roles are more, not less, stringent than those of more broad-based morality, the demands of these roles are uncontroversial in that they never override, but only add to, the dictates of broad-based morality. Had Dr. Roma and Ms. Veronica been in a nonprofessional setting, Dr. Roma might have been free to respond to Ms. Veronica's seductive suggestion. But the greater demands imposed by the medical role prevent him from doing so, as he explains. Indeed, his internal awareness of temptation triggers a contrary response, one that definitively and unhesitatingly respects the proper professional boundary. Some theorizing distinguishes moral virtues from other valuable or useful character traits. However, within a professional setting that involves role-specific duties, any trait that is conducive to the goal or good of that practice—here health and healing—*acquires the status* of a moral virtue.[20] Practitioners' virtues may, in this sense, be said to be constituted by their roles. Dr. Roma's restraint is itself an exhibition of virtue, not merely of good judgment or some form of prudence. It is morally incumbent on Dr. Roma to avoid Ms. Veronica's provocation.

Moral Psychology as Including Temptations and Weaknesses
Virtue-focused traditions account for the whole moral psychology of ethical responses, emphasizing that each virtue is opposed to—and helps ward off—a particular, matching temptation or vice. Possessing empathy will help prevent a person from succumbing to indifference toward others; the virtue of kindness will ward off cruelty; and so on.

The following conversation continues after the immediately preceding one involving the professional model in need of a taxi:

Ms. Veronica: Oooh. That feels like a rejection.
Dr. Roma: I'm sorry, it wasn't meant that way. You know, you have mentioned that over the course of your depression, you've felt that men have either wanted you as their "party doll" or ignored you as a "bimbo" [her terms from prior visits], and I wonder if you've given more thought to getting into psychotherapy around this issue, as we've discussed before. You've mentioned that you've had friends who have found Dr. English very helpful.

Here, Dr. Roma needs not only to rebuff Ms. Veronica's advances, but to do so without compromising the relationship he has formed with her or doing anything to threaten her already fragile sense of her own sexuality. His efforts to show sympathy for Ms. Veronica's feelings about past sexual exploitation, while at the same time refusing her advances, stem from his own understanding of, and sensitivity to, her insecurities around sexual issues. Against this background, Dr. Roma will presumably be able both to ward off his own growing feelings toward Ms. Veronica and to deal with the countertransference. These two conversations with Dr. Roma and Ms. Veronica illustrate our introductory point about the virtue-laden quality of clinical methods, practices, and techniques. For example, while dealing with countertransference is a technical practice aimed at therapeutic goals (which are themselves value laden), dealing with countertransference is also itself virtue laden in that it calls for the clinician to inhibit impulses, think prudently, and place the patient's behavior and his own response into the larger therapeutic context. In this sense, countertransference management is one of the tasks of a virtuous clinician and reflects virtues such as prudence, empathy, patience, restraint, and (see below) *phronesis*.

Following the model by which virtues are a remedy against specific temptations, there will always be situation-specific temptations to which specific role-constituted virtues correspond, and against which they serve to protect. Features of the psychiatry setting—such as the vulnerabilities of patients, the privacy of the arrangements governing therapeutic sessions, the personal and intimate material often discussed, and the heightened power imbalances between practitioner and client—seem to impose extra moral demands on practitioners and to magnify the likely temptations. The most obvious here are temptations to engage in sexual misconduct. Less obvious temptations include "power trips," such as that of "playing God" or the vicarious satisfaction from hearing another person's intimate and personal story. Other examples include the temptations to exploit the situation by indulging bias, whimsy, narcissism, and prejudice to preserve one's own self-esteem and psychological unity at the expense of the patient. Temptations like these are as much part of psychiatric practice as are occasions inviting the more commonly acknowledged vices (e.g., involving sexuality). These various temptations are a routine dimension of clinical practice, place corresponding moral demands on practitioners, and typically require the exercise of moral virtues.

Phronesis

Many virtues are demanded by the practice of psychiatry, including many ordinary qualities, such as trustworthiness and empathy, that are required in everyday settings as well. An enumeration is beyond the scope of this discussion. However, those writing about the character of "the good doctor" have often noted the vital part played by the virtue Aristotle identified as *phronesis*, usually translated as practical wisdom.[21] *Phronesis* is the set of capabilities that allow us to deliberate about things with ends or goals in mind, and to discern and enact right action, thus acknowledging the complexities involved in practical realities. The clinician must combine theoretical knowledge with the particularities of individual cases, a combination that calls for a grasp of particulars, cleverness (in the ability to find what is needed to achieve an end or goal), perception (in order to notice facts in a situation), and finally, understanding—good, practical commonsense.

The setting for the following conversation was an examination room (with the door open) in a hospital's emergency department.

Mr. Buck (fidgeting and restless as he then takes out a sizable pocket knife and starts rolling it around in his hands): Now that I've told you my name and address and such crap, you probably want to know why I came in, right?

Dr. Douglas: *What's going on here?! He's not obviously paranoid or psychotic,*
but . . . Sure.
Mr. Buck (opening and closing the knife): I've had thoughts about killing
people. They're just pissing me off all the time. Anything they say . . . the people
at work, the supervisor, even my buddies.
Dr. Douglas: *Okay, violence is driven often by narcissistic injury, so perhaps I*
should admit my own vulnerability. Mr. Buck, your playing with that knife is
really making me nervous and making it hard for me to concentrate on what
you're saying. Would you mind putting it away?
Mr. Buck (surprised; puts knife back into pocket): Sorry. Okay.
Dr. Douglas: Thanks. You were saying that that you were having violent
thoughts about people at work. Can you tell me more about that?
Mr. Buck: Sure, but can I have a cup of coffee?
Dr. Douglas: Sure. How many cups have you had today?
Mr. Buck: About forty.
Dr. Douglas: *Could this guy's caffeine poisoning be driving his irritability?* On
second thought, I'm wondering if your coffee drinking is making you irritable.
Would you mind if I brought you some juice instead?
Mr. Buck: Okay. Usually coffee mellows me out, so since these thoughts have
started, I've been drinking more. No kidding—you think it's the coffee!?

After completing his assessment and allowing the effects of Mr. Buck's
caffeinism to subside, Dr. Douglas discharged the patient to outpatient
follow-up.

Dr. Douglas exhibited considerable clinical elegance here. His insight
that caffeine poisoning might be the source of Mr. Buck's alarming
behavior achieved several ends. He adroitly diffused an immediately
dangerous situation and then made a provisional diagnosis, while at the
same time gratifying his patient's wish for something to drink. His
response exhibited perception (in seeing where the problem lies) and
understanding (in discerning its immediate solution)—the core traits that
are associated with *phronesis*.

The task of *phronesis* lies, in part, in determining which other virtues
will be applicable in any particular circumstances. The challenge is often
adjudicative in that one needs to achieve a balance among various
virtues. Conflicting impulses within a person present some of the hardest
cases here; *phronesis* will be required to resolve the dilemma. Similarly,
confronted with another sort of ethical dilemma, where the dual roles
undertaken by the practitioner are in conflict, we can suppose that good
practical sense or judgment—which we have characterized as *phronesis*—
would permit an ethical solution. In the above case, if his patient's erratic
and violent responses had escalated and if the knife had remained
unsheathed, then Dr. Douglas may have been required to make a different

decision. At the cost of the relationship that he had achieved with this patient, Dr. Douglas's role as protector of public safety may have culminated in his having Mr. Buck apprehended and treated involuntarily. This alternate scenario illustrates a common situation confronted by psychiatrists who work with potentially dangerous patients; the notion of *phronesis* seems to capture the requisite capacity to judge whether and when a situation might carom out of control.

The importance of adopting a pragmatic approach to psychiatric practice, recently emphasized by David Brendel, provides another example of the value of *phronesis* to psychiatric practice.[22] Mental disorders are complex, Brendel explains, and "treating them usually occurs in the face of significant uncertainty." When there is sound empirical evidence for the efficacy of a treatment, "clinical ethics demands that the evidence be heeded. But in cases where there is less certainty (or no relevant empirical evidence at all), clinical decision making should not be wedded to any particular theory at the expense of concrete, practical considerations." The pragmatic judgments described here exemplify *phronesis*; if, as Brendel suggests, psychiatric practice is unusually complex and uncertain, then the demand for *phronesis* will arguably be greater in this clinical setting than in many others.

Part 2: Questions about Teaching the Virtues Required in Psychiatric Practice

Three questions have been raised that pertain to teaching the virtues required in psychiatric practice. The first of these is whether virtue *should* be taught—that is, whether this kind of training in values and character is appropriate. The second, one of the oldest ever asked in philosophy, is whether virtue *can* be taught. The third is *how* it might be taught.

Some have claimed that while students of medicine should be taught knowledge and skills, it is "counterproductive, presumptuous and futile to try to make students better persons."[23] We disagree. The implied distinction here between an education that includes teaching values and virtues and one that is neutral and value free is not one that bears up under closer examination. Writing of medical humanities training, Loretta Kopelman points out that it is impossible to analyze, justify, explain, criticize, or teach from an entirely neutral or value-free stance.[23] Values are inescapable, influencing every aspect of the curriculum, including "what theories, issues, readings, and skills are presented, thereby shaping students' beliefs, views, and values." Rather than pretending to avoid them, Kopelman believes instructors should try to *identify* and *justify* the values involved. Without digressing into a long discussion of the controversial area of moral education, we offer the following case, which illustrates how an educational focus on role-constituted virtues and obligations can awaken and reorder students' preexisting moral understandings.

The following is a small-group discussion among first-year medical students about student cheating:

Mark: Look, if a student wants to copy on an exam, that's his problem. I'm not my brother's keeper.
Dr. Elder: We heard from Mary that the hassle of reporting a classmate's cheating is high. You could be challenged, you'd be labeled a rat, etc. So why do we as young doctors consider doing it at all?
Mary (hesitant):   Public trust.
Dr. Elder: Tell us more what you mean, Mary.
Mary: The public trust. If doctors don't police themselves, then the public will think we're jerks like everyone else.
Dr. Elder (chuckling):   You don't really think everyone else is a jerk?
Mark: I get it. The bar is higher for us.

Once we recognize the nature of professional role morality, outlined earlier, the unsustainability of the claim that character training is *inappropriate* can be illustrated in a slightly different way as well. The distinction between capabilities that are skills and those that are virtues does not hold up. Within role morality the goals and goods of the practice—mental health and healing, in psychiatry—determine the whole nature of the enterprise. Doctors are supposed to be trustworthy, as in the case above. Similarly, psychiatrists must achieve a successful alliance with the patient because that relationship is necessary for healing; as a precondition for effecting that alliance, feeling and communicating empathy must be construed as a valued virtue, not a value-neutral skill.

The second of the questions above—whether virtue *can* be taught—is one first raised in Plato's *Protagoras*, in the context of Socrates' observation that there were no expert teachers of virtue. Aristotle's response, though one that is not universally accepted, was that virtues can be acquired and strengthened through habituation. Recent discussion has noted that the subcapabilities underlying the acquisition of virtues include moral reasoning and sensitivity, which can both be enhanced through training and practice.[24–28] Indeed, each of the virtues is itself a heterogeneous collection of states and traits, many of which, like attention and sensitivity, are elements in any number of everyday activities and in various types of formal and informal learning.

Because it has been recognized that subcapabilities such as moral reasoning and sensitivity can be enhanced through training, such traits have been the focus of considerable recent attention within the domain of moral education. Moral reasoning skills can be taught, for example, through discussion of moral dilemmas and case materials in a classroom or group setting; other techniques involve cooperative games, role playing, simulation exercises of various types, and journal keeping. Some of these methods are aimed at the specific subcapabilities that make up particular virtues, whereas others have been employed in order to instill the desired virtue more directly. Thus, efforts at empathy training, now widely employed in a range of settings, are often designed to stimulate the imagination—again, through simulation, role playing, exposure to literary and cinematographic works, journal keeping, and other forms of self-discovery and self-monitoring.[26,27]

The virtues required for psychiatric practice are a diverse group, as we have seen, and one particular way of distinguishing among them has significant implications for how they are learned. Trustworthiness, a key practitioner's virtue, requires habituation not unlike that employed when we instill any habit—that is, regular, attentive practice. To habituate hand washing, we must remember to do it regularly until it becomes unthinking and routine. Similarly, taking care to act in a trustworthy way at all times will bring about trustworthiness. This is not to imply that trustworthiness will be easy to acquire or that it will not call for alertness, self-control, sensitivity, and several other capabilities. But the method of acquiring it is direct because the components of trustworthiness are responsive to self-discipline and to ongoing efforts of resolve.

For some virtues such as empathy, however, which is primarily affective in character, we cannot voluntarily invoke the appropriate response, and we therefore cannot habituate it directly—that is, by practicing to do it. Acquiring such virtues depends on a different model. The tendency to respond with empathy must be engendered *indirectly*—for example, by practicing certain habits of mind such as imaginatively placing ourselves in the situation of other persons, by engaging in allied forms of simulation, or by paying close attention to the details of the others' hardships or plights.

Also part of traditional conceptions of moral education is the emphasis on exposure to role models, whether real or imaginary. It is widely supposed that through immediate contact or literary depictions, the learner will adopt and internalize the virtues thereby observed in respected figures. The importance of this sort of learning has long been recognized in the apprenticeship, or practice-based, model of medical education. Examples and exemplars offer learners a concrete personification to guide their practice.

In conclusion, then, the role-generated virtues of psychiatric practice should and can be taught. This claim is in no way incompatible with the presupposition that these virtues depend upon natural, affective, and social tendencies that have been appropriately shaped during childhood. Nor is the claim incompatible with the fact that trainees will almost certainly possess differing aptitudes for such learning—aptitudes that reflect differences with respect to those same tendencies, not to mention the process of their own moral education. The implications for the training, and perhaps even selection, of psychiatric residents are undoubtedly significant, and it may well be that, whether consciously or not, these factors are already being taken into account in selecting residents and subsequently evaluating their performance. In any event, an ethical approach that focuses on the character of the practitioner—while not, perhaps, sufficient by itself—is a necessary and important ingredient in ensuring that the professional goals and goods of medicine are upheld and honored in psychiatric practice.

References

1. Kupperman, J. J. (1991). *Character*. New York: Oxford University Press.

2. McKinnon, C. (1999). *Character, virtue theories and the vices*. Boulder, CO: Broadview.

3. Peterson, C., & Seligman, M. (2004). *Character strengths and virtues: A handbook and classification*. New York: Oxford University Press.

4. McDowell, J. (1979). Virtue and reason. *Monist, 62*(3), 49–72.

5. Pincoffs, E. (1986). *Quandaries and virtues: Against reductivism in ethics*. Lawrence: University of Kansas Press.

6. Oakley, J. (1996). Varieties of virtue. *Ethics, 9*, 128–152.

7. Crisp, R. (Ed.). (1996). *How should one live? Essays on the virtues*. New York: Oxford University Press.

8. Crisp, R., & Slote, M. (1997). Introduction. In R. Crisp & M. Slote (Eds.), *Virtue ethics* (pp. 1–25). New York: Oxford University Press.

9. Hursthouse, R. (1999). *On virtue ethics*. New York: Oxford University Press.

10. Foot, P. (1978). *Virtues and vices*. Berkeley: University of California Press.

11. Stohr, K., & Heath, C. (2002). Recent work in virtue ethics. *American Philosophical Quarterly, 39*, 49–72.

12. Nussbaum, M. (1999). Virtue ethics: A misleading category. *Journal of Ethics, 3*, 163–201.

13. Beauchamp, T., & Childress, J. (2001). *Principles of biomedical ethics* (5th ed.). New York: Oxford University Press.

14. Slote, M. (2004). *Ethical theory and moral practice*. New York: Springer.

15. Chambers, T. (1999). *The fiction of bioethics*. NewYork: Routledge.

16. Radden, J., & Sadler, J. (2010). *The virtuous psychiatrist: Character ethics in clinical practice*. New York: Oxford University Press.

17. Tong, R. (1998). The ethics of care: A feminist virtue ethics of care for healthcare practitioners. *Journal of Medicine and Philosophy, 23,* 131–152.

18. Tong, R. (1997). Feminist perspectives on empathy as an epistemic skill and caring as a moral virtue. *Journal of Medical Humanities, 18*(3), 153–168.

19. Churchill, L. (1989). Reviving a distinctive medical ethics. *Hastings Center Report, 19*(3), 28–34.

20. Oakley, J., & Cocking, D. (2001). *Virtue ethics and professional roles*. Cambridge: Cambridge University Press.

21. Aristotle; T. Irwin (Trans.). (1985). *Nichomachean ethics*. New York: Hackett.

22. Brendel, D. (2006). *Healing psychiatry*. Cambridge, MA: MIT Press.

23. Kopelman, L. (1999). Values and virtues: How should they be taught? *Academic Medicine, 74,* 1307–1310.

24. Hoffman, M. (2000). *Empathy and moral development: Implications for caring and justice*. Cambridge: Cambridge University Press.

25. Rajczi, A. (2003). Why are there no expert teachers of virtue? *Educational Theory, 53,* 389–400.

26. Gordon, R. (1998). Sympathy, simulation, and the impartial spectator. *Ethics, 105,* 743–763.

27. Charon, R. (2001). Narrative medicine: A model for empathy, reflection, profession, trust. *Journal of the American Medical Association, 286,* 1897–1902.

28. Larson, E. B., & Yao, X. Y. (2005). Clinical empathy as emotional labor in the patient-physician relationship. *Journal of the American Medical Association, 293,* 1100–1110.

II

Capacity, Coercion, and Consent

One of the key tasks that mental health care professionals are asked to perform is to assess the capacity of persons to be autonomous. Do those in their care have the ability to make decisions about their health care, finances, and day-to-day decisions about accepting specific treatments?

Competence is determined relative to one's ability to perform a given set of tasks. To refuse or consent to treatment, a person must understand what she is refusing and the consequences of refusing. She must be mentally capable of making a rational decision that takes these understandings into account. The patient cannot be deciding under threat of punishment or retaliation. Mental health professionals are often asked to determine if a patient has the intellectual and emotional capacity to carry out these tasks.

One way to minimize the impact of such assessments is to use advance directives. These documents, familiar from end-of-life-care situations in hospitals, permit a person to document his or her wishes and values while competent and able to communicate. Psychiatric patients could also make use of these directives when competent to assist health care providers if and when they become incompetent. While a determination of incompetency would still be necessary to trigger an advance directive, it would then provide the best window into what the patient would want.

Paul Appelbaum notes that there have been challenges when psychiatric advance directives are created. Patients may state that they refuse all treatment should they become incompetent due to mental illness. They can insist on this even if there are effective and safe treatments that could be used to restore competency and even if they meet the legal standard to permit involuntary treatment.

Appelbaum notes that most patients do not use advance directives to reject care when they are incompetent. Rather, they try to provide guidance about what sorts of care they wish and what values they would like care providers to consider. Since patients do have the right to complete advance directives if they are competent, including the selection of a surrogate decision maker, discussing this option with patients while they are competent is important. It is also important to note that a health care provider can try to persuade a patient not to write an advance directive in a way that would preclude absolutely all treatment under every circumstance. And although Appelbaum focuses on the role of psychiatrists here, more and more of these kinds of conversations will (and should) happen between patients and other behavioral health care providers.

Arthur Caplan argues that while respect for autonomy is a commendable value in both physical medicine and mental and behavioral health care, autonomy does not make sense in all contexts. Addiction, for example, is a disease that may not render the addict manifestly incompetent. But a person under the sway of addiction may be unable to seek or comply with treatment. Caplan suggests giving greater leeway to compel treatment known to have a high probability of effectiveness if it can be done in a relatively short period of time. If after a week or two of involuntary therapy, a patient still resists or declines more, then that wish would have to be effective. The moral idea behind this type of involuntary treatment is that some addicts, although not incompetent, might be restored to greater states of capacity and competency if they can be given enough time to have the power of their addiction broken.

Anorexia is another mental illness in which those afflicted are often not manifestly incompetent. They are oriented to time and place, can reason and plan, and seem to fully understand the risks and consequences of their choices. Gans and Gunn argue that the decision to respect an anorexic person's refusal of food sometimes ought to be honored in other situations, though not for reasons similar to those Caplan gives. They note there is a difference between listening to a twenty-year-old woman who has been starving herself in private for a year and heeding the denial of further care from a fifty-year-old patient, diagnosed with chronic anorexic nervosa, who has proven untreatable and has exhausted the resources and patience of the area hospitals, clinics, practitioners, and family. The latter patient may be someone at the end stage of anorexia who understands the futility of available treatment and does not wish to endure it any longer. The younger patient may not benefit from therapy, but until she is given a chance to try it, her refusal perhaps is less worthy of respect. Gans and Gunn understand the danger in pronouncing every patient with anorexia someone whose decisions do not merit respect, because no one has shown that every anorexic person is necessarily incompetent.

George Szmukler examines the challenge that personality disorders pose to competency determination and suggests examining four elements of capacity to determine competency to accept or refuse treatment. The person must possess an understanding of the nature of the disorder and the benefits and risks associated with treatment, an appreciation that they suffer from a disorder and that treatment would be of possible benefit, the ability to reason with this information as shown by their ability to explain the consequences that will ensue from the choices they have, and the ability to make a choice.

It is important to note that in the discussion of assessing capacity, the trigger for such assessments ought not simply be refusal to comply with the recommended treatment. Patients who agree quickly or show no interest in their care may well have impaired competence. Competency is decision specific; determining that a patient cannot make a choice among medications does not mean they are incapable of deciding what they would like to watch on television or eat for dinner.

5

Psychiatric Advance Directives and the Treatment of Committed Patients

Paul S. Appelbaum

Advance directives have been one of the more promising innovations in recent years to give patients a greater voice in their psychiatric treatment (1). Completed when patients are competent, advance directives allow patients to appoint proxy decision makers and to make choices about particular treatments, all to take effect should patients later become incompetent to make decisions for themselves. Advance directives have been hailed as a way of encouraging patients and treaters to discuss future contingencies and to negotiate mutually acceptable approaches to care (2,3). All states have statutes that govern the use of advance directives, which can be applied to general medical and psychiatric care, and many states now have special provisions for advance directives for psychiatric care per se.

However, mental health professionals have always been concerned that advance directives could also be used in a less collaborative way. One of the earliest proponents of advance directives, Thomas Szasz—a fierce critic of psychiatric diagnosis and treatment—suggested that people with mental disorders use advance directives to preclude future treatment, especially treatment with medications (4). As Szasz saw it, if advance directives represented the unalterable choices of competent patients, there would be no way to override the preferences embodied in the directives. This suggestion raised the prospect of a class of patients who would be permanently untreatable, even if they later became psychotic and were hospitalized involuntarily. Now, in the wake of a decision by the U.S. Court of Appeals for the Second Circuit, that prospect seems closer to materializing.

The case, *Hargrave v. Vermont,* grew out of a complaint filed in 1999 on behalf of Nancy Hargrave, a woman with a history of paranoid schizophrenia and multiple admissions to the Vermont State Hospital (5). Hargrave had completed an advance directive—known in Vermont as a durable power of attorney for health care, or DPOA—in which she designated a substitute decision maker in case she lost competence and in which she refused "any and all anti-psychotic, neuroleptic, psychotropic, or psychoactive medications." The major national law firm that represented Hargrave immediately filed suit to block the state of Vermont from overriding her advance directive should she ever again be involuntarily committed and obtained certification to represent the entire class of patients in similar situations.

Hargrave's target was Act 114, a 1998 Vermont statute that attempted to address the dilemma inherent in psychiatric advance directives. Although advance directives were intended to facilitate patients' participation in treatment decisions, they have, as noted, the potential to prevent all treatment, even of patients who are ill enough to qualify for civil commitment under the prevailing dangerousness standards. To mitigate this prospect, the Vermont legislature allowed hospital (or prison) staff to petition a court for permission to treat an incompetent involuntarily committed patient, notwithstanding an advance directive to the contrary. Before the court could authorize nonconsensual administration of medication, it had to allow the terms of the patient's advance directive to be implemented for forty-five days. So a patient like Hargrave, who had declined all medications, would be permitted to go unmedicated for a forty-five-day period, after which the court could supersede the patient's refusal of treatment.

The core of Hargrave's challenge to the statute was based on Title II of the Americans with Disabilities Act (ADA), which requires that "no qualified individual with a disability shall, by reason of such disability, be excluded from participation in or be denied the benefits of the services, programs, or activities of a public entity, or be subjected to discrimination by any such entity" (6). Hargrave claimed that she and other members of her class were being discriminated against on the basis of mental disorder, given that only committed persons with mental illness could have their advance directives overridden under Act 114. And the public "services, programs, or activities" from which she was being excluded was the state's durable power of attorney for health care itself.

In response, the state of Vermont offered three arguments. First, because Hargrave had been involuntarily committed, Vermont claimed that she qualified under an exclusion to the ADA for persons who pose a "direct threat." Next, the state contended that the plaintiff was not being discriminated against on the basis of disability, because anyone who completed an advance directive was susceptible to having his or her choices superseded (the state has an alternative override mechanism that involves judicial appointment of a guardian), and in any event, it was the status of being civilly committed, not being mentally ill, that was the point of distinction here. Finally, Vermont looked to a federal regulatory provision that allows a public entity to continue existing practices, despite an ADA challenge, if the change being called for would "fundamentally alter the nature of the service, program, or activity" (7).

The Second Circuit, like the U.S. District Court that had originally heard the case, failed to find any of these contentions persuasive. With regard to the claim that Hargrave and other involuntarily committed patients constitute a direct threat, the three-judge panel noted that not all committed patients would be a threat to others, as required under the ADA, because many were hospitalized for danger to self. Even persons who were found to be dangerous to others at the time of commitment, the court held, could not be presumed still to be dangerous when override of their advance directives was sought. The court was similarly unpersuaded that some condition other than mental illness was the basis for the differential treatment, given that Act 114 applied only to persons with mental illness. And allowing advance directives to stand as written, the court decided, even when patients were committed, does not fundamentally alter the advance directive statute (although it might affect the provision of psychiatric treatment to involuntary patients), which the court held was the proper point of reference. Hence the court concluded that Act 114 violated the ADA and enjoined its enforcement.

Hargrave, then, stands for the proposition that the state, having established a statutory basis for medical advance directives, cannot exclude involuntarily committed psychiatric patients from its coverage. Although the Second Circuit's opinion applies directly only to Vermont and New York, it is an influential court, and its opinion may well be echoed in other circuits around the country. Advance directives may now constitute an iron-clad bulwark against future involuntary treatment with medication—except in emergencies—even for incompetent, committed patients and even when the alternative is long-term institutional care.

In many respects, *Hargrave* represents a continuation of the battle over the right of psychiatric patients to refuse treatment that began in the 1970s. Indeed, the list of amici who filed briefs in support of *Hargrave* reflected the coalitions that were formed to push for a right to refuse treatment in the 70s. But that battle ended ambiguously. Although some states were compelled by the courts to permit even committed patients to refuse medication unless they were found incompetent by a judge, other states still allow the treating physician—sometimes after a second opinion has been obtained—or a panel of clinicians to override refusal on clinical grounds (8). Even in states that require findings of incompetence and substituted judgment as to whether the patient, if competent, would have accepted the treatment, the vast majority (typically more than 90 percent) of cases that are adjudicated end with the court authorizing involuntary treatment with medication. The sense of many experienced observers is that when patients are psychotic and treatment seems clearly indicated, the courts find a way to justify administration of medication, sometimes despite the legal criteria (8).

If adopted more widely, however, *Hargrave* would appear to provide a tool whereby patients who are determined to avoid treatment with medications would be able (except in emergencies) to completely preclude such treatment. A reviewing court would be bound to honor the terms of the now-incompetent patient's advance directive and order that treatment be withheld. Judges or quasi-judicial decision makers would no longer have the discretion to apply "commonsense" criteria—for example, that patients with flagrant psychosis should be treated if possible—to mandate medication. Today, few severely ill committed patients avoid treatment with medications, regardless of the legal standard in their jurisdiction. *Hargrave* could change that. If large numbers of patients were to complete advance directives such as Nancy Hargrave's, declining all medication, hospitals might well begin to fill with patients whom they could neither treat nor discharge.

Are there legal mechanisms that could avoid this outcome without running afoul of the ADA? In the *Hargrave* case, the court itself noted that nothing in this decision precludes statutory revisions that do not single out persons who are disabled because of mental illness—for example, revisions that increase the competency threshold for executing a DPOA or that allow the override of the DPOA of any incompetent person whenever compliance with the DPOA would substantially burden the interests of the state. However, it is doubtful that raising the competence threshold would have much impact, and the court's suggestion regarding "interests of the state" that might warrant overriding any person's advance directive is, frankly, enigmatic.

But perhaps a clever legislator can find an opening here to blunt the impact of the decision. And there is no guarantee that other circuits, or even ultimately the U.S. Supreme Court, would necessarily agree with the Second Circuit's analysis. Of course, were the level of concern sufficient, it would always be possible for Congress to amend the ADA to exclude the class of persons at issue. Congress, though, is typically reluctant to tinker with major legislation, and the disability rights community would likely oppose firmly any amendment of the ADA.

Because the ultimate scope and impact of *Hargrave* may not be known until a decade from now, it is worthwhile to consider the possible effect of the decision on the use of advance directives for psychiatric treatment. Current research suggests that most patients who complete advance directives do not use these directives to decline all treatment with medication but rather to indicate preferences among alternative treatments or to inform future treaters of particular concerns—for example, the care of their pets while they are hospitalized. Although *Hargrave* may stoke some enthusiasm for advance directives among patients who are opposed to receiving any medication, it remains to be seen how common the phenomenon will become. Studies now under way will tell us more about the utility of advance directives in psychiatry—for example, whether, given the current state of the mental health system, advance directives actually have an impact on subsequent care (9). At a minimum, however, it seems likely that *Hargrave,* as it becomes more widely known, will chill enthusiasm for psychiatric advance directives among many clinicians. Because clinicians' suggestions that patients consider completing advance directives probably play an important role in encouraging the completion of such directives (10), *Hargrave*'s legacy may be to inhibit the use of this once-promising tool.

References

1. Appelbaum, P. S. (1991). Advance directives for psychiatric treatment. *Hospital and Community Psychiatry, 42,* 983–984.

2. Srebnik, D. S., & LaFond, J. (1999). Advance directives for mental health treatment. *Psychiatric Services (Washington, D.C.), 50,* 919–925.

3. Swanson, J. W., Tepper, M. C., Backlar, P., et al. (2000). Psychiatric advance directives: An alternative to coercive treatment? *Psychiatry, 63,* 160–177.

4. Szasz, T. (1982). The psychiatric will: A new mechanism for protecting persons against "psychosis" and psychiatry. *American Psychologist, 37,* 762–770.

5. *Hargrave v. Vermont.* (2003). 340 F.3d 27 (Second Circuit).

6. Americans with Disabilities Act, USC Title 42, Section 12132.

7. Code of Federal Regulations, Title 28, Section 35.130 (b)(7).

8. Appelbaum, P. S. (1994). *Almost a Revolution: Mental Health Law and the Limits of Change.* New York: Oxford University Press.

9. Papageorgiou, A., King, M., Janmohamed, A., et al. (2002). Advance directives for patients compulsorily admitted to hospital with serious mental illness: Randomised controlled trial. *British Journal of Psychiatry, 181,* 513–519.

10. Srebnik, D. S., Russo, J., Sage, J., et al. (2003). Interest in psychiatric advance directives among high users of crisis services and hospitalization. *Psychiatric Services (Washington, D.C.), 54,* 981–986.

6

Denying Autonomy in Order to Create It: The Paradox of Forcing Treatment upon Addicts

Arthur L. Caplan

The Primacy of Autonomy in Provider-Patient Relationships

American bioethics affords extraordinary respect to the values of personal autonomy and patient self-determination [1]. Many would argue that the most significant achievement deriving from bioethics in the past forty years has been to replace a paternalistic model of health provider-patient relationships with one that sees patient self-determination as the normative foundation for practice. This shift away from paternalism toward respect for self-determination has been ongoing in behavioral and mental health as well, especially as it is reflected in the "recovery movement" [2–4].

As a result of the emphasis placed on patient autonomy, arguments in favor of mandatory treatment are rare and often half-hearted. Restrictions on autonomy are usually grounded in the benefits that will accrue to others from reining in dangerous behavior [5]. However, anyone who wishes to argue for forced or mandated treatment on the grounds that society will greatly benefit is working up a very steep ethical hill.

A person has the fundamental right, well established in medical ethics and in Anglo-American law, to refuse care even if such a refusal shortens their own life or has detrimental consequences for others. Therefore, while the few proponents of mandatory treatment for those afflicted with mental disorders or addictions are inclined to point to the benefit such treatment could have for society, it is exceedingly unlikely that any form of treatment that is forced or mandated is going to find any traction in American public policy on the basis of a consequentialist argument, great as those benefits might be.

However, is benefit for the greater good the only basis for arguing for mandatory treatment? Can a case be made that acknowledges the centrality and importance of autonomy but would still deem ethical mandatory treatment for addicts? I think it can.

Infringing Autonomy to Create Autonomy

People who are truly addicted to alcohol or drugs really do not have the full capacity to be self-determining or autonomous. Standard definitions of addiction cite loss of control, powerlessness, and unmanageability [6]. An addiction literally coerces behavior. An addict cannot be a fully free, autonomous agent precisely because they are caught up in the behavioral compulsion that is addiction. If this is so, at least for some addicts, then it may be possible to justify compulsory treatment involving medication or other forms of therapy, if only for finite periods of time, on the grounds that treatment may remove the coercion causing the powerlessness and loss of control.

Addicts, just like many others with mental illnesses and disabilities, are not incompetent. Indeed, to function as an alcoholic or cocaine addict, one must be able to reason, remember complex information, set goals, and be oriented to time, place, and personal identity, but competency by itself is not sufficient for autonomy. Being competent is a part of autonomy, but autonomy also requires freedom from coercion [7]. Those who criticize mandatory treatment on the grounds that an addict is not incompetent and thus ought not be forced to endure treatment are ignoring this crucial fact. Addiction, bringing in its wake, as it does, loss of will and control, does not permit the freedom requisite for autonomy or self-determination.

If a drug can break the power of addiction sufficiently to restore or reestablish personal autonomy then mandating its use might be ethically justifiable. Government, families, or health providers might force treatment in the name of autonomy. If a drug such as naltrexone is capable of blocking the ability to become high from alcohol, heroin, or cocaine [8,9], then it may release the addict from the compulsive and coercive dimensions of addiction, thereby enhancing the individual's ability to be autonomous. If a drug or therapy can remove powerlessness and loss of control from the addict's life, then that fact can serve as an ethical argument allowing the mandating of treatment. If naltrexone or any other drug can permit people to make choices freed from the compulsions or cravings that would otherwise control their behavior completely, then it would seem morally sound to permit someone who is in the throes of addiction to regain the ability to choose, to be self-governing, even if the only way to accomplish this restoration is through a course of mandated treatment.

Of course, it would not be ethical to force treatment upon anyone if there were significant risks involved with the treatment, but new drugs, such as naltrexone, appear safe and effective for those addicted to heroin, and perhaps cocaine, and should also prove so for alcoholics. The mechanisms behind the drug are well understood [8,9], and in some populations, this drug has been used for a long time to reduce the cravings of addiction safely and effectively. Mandating treatment requires that the intervention carry minimal risk as the patient cannot consent, but some interventions may be able to meet this admittedly difficult standard.

Nor would it make moral sense to force treatment upon someone, restore their autonomy successfully, and then continue to force treatment upon them in their fully autonomous state. The restoration of autonomy is the end of any moral argument for mandatory treatment.

Similarly, efforts to restore autonomy would not justify continuous, open-ended use of drugs or therapy in addicts. There must be some agreed-upon interval, after which treatment must be acknowledged to have failed and other avenues of coping with addiction to alcohol or drugs pursued.

Precedents for Mandating Treatment in the Name of Autonomy

Interestingly enough, despite the emphasis on autonomy in law and ethics in American health care, there are situations where the ethical acceptability of the rationale of autonomy restoration in permitting mandatory treatment is already accepted. Consider what occurs in rehabilitation medicine. The short-term infringement of autonomy is tolerated in the name of long-term creation or restoration of autonomy.

Patients, after devastating injuries or severely disfiguring burns, often demand that they be allowed to die. They say: "Don't treat me," or they may insist that "I can't live like this." In evaluating their requests, no one would be able to question seriously their competency. They know where they are. They know what is going on. However, staff in rehabilitation and burn units almost always ignore these initial demands. Patient autonomy is not respected. Why?

What rehabilitation experts say is that they want to allow an adaptation to the new state of affairs: to the loss of speech, amputation, facial disfigurement, or paralysis. They know from experience that if they do certain things with people—train them, counsel them, teach them adaptive skills—they can encourage them to start to "adjust" [10].

There are, admittedly, still people who say at the end of a run of rehabilitation: "I don't want to live like this." The suicide rate is higher in these populations. Nevertheless, at least initially, rehabilitation specialists will say that they have to force treatment on patients because they know from experience that they can often encourage them to accept their new state of affairs. The normal practice of rehabilitation immediately after a severe injury is to mandate treatment, ignore what patients have to say, and then see what happens. If they still do not want treatment after a course of rehabilitation, then their wishes will be respected [10].

The rehabilitation model is precisely the model to follow in thinking about the mandatory use of a drug such as naltrexone for the treatment of addiction. The moral basis for mandating treatment is for the good of the patient by rebirthing their autonomy. How long and whether someone ought to be able at some point to say, "I've done this for six months, I'm finished, I want to get high again," is a challenging problem, but it is not the key one. The key moral challenge is to open the door to temporary mandatory treatment. That can be achieved, ironically, on the grounds of autonomy. It may press current ethical thinking to the limit, but mandating treatment in the name of autonomy is not as immoral as many might otherwise deem forced treatment to be [7]. Once competency and coercion are distinguished, it is clear that both are requisite for autonomy. Mandatory treatment that relieves the coercive effects of addiction and permits the recreation or reemergence of true autonomy in the patient can be the right thing to do.

References

1. Beauchamp, T. L., & Childress, J. (2008). *Principles of Biomedical Ethics* (5th ed.). New York: Oxford University Press.

2. Sheldon, K., Williams, G., & Joiner, T. (2003). *Self-Determination Theory in the Clinic*. New Haven, CT: Yale University Press.

3. Cook, J. A., & Jonikas, J. A. (2002). Self-determination among mental health consumers/survivors: Using lessons from the past to guide the future. *Journal of Disability Policy Studies, 13*, 87–96.

4. The White House. (2007). *The President's New Freedom Initiative: The 2007 progress report*. Available at http://www.cartercenter.org/documents/1701.pdf (accessed September 14, 2008).

5. Silber, T. J. (1989). Justified paternalism in adolescent health care: Cases of anorexia nervosa and substance abuse. *Journal of Adolescent Health Care, 10*, 449–453.

6. Goodman, A. (1990). Addiction: Definition and implications. *British Journal of Addiction, 85*, 1403–1408.

7. Caplan, A. L. (2006). Ethical issues surrounding forced, mandated or coerced treatment. *Journal of Substance Abuse Treatment, 31*, 117–120.

8. Comer, S., Sullivan, M. A., Yu, E., Rothenberg, J. L., Kleber, H. D., Kampman, K., et al. (2006). Injectable, sustained release naltrexone for the treatment of opioid dependence. *Archives of General Psychiatry, 63,* 210–218.

9. Krystal, J. H., Cramer, J. A., Krol, W. E., Kirk, G. F., & Rosenheck, R. A. (2001). Naltrexone in the treatment of alcohol dependence. *New England Journal of Medicine, 345,* 1734–1739.

10. Caplan, A. L., Haas, J., & Callahan, D. (1990). Ethical and policy issues in rehabilitation medicine. In B. Duncan & D. Woods (Eds.), *Ethical Issues in Disability and Rehabilitation* (pp. 135–154). New York: World Institute on Disability.

7

End-Stage Anorexia: Criteria for Competence to Refuse Treatment

Margery Gans and Willam B. Gunn Jr.

1 Introduction

Anorexia nervosa is a complex disorder that primarily afflicts women. It can be fatal; the mortality rate is thought to be between 6 and 20 percent (Griffiths & Russell, 1998; Mitchell, Pomeroy, & Adson, 1997). A central symptom of anorexia nervosa is the patient's conviction that, no matter how emaciated she becomes, she is "fat." To be "fat" is to be "bad." She therefore severely restricts her food intake, even to the point of starvation. Unless she is "thin," her life is meaningless and she is worthless or bad (Orbach, 1986; Shelley, 1997). Even when a patient's health deteriorates to the degree where death is imminent, she may refuse treatment. If she refuses treatment, her treaters and family must decide whether to override her refusal, disrespect her autonomy, and risk the therapeutic alliance even without a guarantee that treatment will be effective, or respect her wish and risk her death. Or, weighing the conditions, they may override her refusal and reverse the effects of starvation, save her life, and launch her on the road to recovery (cf. Griffiths & Russell, 1998, pp. 130–131).

In this article, we will introduce a case in which the central question was the competence of a woman in the end stages of anorexia nervosa to refuse treatment when she knew that death was a likely outcome. Then we will identify the major issues relevant in this situation: the nature of anorexia nervosa, the notion of competence, and the complications inherent in determining competence to refuse life-saving treatment in a patient diagnosed with anorexia nervosa. Finally, we will identify the criteria we used to determine competence in this patient and describe the process we used to assess her competence.

2   The Case: Referral

The case was referred for evaluation in May 1998. At this time, the patient, Mrs. Black (not her real name), was a forty-four-year-old married female with two children, a son aged twenty and a daughter aged seventeen. Mrs. Black had a twenty-five-year history of anorexia nervosa. At the time of the evaluation, she suffered from anorexia nervosa and related medical complications. She was living in a hospice connected to the hospital at which she had received much of her treatment over the years, admitted by her physician who felt she might have less than six months to live. No further treatment for the anorexia nervosa was being administered.

The referral for an evaluation was generated when Mrs. Black requested the option to refuse life supports the next time her medical condition deteriorated. In 1997, she had previously been twice on life support systems. Following these episodes she decided that she would refuse such measures in the future. Her husband, at the time her legal guardian, was "in agreement with her intention and requests an evaluation to be certain that [his wife] is competent to make this decision." The ethics committee of the hospital was concerned about this decision and Mr. Black's support. Their concern prompted a request for an evaluation by Mr. Black to determine his wife's competence to make this decision to refuse life support systems.

3   Anorexia Nervosa: An Overview

3.1   Description
Anorexia nervosa has been described in the literature since the seventeenth century (Silverman, 1997). Its incidence seems to have risen in the last half of the twentieth century and has not abated in the twenty-first century (cf. Draper, 2000). The *Diagnostic and Statistical Manual* IV-TR defines *anorexia nervosa* as:

• A refusal on the part of the patient to maintain body weight at or above a minimally normal weight for age and height, for example, less than 85 percent of what's expected

• An intense fear of gaining weight or becoming fat, even though underweight

• A disturbance in the way in which one's body weight or shape is experienced

• Undue influence of body weight or shape on self-evaluation, or denial of the seriousness of the current low body weight

• In patients who are postmenarcheal, amenorrhea, defined as the absence of three consecutive periods

Two types are identified, restricting and binge-eating/purge type. In the first, the anorexic restricts food intake only. In the latter, the anorexic complements restricting with binge eating and purging cycles (American Psychiatric Association, 2000).

The severity of anorexia can range from a mild, possibly transient experimentation with restricting food intake, akin to extreme dieting, and a mildly distorted body image, to a lifelong course of starvation accompanied in the binge/purge type by, for example, vomiting, laxative abuse, and/or excessive exercise. A patient diagnosed with anorexia nervosa may also engage in obsessive, compulsive activities related to food and exercise, and social withdrawal secondary to utter preoccupation with the disorder. In severe and chronic cases, medical complications set in and are exacerbated by the continuing abuse of the body so that damage to internal organs, teeth, and bones can become irreversible. For these women, death can become a real probability. For example, heart failure may occur secondary to electrolyte imbalance. There may be failure of other internal organs or a complex combination of physical impairments (Kaplan & Woodside, 1987; Mitchell et al., 1997).

As noted in the DSM IV-TR, the starvation in anorexia nervosa is complicated by the fact that the patient is willfully restricting food and, in many cases, does not perceive herself as "sick" (Beumont & Vandereycken, 1998). Rather, because of her distorted body image and her investment in being "thin," she resists treatment, defies treaters, and pursues her course of starvation relentlessly, despite its physical and medical consequences. The disorder is existential, in that the patient derives her fundamental meaning and satisfaction, her reason to live, from her efforts to become "thin" (Binswanger, 1958; Bruch, 1973, 1988). She may describe the anorexia nervosa as her "best friend" (Shelley, 1997). And since her body image is severely distorted, she never experiences herself as thin enough and so the disorder is not self-limiting (Dresser, 1984a).

3.2   Theories of Anorexia

Theories of anorexia nervosa have struggled to explicate the meaning of the disorder, to decode the "message" that it seems these determined young women are trying to convey. Early psychoanalytic theory focused on anorexia nervosa as an expression of a young woman's fear of sexuality, of adult womanhood, and its demands as represented by pregnancy and motherhood. It suggested a fixation at the oral level of development. The patient diagnosed with anorexia nervosa rejects oral intrusions and keeps her body childlike and undeveloped, thereby rejecting gifts from the mother (e.g., food) as well as her own potential as a physically developed woman (Bemporad & Herzog, 1989; Bruch, 1973). Family therapists interpreted the refusal to eat as a cry for autonomy in a family system in which the young women are intruded upon and overcontrolled by ambitious and insensitive parents (Minuchin, Rosman, & Baker, 1978; Stierlin & Weber, 1989). The child is unconsciously set up to meet the parents' impossible-to-fulfill needs and expectations. Finding herself in a double bind about which she cannot speak because of the family prohibitions, the patient acts out this bind by being both an overly compliant "good" and "thin" girl and a rebellious, difficult, angry daughter who refuses to eat (Selvini Palazzoli, 1974). More recently, there has been a feminist perspective that sees in anorexia nervosa an exaggeration of the distorted body image that is presented to young women as an ideal through advertising, the media, and their families. From this point of view, in addition to being a serious psychological and medical problem, anorexia nervosa is also a statement on the culture that focuses attention on the destructive aspects of our portrayals of women (Fallon, Katzman, & Wooley, 1994).

Bruch (1973, 1988), a pioneer in the study and treatment of anorexia nervosa during the early 1970s, synthesized these views and influenced treatment methods. She saw anorexia as an effort on the part of the individual to define her own identity and assert herself. At her core is a profound self-loathing, which the patient diagnosed with anorexia nervosa attempts to assuage by being thin (Orbach, 1986). Bruch argues that, for treatment to succeed, it is critical that the therapist cooperate with the patient to restore or create her sense of self, and work with her to achieve and experience autonomy. If the focus on weight gain takes precedence over patient autonomy and choice, it can result in therapeutic rupture and setbacks. To intervene and force the patient to accept treatment she is not ready for, especially insofar as it means weight gain or capitulation to others' priorities, is to betray the patient's need for autonomy (see also Beumont & Vandereycken, 1998; Griffiths & Russell, 1998; Strober, 1997).

This therapeutic respect for the patient's autonomy is critical even when the anorexia nervosa has progressed to a life-threatening condition. If anorexia is, for the patient, a means to an authentic and worthwhile life, then giving up the anorexia—gaining weight—can mean giving up the reason for living (Beumont & Vandereycken, 1998; Shelley, 1997). A refusal of treatment that in another patient might look "suicidal" may, for the patient diagnosed with anorexia nervosa, be an affirmation of the only life she can conceive of living (Shelley, 1997, chap. 4).

Treaters, on the other hand, feel the moral and ethical obligation to treat the life-threatening aspects of anorexia, even if "saving the patient's life," conflicts with the patient's view of what constitutes a life worth living. The ethical decision-making process is not straightforward (Carney, 2001; Draper, 2000; Dresser, 1984a, 1984b; Fost, 1984; Goldner, Birmingham, & Smye, 1997; MacDonald, 2002; Tiller, Schmidt, & Treasure, 1993; Vandereycken, 1998). Hébert and Weingarten (1991) point out that a caregiver's decisions may be colored by the level of frustration the patient has generated during hospitalizations. They report a case in which, in the face of repeated treatment refusal and disruption on the unit, treatment was withdrawn. The authors warn that under these conditions, treaters' "transference" may lead to a premature withdrawal of treatment because of their own negative feelings. Some argue that it is never acceptable to stop treatment (Levinsky, 1984) no matter how disruptive the patient, while others ask, "Are there no limits to what we must accept from patients?" (Levine, 1999, p. 760). If, however, the illness has become "'intractable' and [is] causing 'desperate and unbearable suffering,'" are even aggressive and intrusive treatments justified regardless of the patient's wishes? (Vandereycken, 1998, pp. 1–2). If so, are there any limits to what treatments are acceptable (MacDonald, 2002)? There are case reports of the positive outcome of enteric feeding (Neiderman, Zarody, Tattersall, & Lask, 2000) and nasograstric refeeding (Robb et al., 2002) with initially resistant patients. Others argue that forced hospitalization and treatment may destroy the therapeutic relationship that is critical to recovery and sabotage the lifesaving goals of treatment (Dresser, 1984a, 1984b; Dresser & Boisaubin, 1986). Strober (1997) points out:

If the patient's physical health is restored—the undeniable hope of all who gaze upon her with revulsion and panic—she is left feeling profoundly inadequate and psychologically imperiled by comparison. (p. 229)

However, if the patient diagnosed with anorexia nervosa dies, there will be no chance of recovery.

In these extreme situations, some patients assert their right to refuse treatment, even knowing that death may be the outcome. If this right is respected, treatment may continue without aggressive interventions, treatment may be suspended, or, in the case of severe and chronic anorexia, palliative care may be instituted. Arguments have been made for both palliative care and coerced aggressive treatment (Draper, 2000; Dresser, 1984a, 1984b; Dresser & Boisaubin, 1986; Fost, 1984; Goldner, 1989; Goldner et al., 1997; Griffiths & Russell, 1998; Neiderman et al., 2000; Robb et al., 2002). Respecting the patient's right to refuse treatment when the stakes are this high turns on the question of her competence to make that decision.

4   Competence to Refuse Treatment

Competence in general is determined by one's ability to perform a given set of tasks. To refuse or consent to treatment, a person must be competent to do so voluntarily. The patient must understand what she is refusing and the consequences of refusing. She must be mentally capable of making a rational decision, which takes these understandings into account (Roth, Appelbaum, Sallee, Reynolds, & Huber, 1982).

Appelbaum and Grisso (1988) enumerate four criteria for assessing competence, namely:

- The person must be able to understand and communicate the choices available.
- She must understand the information relevant to making the decision.
- She must appreciate the situation and the consequences of her consent or refusal to treatment.
- She must demonstrate during this process that she can manipulate information rationally (see also Appelbaum, Lidz, & Meisel, 1987).

Appelbaum and Grisso (1988) write:

In summary, the assessment of competency to consent to or to refuse treatment appears to require among other elements a consideration of the accuracy of the patient's "appreciation" of the nature of his or her situation. (p. 1638)

Gutheil and Bursztajn (1986) stress that cognitive understanding may need to be supplemented by "appreciation," that is, an emotional grasp of the consequences of her decision.

4.1   Competence in the Patient Diagnosed with Anorexia Nervosa

Assessing competence can be complicated with a patient diagnosed with anorexia nervosa because often such individuals, who are not severely compromised by starvation, appear quite competent in areas of life that are not influenced by the obsession with food and/or body weight. Gutheil and Bursztajn (1986) describe these patients as "globally competent," with a "subtle" or "focal" incompetence in one area (Roth et al., 1982). They write:

The competence of patients with classical anorexia is inherently suspect in the narrow area of self-nutrition (that is the essence and defining feature of the disease), clinicians must carefully document and forthrightly present the body image distortions such as those described, together with their impact on impairing decisions about eating. (Gutheil & Bursztajn, 1986, p. 1022)

This argument is often used to declare such patients incompetent a priori on the basis of their anorexia (Lewis, 1999).

Some experts argue, however, that conditions exist in which it may make sense to respect the patient's right to refuse treatment, even when the outcome may be death. They argue that, among other things, chronicity, severity, the presence of irreversible damage, the number of treatments attempted, in combination with a patient's demonstrated competence to appreciate her situation, need to be considered (Draper, 2000; Dresser, 1984a, 1984b).

Draper (2000) cites the patients who

have been afflicted beyond the natural cycle of the disorder (which is between one and eight years); have already been force-fed on previous occasions; are competent to make decisions concerning their quality of life; have insight into the influence which their anorexia has over some aspects of their lives, and are not at death's door. (pp. 122–123)

There is a difference between the twenty-year-old woman who has been starving herself in private for a year with no treatment and the fifty-year-old patient, diagnosed with chronic anorexic nervosa, who has exhausted the resources and patience of the area hospitals, clinics, and practitioners. In the natural cycle of the disorder, the latter patient represents someone at the "end stage" of anorexia. Is there a point, when someone is in the end stages, that practitioners abandon the hope that the patient will be restored to competence? How is the end stage determined? Is it necessary to send this patient to internationally known centers for treatment? And, if so, who should pay? The attempts to restore competence may mean the use of almost unlimited resources because there is no known "cure" (see Griffiths & Russell, 1998). And yet death is irreversible, and we cannot, with complete certainty, know whether one more trial of treatment might have worked.

As Draper (2000) points out, however, the issue is not how much treatment to impose but when to respect the patient's right to refuse further treatment, that is, when to respect her autonomy and how to determine whether and when she is competent to make this decision. Dresser (1984a, 1984b) and Dresser and Boisaubin (1986) agree that an argument can be made for respecting the patient's decision provided she can demonstrate an understanding of the situation and her life is not endangered. The more disturbing decision is to be made when her life *is* endangered.

Then the question becomes, Is there some point at which the patient diagnosed with anorexia nervosa resembles, and deserves the same rights as, any chronically ill person with a terminal disease who opts to refuse further treatment? Can a patient diagnosed with anorexia nervosa ever be trusted to make decisions about her own treatment once her situation is life threatening? Can she choose to die rather than to live a life that to her is unbearable, even if that decision seems irrational to those around her?

The distinction between irrational and incompetent is significant. The law gives permission to commit irrational acts. However, the consequences, potential harm, and competing interests of all affected, including the family and society, need to be taken into account (Carney, 2001; Dresser, 1984a, 1984b). In this culture we have determined that the decision to die by refusing treatment is permitted as long as the patient is deemed competent, even if irrational. Draper (2000) addresses the issue of incompetence versus the irrationality of the patient diagnosed with anorexia nervosa. She writes:

> There are two justifications for associating irrationality with incompetence in the case of anorexia. One is that the desire not to eat undermines an even stronger desire not to die. Another is that the desire not to eat might itself be an involuntary one, grounded in some other deeply held, but false, belief about their body image—usually that they are "fat." (p. 129)

With regard to the desire not to eat, she points out, we do not generally interfere with the bizarre, even if life-threatening, eating habits of the extreme overeater. We consider their behavior "irrational" but do not declare them incompetent on the basis of it.

Are there conditions in which the patient's decision might be judged "irrational" but not "incompetent"? Are there even situations in which the decision to refuse treatment might be both rational and competent? What if, as Draper (2000) poses, "the quality of her life was so poor that the therapy was no longer of benefit to her, or that it was on balance more of a burden than a benefit?" (p. 122).

Would this necessarily be an "irrational" decision? In this case, the assessment of quality of life by the patient diagnosed with chronic anorexia nervosa might trigger an evaluation for competence rather than the automatic assumption that, by virtue of her illness, she is incompetent. Draper (2000) notes that the patient may prefer to "take her chances with death" (p. 131). She concludes that if they are not at death's door, or starving to the point of cognitive impairment, then "sufferers are actually as competent as anyone else to make decisions about the quality of their lives" (p. 133).

Two dangerous precedents loom. One is that allowing the patient to refuse treatment when her beliefs continue to distort her evaluation of her own health may open a door to sanctioning the premature death of patients who, with more vigorous intervention, even against their will, might be restored to competence (Neiderman et al., 2000; Robb et al., 2002; Tiller et al., 1993; Vandereycken, 1998). Competence in this case is an awareness of, and loss of tolerance for, the illness, resulting in a wish to live. The second dangerous precedent lies in applying the determination of incompetence to all patients diagnosed with anorexia nervosa regardless of their individual circumstances and capacities. It undermines the tension we value between individual autonomy and public safety. It would mean, as Dresser (1984a) argues, that because the patient's behavior of starving herself appears to laypeople as "unreasonable and irrational," then every patient diagnosed with anorexia nervosa could be deemed "legally incompetent on grounds of emotional denial, thus exposing all anorexic individuals to involuntary treatment" (p. 48).

If we are willing to allow for the possibility that a patient who met certain criteria, for example, a long and chronic illness, multiple treatment failures, poor quality of life, possible irreversible medical complications, could be competent to refuse treatment, then how would that particular competence be determined? Two questions need to be explored: What conditions would have to prevail to trigger such an evaluation at all, and what are the standards for competence that one would use in such a situation? These questions were raised in the case that was introduced. We will now present the full case and follow with the discussion of the competence evaluation.

5 Case Study

5.1 Relevant History

The patient, "Mrs. Black," was the eldest of three siblings. Her father died in 1983, and she was not close to her siblings. Her mother was living and remained closely involved with her daughter's care.

Mrs. Black reported that in childhood, her father sexually, emotionally, and physically abused her. Other family members did not corroborate this. The patient claimed not to remember this abuse until she underwent hypnosis in the 1980s when she recalled the sexual abuse and also her father's abuse around food. She reported that "she was obese as a child and that her father forced her to chew her food and spit it into a plastic bag at the table, prohibiting her from swallowing." The patient also recalled that others in the family were abused by her father, including her mother. These incidents of abuse occurred chiefly when her father had been drinking. The patient's mother agreed that the father had been "verbally abusive," especially when he had been drinking, but believed that the abuse had been directed primarily at her.

Mrs. Black graduated from college with a degree in education and taught in the public schools for seventeen years. She was married to her husband when she was twenty-one years old. She reported that she continued to spend a lot of time at her parents' house and that she "cooked dinner for them 'every single night' and that her husband permitted this concentration of attention on her parents." Mr. and Mrs. Black had two children.

5.2 History of the Anorexia Nervosa

Mrs. Black reported that her anorexia began in college. In high school she was at her highest weight of 155 pounds. She is 5 feet 2 inches tall. In college, in an effort to lose weight and control her intake, she began taking laxatives and restricting the amount and variety of what she ate. She kept her anorexia a secret from friends and family "for years" and reported that she took "100 laxatives a day for years" except when she was pregnant with each child. During each pregnancy, she ate normally, stopped taking laxatives, and stopped smoking. After the birth of each child, she resumed her laxatives and continued through at least the mid-1990s. During one inpatient hospitalization in 1991, she admitted to sneaking laxatives in. She was discharged from her primary physician's care when she lied about taking laxatives. Her potassium levels and incidents of dehydration in 1996 and 1997 indicated that she probably continued to take them, despite her denials. She denied vomiting when interviewed, but the record showed that she had had oral surgery to replace her teeth with dentures following enamel damage due to vomiting.

In recent years, Mrs. Black's weight fluctuated between 75 and 90 pounds. Records from 1996 through 1998 showed an average daily caloric intake of approximately 300, ranging from 200 to 1200. She also had, for one year, a gastronomy tube and required the assistance of her mother and her husband to consume nutritional supplements. In the fall of 1997, her weight rose to the low 90s and she was "miserable" and felt "very fat."

In 1996, Mrs. Black had episodes of confusion and disorientation "of multidetermined origins." She was in and out of the hospital every few weeks and was referred in December to the Ethics Committee to determine whether her guardianship should be changed from her husband to a "more neutral party." The question remained open; guardianship was not changed. In 1998, her primary care physician felt she had a limited amount of time to live and that all efforts that Mrs. Black would cooperate with had been made to restore her health. Palliative care was considered to be the only option. Mrs. Black was admitted to the hospice with the understanding (per hospice regulations) that she had less than six months to live. She was quite content at the hospice.

5.3   Other Psychiatric Issues

Mr. Black reported that she "went downhill" after her father's death in 1983 and that her chief observable symptoms were of obsessive-compulsive disorder. She focused on cleaning, washing, and throwing food away if used or opened. She was prescribed Afranil; the symptoms abated and did not return. She was treated for depression at Hospice House.

5.4   Medical History

Mrs. Black had a number of medical problems associated with her anorexia. In 1984 she suffered from mononucleosis. In subsequent years, she was treated for circulatory problems, headaches and numbness, severe back pain, kidney stones, bleeding ulcers, and pancreatitis. The pancreatitis resulted in liver dysfunction for which she required a liver stent to drain excess bile. Due to low weight and her weakened condition, it had become increasingly difficult to change the stent. She had also been diagnosed with central pontine myelinolisis (CPM), a nutritional neuropathy resulting in stroke-like symptoms that affect cognitive functioning. She may also have had nutritional cardiomyopathy. Over the years, she had repeated incidents of low potassium and unbalanced electrolytes, dehydration, and tachycardia. She developed chronic hip and leg pain following a fall in January 1998 and was confined to a wheelchair. At the time of the evaluation, she was no longer able to walk unassisted. She continued to smoke at least one packet of cigarettes a day.

She admitted to abusing over-the-counter drugs, including Dexatrim, between 1987 and 1992. Progress notes in 1997 and 1998 indicated the suspicion that she was seeking painkilling drugs in higher-than-therapeutic doses. At the time of the evaluation she was taking medication for her edema and morphine for chronic pain. She had been taken off 150 milligrams of Zoloft because of metabolic problems.

5.5   Treatment History

Mrs. Black was first hospitalized for anorexia nervosa in 1989. She was also diagnosed with obsessive-compulsive disorder and post-traumatic stress disorder.

Mrs. Black began treatment with her primary care physician in 1989 after fifteen years of undiagnosed, undisclosed anorexia nervosa. She was not compliant with treatment, and the physician warned her repeatedly prior to 1994 that by continuing to be anorexic, she would one day "cross a line [and] the problem will be permanent." In 1994, he discharged her from his practice when he discovered that she was taking laxatives and diuretics secretly while continuing to take the prescribed potassium—a possibly lethal combination. Mrs. Black had two more doctors before returning to this physician in 1998. One doctor attempted to make a behavioral contract with Mrs. Black. The initial primary care physician was willing to take her back only with the "expressed agreement" that he would see her only if she "came back to die." Otherwise, he felt obliged to make clear that he was "out of suggestions."

Mrs. Black had multiple hospitalizations, both in her community and in nearby large cities, in general psychiatric and specialized eating disorder programs, both short- and longer-term stays. She was also hospitalized numerous times for medical problems. She was on life supports two times. Mr. Black described the last five years as "one medical journey after another."

Mrs. Black also had a series of outpatient therapists. The primary therapist was a therapist with whom she did hypnotherapy and recovered memories of alleged sexual abuse by her father. This therapy was terminated when the patient could not agree to conditions of treatment, including minimum calorie intake and compliance with electrolyte control conditions. She resumed with this therapist a year later. Two years after she was in therapy with a different practitioner, a progress note stated that this psychotherapy "made [Mrs. Black] feel worse." In the mid-1990s, a therapist attempted to treat the family and Mrs. Black with a "tough love" approach and counseled Mr. Black to lock his wife out of the house if she did not comply with the behavioral plan. He was not willing to do this. Other than this, the family reported no ongoing family therapy. At least one hospital in which Mrs. Black was an inpatient routinely offered family therapy; it is not known if this was refused or forgotten. Mr. Black reported that his wife "bowed out" of a recommendation for family therapy. The couple had therapy for approximately one year, but Mrs. Black felt that "nothing changed." Each family member has had some individual counseling; none felt it was especially helpful. No record or interview documented any sustained period of remission except during Mrs. Black's pregnancies, even though in one hospitalization at least she gained weight. Nor is there any record from the patient's therapy of increases in insight or motivation to recover.

5.6   Mrs. Black's Mental Status at the Time of the Interviews

At the time of the evaluation Mrs. Black weighed between 70 and 80 pounds. By request, she was not being weighed in hospice. She was emaciated, unable to walk, and appeared years older than her chronological age. Over a series of interviews, Mrs. Black was in a wheelchair with an intravenous morphine device for her hip and leg pain. She was tired during some interviews, but mentally alert moments before when talking with her family. She showed a range of affect and at times a sense of humor. Her emotions were appropriate to what we discussed—tearful when talking about her children, angry when discussing her feelings of betrayal by her husband. She appeared pessimistic and hopeless about her anorexia, but this was not unrealistic. She denied being actively suicidal and reiterated her wish to die should she need life supports. She had some insight into her illness, but continued to focus on food and weight without awareness of complex psychological issues. She did connect her history of sexual abuse to her anorexia nervosa, but not in any elaborated way. She reported that she continued to be afraid of being "fat" and was not willing to participate in any treatment that involved weight gain.

6   Criteria for Assessing Competence

The need in this case was to design criteria that would test Mrs. Black's competence to refuse life supports. Given that she remained immersed in anorexic thinking, one option was to find a priori that she was incompetent. However, her husband strongly felt that given her history and the family's experience of Mrs. Black, she was competent to make this decision and that a more complex approach to the question was needed. These evaluators and the ethics committee of the hospital agreed.

In line with the standard requirements for establishing competence, two sets of standards were designed: one for cognitive competence and one for emotional competence.[1] In interviewing Mrs. Black, the cognitive and emotional understandings overlapped; this article will make more effort to represent her response to the questions than to keep a neat dichotomy between the two. The assessment also included interviews with family members, treaters, and a review of the records. Information from these sources will also be woven into the discussion.

6.1   Cognitive Competence

Mrs. Black did not think realistically about her refusal to gain weight or her anorexic condition and had not done so for twenty-five years. In fact, she was clear in the evaluation that she felt she would "go back to being my anorexic [self]" if she were to gain strength. Since this cognition was firmly in place, the decision for the purposes of the assessment was made to focus on her cognitive grasp of the consequences of her refusal, that is, likely death. To this end, the following tasks were identified to assess her cognitive understanding:

• Could Mrs. Black understand and appreciate the meaning of death?

• How did others assess her cognitive understanding of death and her capacity to make this decision?

• Could she understand and appreciate the imminence and probability of her death?

• Could she discuss the decision to refuse life supports?

• What were the opinions of others, for example, treaters and family, of Mrs. Black's overall ability to understand and appreciate her decision and its consequences?

• To what extent was she aware of the effects of her anorexia on herself and her family?

The following tasks were identified with regard to Mrs. Black's emotional understanding of the consequences of her refusal:

• Could Mrs. Black appreciate the effects of her death on her family?

• Did her family's views of the effects of her death confirm or disconfirm her understanding?

• Did she have the ability to say good-bye to her family?

• Could she articulate her reasons for her willingness to die?

• Could she, and the family, participate in a family meeting in which these issues were dealt with?

6.1.1   Could Mrs. Black Understand the Meaning of Death?

Given that all these tasks attempt to evaluate an understanding and appreciation that most people might have trouble with, it was important to delineate some features that could indicate a person's capacity to think about death. Therefore, in listening to Mrs. Black's response to the first question, "What is the meaning of death?" we looked for an understanding that death is final (unless some religious belief included afterlife of some sort), that there would be no more "future," and that was qualitatively different from living and not seen as an escape, or a way to find out what others would think or feel after she was dead.

Mrs. Black reported that she thinks about death and its meaning and that she was frightened by it. She had been watching people at the hospice die and understood that there were significant experiences she would forgo by dying, including milestones in her children's lives. She noted that looking forward to particular milestones had helped to keep her alive up to this point and that she "can no longer live two weeks at a time." She described death as an option to living miserably with little to no hope of improvement. She doubted that she could ever live a "normal" life, even if she were to gain weight. She stated that her goal was "comfort and peace," both at the hospice where she was no longer in treatment and in death. She expressed the anorexic paradox: that "'gaining weight' means inducing unbearable feelings that lead to a wish to die." In addition, she understood that her irreversible organ damage would likely make her an invalid for the rest of her life. She only wanted to live if she could "feel good and comfortable." She said: "It is better to die than to live with yourself. . . . I am trying to let myself die."

On a behavioral level, Mrs. Black was engaging in the rituals and actions associated with death. She was active in planning her funeral. At times this seemed to represent a self-dramatization, however, she was in a hospice where this is the practice. She had determined the roles that she wanted her family to play at her funeral. When asked if she was "ready to die," she replied that she was. When asked if she would consider suicide, she said she would not because she had seen its effects in her family when a cousin committed suicide.

6.1.2   How Did Others Assess Her Understanding and Capacity to Make a Decision?

Mrs. Black's family and treaters were interviewed with regard to their assessment of her understanding and appreciation of death and her capacity to make this decision. Family members visited Mrs. Black almost every day. Mr. Black pointed out that his wife had never been reactively suicidal; her decision to refuse life supports has been thoughtful and consistent with her need for control. She has consistently refused forced feedings. He noted that he thought she had "some issues to face," but that she knew what it means to die. Mrs. Black's mother noted that her daughter's thinking was not clouded by medications. She felt that Mrs. Black was "just tired of it" and pointed out that she continues to engage in life-harming behaviors such as smoking. Mrs. Black's mother also recalled one night when Mrs. Black expressed her fear of death and conveyed to her mother a visceral grasp of death as the end. Mrs. Black's son and daughter were also of the opinion that their mother understood that her choice means death. Her son seconded the mother's opinion that his mother would not relinquish "control . . . even if it leads to her death." He felt that his mother was afraid to die and "knows the consequences" of her choices.

Mrs. Black's former treaters documented her long-standing anorexia and refusal to comply with treatment. The workers at the hospice corroborated her adequate mental status, for example, her capacity to perform the activities of daily living and to make decisions about her day-to-day life. They did not feel she was "too confused or disoriented" to make the decision to refuse treatment. They also felt she had issues to work out with her family. The workers noted that Mrs. Black was engaged in some behaviors, for example, buying new clothes and planning short vacations, that might reflect a denial of death; they also confirmed that she was well aware of the nature of hospice care and refused to see a visiting nurse who tried to talk with her about "improvement." Their interpretation was more that Mrs. Black was choosing to "live until she dies."

6.1.3   Understanding and Appreciation of the Imminence and Probability of Her Death

Mrs. Black understood that the hospice entrance requirements included a physician's determining that she had six months or less to live. She herself reported that several doctors had given her a shorter, specific amount of time to live. The doctors denied this. Mrs. Black seemed not only to grasp the imminence of her death, but also wished for it to come sooner. She reiterated several times that she understood that if she does not accept treatment, she will die. She stated that she was not interested in new treatments, saying, "If I were eighteen; if this was a new disease" she might, but not at this stage.

6.1.4   Discussion of the Decision to Refuse Life Supports/ Corroboration by Others

Mrs. Black explained that she refused life supports because she is "just really exhausted." She cites her physical discomfort, including being in a wheelchair, the inadvisability of replacing her liver stent, chronic pain, and her fatigue. As noted, others corroborate Mrs. Black's history of considering death as an option, as well as her exhaustion and refusal to gain weight. A doctor wrote in 1994: "[Patient] does indeed recognize intellectually the seriousness and potential lethality of her anorexia. . . . [B]ut is immobilized in terms of making any changes in her life." By 1996, Mrs. Black had a living will and had indicated that she did not want to be resuscitated. The wish to die is apparent in progress notes through 1997 and 1998.

Mr. Black felt that his wife had perhaps wanted to die for a long time, but had stayed alive "even if only to please others." He had seen for years how she could not make use of the considerable resources offered to her. At this point, he still did not have a theory as to whether she "could not" or "would not," but knew for sure that she had not. Both children and Mrs. Black's mother expressed the awareness that death had been an issue for their mother for a number of years.

6.1.5   Awareness of the Effects of the Anorexia Nervosa on Self and Others

Mrs. Black could describe the history of her anorexia, the damage it had done to her body. She explained that she lost her teeth as a result of the disease. She said that she might gain weight now if she could be guaranteed to "walk and feel good," but added that if her health stabilized, she would resume her anorexic behavior. She had ceased her anorexic behavior when she was pregnant so that she would not hurt her children. She was able to describe how her disease had prevented her from being a fully involved mother with her children, especially in relation to her daughter.

6.1.6   Emotional Functioning with Regard to the Decision to Refuse Life Supports: Appreciation of the Effects of Death upon Her Family/ Family Corroboration

Mrs. Black was asked about the effect of her death on each family member. She spoke most clearly about its effect on her mother; she was least clear about its effect on her daughter. She described her mother as being "devastated . . . she'll be lonely and guilty." In her opinion, her mother was in denial about the seriousness of the situation. Her daughter, she thought, would be "sad," but Mrs. Black could not elaborate. She gave a more nuanced account of its effect on her son and was tearful discussing her husband, saying "[It's been] twenty-one years and I still don't know [how he feels]." This had been a chronic complaint of hers. She indicated that she felt he was an "enabler" and had not been assertive enough in their relationship. She denied that she wished that she now would "fight harder" for her life.

Mr. Black acknowledged being tired, as well as angry. He expressed guilt and regret that he had not "[put his] foot down on different things" and had allowed his wife to be the "controlling person." He, too, had trouble identifying his feelings about his wife's death. He explained that he and his children could not understand how she could have felt and behaved as she did vis-à-vis the anorexia; they saw that she had no choice, that it was "the disease." As guardian, Mrs. Black's husband felt his role had always been to make the decision that she would make, "to make the decision she wants," that is, to refuse life supports. Both children expressed some sense of relief regarding their mother's death. The son was portrayed as "sad" and the daughter as "bitter." The daughter, who noted that her mother had been ill all of her life, felt that her mother's death would ease the burden on her father and allow him to be a more active parent.

6.1.7 Ability to Say Good-Bye/Corroboration by Others

Mrs. Black was unsure of her ability to say good-bye. She felt it would be most difficult to say good-bye to her mother and children. She had written each child a letter, placed in a safe deposit box, to be read following her death. She repeated her theory about her mother's "denial," which will make it hard to say good-bye. The conflict with her husband overshadowed her ability to think about saying good-bye to him. She knows she has not completed this process.

Mr. Black reported that he and his wife have talked about her death frequently. He would like to be "on peaceful terms" with her but recognizes that he is not. He implied that their ongoing conflicts have been impediments to saying good-bye. Mrs. Black's mother agreed that she does not talk with her daughter about death, "maybe because it's unpleasant." She admitted that she may regret not saying good-bye if she does not face it and talk about it now.

The hospice workers corroborated that the family has talked about Mrs. Black's possible death and decision to refuse life supports. However, they disagreed as to the depth of emotion shared by the family. Some felt that Mrs. Black was more sincere than others. All the treaters felt that the family, despite the amount of time they spent together, had little meaningful contact.

6.1.8 Capacity to Articulate Reasons for Dying

Mrs. Black, as noted, articulated a number of reasons for dying, including past as well as present motives. She spoke about her anger with her husband and at one point suggested that her death would be a source of suffering for him in which she would take satisfaction. She was also aware of the burden her illness had placed on her family, in particular her daughter's deprivation of a functioning mother. Specifically, she sees how her incapacitation has interfered with normal family activities, saying, "I'm tired of being a burden and having 'Mummy's sick, we can't do this, we can't do that.'" She hoped that her death would relieve others of guilt. She also recognized that it would increase guilt. She appeared to have both beneficent and punishing motives related to her death.

6.1.9 Family Meeting

Toward the end of the evaluation, a family meeting was planned to include Mrs. Black's nuclear family and her mother. A family therapist who had met the family and knew the history of the case, and who was available to follow the family, provided support and facilitation, while the interviewer assessed the family's capacity to explore the above questions while sitting together. The meeting was very emotional; it was clear that everyone in the family, more and less willingly, understood that Mrs. Black could die if she refused treatment and that she was refusing treatment. The issues that each discussed individually were evident at the meeting.

Each person expressed his or her feelings about the cost to the family of this illness. Mrs. Black expressed again her anger and frustration with her husband as well as some regret that their problems had not been dealt with earlier. Mr. Black reiterated a wish to have an "'answer' to the 'mystery' of the anorexia and how his wife could be choosing to die." Mrs. Black's son stressed again the role the "illness" played in the situation, relieving his mother of some of the responsibility for her choice. Mrs. Black's daughter emphasized her mother's suffering, saying, "I think now she wants to [die], she's sick of everything." As predicted by others, Mrs. Black's mother had the most difficult time addressing the finality of her daughter's choice, asking as she had before if the anorexia could be reversible.

Mrs. Black was unable to stay in the room for the whole interview, leaving for the last half-hour and returning at the end for closure. Her discomfort in the meeting suggested that she had not been able to say good-bye to each family member in a way that "acknowledges the effects of her death on that person and seeks to make some amends for the conflicts and hard feelings of the past and present." Mrs. Black's mother may have been correct when she said she would have trouble after her daughter's death because she was not able to face her impending death beforehand. Given the capacity for denial of death in any family, and for denial in families of patients diagnosed with anorexia nervosa in particular, it appeared that family members were able to grasp the reality of impending death, talk about it in an emotionally genuine way among themselves, and not bury or deny the particularity of each person's relationship with Mrs. Black.

6.1.10   Decision with Regard to Competence to Refuse Lifesaving Treatment

The report concluded that Mrs. Black exhibited the cognitive capacities necessary to make the decision to refuse life supports, but not all of the emotional capacities. In particular it was felt that she had not been able to say good-bye with her family and that the acrimony between herself and her husband were obstructing this process. It was recommended that follow-up family and couples' sessions be scheduled with the family therapist so that these areas could be addressed. It was also noted that Mrs. Black might be helped to develop a more complex view of the effect of her death on her daughter. Since Mrs. Black had been able to appreciate some of the unique effects of her illness on her daughter, as opposed to her son, it was not clear whether this gap had to do with her exhaustion during the interview or her failure to appreciate the effects. Part of the difficulty of Mrs. Black's good-byes with her mother was attributed to her mother's denial of the severity of the situation. This denial appeared to have a long history and is not unusual in an anorexic family; Mrs. Black identified it. The recommendations were for family counseling around these issues and for postmortem family counseling.

7.   Postscript to the Case

Mrs. Black died in May 1999. In July 2001, the family agreed to meet with the interviewer and the therapist who facilitated the family meeting to discuss their feelings about the evaluation process and their experiences leading up to and following the death of their mother. All members of the family—husband, son, and daughter—expressed their conviction that Mrs. Black was not going to get better and that there was no wish to attempt further intervention. They also felt that they had been able to say good-bye and that her death was a relief and allowed them all to go on with their lives.

8   Summary and Conclusions

A debate goes on concerning whether a patient diagnosed with anorexia nervosa can be assessed for competence if she wishes to refuse lifesaving treatment. Some argue that the diagnosis automatically condemns the patient to incompetence with regard to any decision that is related to issues of food, eating, and weight. Others argue that, given certain conditions, an assessment of competence can be triggered. There has not before, however, been a set of criteria by which that assessment might be made. This case illustrates both the conditions in which an assessment of competence is required for a severe and chronic patient wishing to refuse lifesaving treatment and the criteria for assessing that patient's competence.

The conditions we deemed significant included:

• Mrs. Black was an end-stage patient with a long and chronic history, without remissions
• Multiple treaters and interventions, including inpatient and outpatient care
• Significant treatment noncompliance over the years
• Significant and irreversible medical problems
• A consistent wish to refuse treatment over a period of time
• A subjective assessment on the part of Mrs. Black that the quality of her life was poor
• An objective assessment by treaters and family members that Mrs. Black's quality of life was poor
• Adequate mental status at the time of the evaluation
• Family involvement in the decision
• Treater involvement in the decision
• The concern of a hospital ethics committee

The interests of the patient, the family, and the community were taken into account. With these conditions met, the authors agreed with the

Ethics Committee and the family that an assessment of competence was called for. The criteria created were designed to focus on the specific competencies of the awareness of the nature and consequences of anorexia, awareness of the possibility of death, an appreciation of death, and the capacity to say good-bye to loved ones. Given that it is complicated for any of us to understand the meaning and imminence of death, the authors felt that this patient and her family met the criteria for competence.

There is always the danger that some patients diagnosed with anorexia nervosa who refuse lifesaving treatment will foreclose on the possibility of enough recovery from the condition to rekindle a desire to live. It is for this reason that the evaluators gathered data from all involved, interviewed Mrs. Black and her family multiple times, and required a family meeting to confront the issues. This template for assessing competence holds the bar very high and, in doing so, aims to safeguard both the right of the patient diagnosed with chronic and severe anorexia to choose to refuse treatment and the right of the temporarily despairing and angry patient the right to live, recover, and change her mind.

Note

1. The authors thank Dr. Thomas Gutheil, Director of the Program in Psychiatry and the Law, Massachusetts Mental Health Center, for his invaluable assistance in defining the standards.

References

American Psychiatric Association. (2000). *Diagnostic and statistical manual of mental disorders* (4th ed.). Washington, DC: Author.

Appelbaum, P. S., & Grisso, T. (1988). Assessing patients' capacities to consent to treatment. *New England Journal of Medicine, 319,* 1635–1638.

Appelbaum, P. S., Lidz, C. W., & Meisel, A. (1987). *Informed consent: Legal theory and clinical practice.* New York: Oxford University Press.

Bemporad, J. R., & Herzog, D. B. (Eds.). (1989). *Psychoanalysis and eating disorders.* New York: Guilford Press.

Beumont, P., & Vandereycken, W. (1998). Challenges and risks for professionals. In W. Vandereycken & P. Beumont (Eds.), *Treating eating disorders: Ethical, legal and personal issues* (pp. 1–29). New York: New York University Press.

Binswanger, L. (1958). The case of Ellen West. In R. May, E. Angel, & H. F. Ellenberger (Eds.), *Existence: A new dimension in psychiatry and psychology* (pp. 237–264). New York: Simon and Schuster.

Bruch, H. (1973). *Eating disorders: Obesity, anorexia nervosa, and the person within.* New York: Basic Books.

Bruch, H., D. Czyzewski & M. A. Suhr. (1988). *Conversations with anorexics.* New York: Basic Books.

Carney, T. (2001, July 1–6). *Regulating anorexia?* Paper delivered at the 26th Congress of the International Academy of Law and Mental Health, Montréal.

Draper, H. (2000). Anorexia nervosa and respecting a refusal of life-prolonging therapy: A limited justification. *Bioethics, 14*(2), 120–133.

Dresser, R. (1984a). Feeding the hunger artists: Legal issues in treating anorexia nervosa. *Wisconsin Law Review, March/April,* 297–374.

Dresser, R. (1984b). Legal and policy considerations in treatment of anorexia nervosa patients. *International Journal of Eating Disorders, 4*(3), 43–51.

Dresser, R. S., & Boisaubin, E. V., Jr. (1986). Psychiatric patients who refuse nourishment. *General Hospital Psychiatry, 8,* 101–106.

Fallon, P., Katzman, M. A., & Wooley, S. C. (Eds.). (1994). *Feminist perspectives on eating disorders.* New York: Guilford Press.

Fost, N. (1984). Food for thought: Dresser on anorexia. *Wisconsin Law Review, March/April,* 375–384.

Goldner, E. (1989). Treatment refusal in anorexia nervosa. *International Journal of Eating Disorders, 8*(3), 297–306.

Goldner, E. M., Birmingham, C. L., & Smye, V. (1997). Addressing treatment refusal in anorexia nervosa: Clinical, ethical, and legal considerations. In D. M. Garner & P. Garfinkel (Eds.), *Handbook of treatment for eating disorders* (pp. 450–461). New York: Guilford Press.

Griffiths, R., & Russell, J. (1998). Compulsory treatment of anorexia nervosa patients. In W. Vandereycken & P. Beumont (Eds.), *Treating eating disorders: Ethical, legal and personal issues* (pp. 127–150). New York: New York University Press.

Gutheil, T. G., & Bursztajn, H. (1986). Clinicians' guidelines for assessing and presenting subtle forms of patient incompetence in legal settings. *American Journal of Psychiatry, 143,* 1020–1023.

Hébert, P. C., & Weingarten, M. A. (1991). The ethics of forced feeding in anorexia nervosa. *Canadian Medical Association Journal, 144*(2), 141–144.

Kaplan, A. S., & Woodside, D. B. (1987). Biological aspects of anorexia nervosa and bulimia nervosa. *Journal of Consulting and Clinical Psychology, 55*(5), 645–653.

Levine, D. Z. (1999). When the doctor's master is a bully. *American Journal of Kidney Diseases, 34*(4), 759–760.

Levinsky, N. G. (1984). The doctor's master. *New England Journal of Medicine, 311,* 1573–1575.

Lewis, P. (1999). Feeding anorexic patients who refuse food. *Medical Law Review, 7*(1), 21–37.

MacDonald, C. (2002). Treatment resistance in anorexia nervosa and the pervasiveness of ethics in clinical decision making. *Canadian Journal of Psychiatry, 47*(3), 267–270.

Minuchin, S., Rosman, B. L., & Baker, L. (1978). *Psychosomatic families: Anorexia nervosa in context.* Cambridge, MA: Harvard University Press.

Mitchell, J. E., Pomeroy, C., & Adson, D. E. (1997). Managing medical complications. In D. M. Garner & P. E. Garfinkel (Eds.), *Handbook of treatment for eating disorders* (2nd ed.) (pp. 383–393). New York: Guilford Press.

Neiderman, M., Zarody, M., Tattersall, M., & Lask, B. (2000). Enteric feeding in severe adolescent anorexia nervosa: A report of four cases. *International Journal of Eating Disorders, 28,* 470–475.

Orbach, S. (1986). *Hunger strike: The anorexic's struggle as a metaphor for our age.* New York: Norton.

Robb, A. S., Silber, T., Orell-Valente, J. K., Valadez-Meltzer, A., Ellis, N., Dadson, M. J., et al. (2002). Supplemental nocturnal nasogastric refeeding for better short-term outcome in hospitalized adolescent girls with anorexia nervosa. *American Journal of Psychiatry, 159*(8), 1347–1353.

Roth, L. H., Appelbaum, P. S., Sallee, R., Reynolds, C. F., & Huber, G. (1982). The dilemma of denial in the assessment of competency to refuse treatment. *American Journal of Psychiatry, 139*(7), 910–913.

Selvini Palazzoli, M. (1974). *Self-starvation: From individual to family therapy in the treatment of anorexia nervosa.* New York: Jason Aronson.

Shelley, R. (Ed.). (1997). *Anorexics on anorexia.* London: Jessica Kingsley.

Silverman, J. A. (1997). Anorexia nervosa: Historical perspective on treatment. In D. M. Garner & P. E. Garfinkel (Eds.), *Handbook of treatment for eating disorders* (2nd ed., pp. 3–10). New York: Guilford Press.

Stierlin, H., & Weber, G. (1989). *Unlocking the family door.* New York: Brunner/Mazel.

Strober, M. (1997). Consultation and therapeutic engagement in severe anorexia nervosa. In D. M. Garner & P. Garfinkel (Eds.), *Handbook of treatment for eating disorders* (2nd ed., pp. 229–247). New York: Guilford Press.

Tiller, J., Schmidt, U., & Treasure, J. (1993). Compulsory treatment for anorexia nervosa: Compassion or coercion? *British Journal of Psychiatry, 162,* 680–697.

Vandereycken, W. (1998). Whose competence should we question? *European Eating Disorders Review, 6*(1), 1–3.

8

"Personality Disorder" and Capacity to Make Treatment Decisions

George Szmukler

Can patients with a personality disorder, by virtue of that condition alone, lack decision-making capacity? This question has been posed in discussions considering the practicability of an impaired capacity (or decision-making) criterion in mental health legislation[1,2] and recently in an interesting case report,[3] in which a patient with a personality disorder was refusing treatment despite having a dangerously low hemoglobin level as a result of self-cutting. The problem arises most acutely when patients with a personality disorder present in crisis with threats of self-harm, especially suicide, or of harming others.

In their case report, Winburn and Mullen consider the capacity of the patient to make a decision about a blood transfusion for blood loss.[3] The role of personality disorder was seen as impairing the patient's ability to give informed consent, because her "refusal was a manifestation of her tendency to adopt a contrary and self-destructive stance in response to clinical advice," which in turn was a manifestation of her disturbed relationship with clinical staff. It was judged that this interaction was such "that she was considered unable to choose to behave otherwise." The case report did not consider the patient's capacity to make a decision about treatment for her personality disorder, although this might be considered an integral aspect of the "disorder" underlying the presenting clinical problem.

One can speculate about how a personality disorder might impair decision-making capacity. To my knowledge, this question has not been specifically addressed. On the face of it, there appears to be a number of possibilities. The type of presentation most commonly calling into question a person's capacity is one in which he or she expresses powerful suicidal ideas. An associated state of prominent emotional distress or arousal might overwhelm the ability to understand information, or to "appreciate" the nature of the situation in which the person finds themselves, or to reason. Or the person may, in an apparently calm state, claim there is no alternative to suicide. This may be in reaction to problems that may appear to others, on the surface at least, to be quite soluble. Or the suicidal intention, or impulse, may appear to be beyond the person's control, to arise from an inner disturbance the subject finds difficult to describe or characterize. Here one might consider there may be underlying difficulties involving "appreciation" or reasoning. Matters may be more complex still when there is a suspicion that the threats of self-harm are directed at achieving an unacknowledged end, of which, perhaps, the author of the threats, himself or herself, seems unaware. On top of that, the person may, especially in an emergency psychiatric setting, reject offers of treatment, raising the question of an involuntary admission to hospital to ensure the person's safety. The anxieties raised under these circumstances can be considerable.

Even in the absence of any specification of the underlying psychological mechanisms, there seems enough in such presentations that is "non-understandable" to make the question of capacity pertinent. It may turn out that it is not possible, in some fundamental sense—perhaps because of the particular nature of the personality disorder—to assess capacity meaningfully (unless there is another, associated mental disorder such as depression).

While working in the emergency clinic at the Maudsley Hospital, we grappled with the place of capacity in the management of persons with personality disorder. Quite commonly patients with personality disorder presented who feared harming themselves or who expressed an intention to do so. We reviewed in detail two such patients who presented consecutively to the clinic as an emergency, both young women in their twenties with a primary diagnosis of personality disorder associated with serious threats of suicide and who were reluctant to accept offers of treatment. Both had a number of previous similar presentations and had self-harmed in the past. Intoxication with drugs or alcohol was not present at the time of assessment.

Assessing treatment decision-making capacity was clearly relevant to whether patients such as these could be treated involuntarily for physical complications following self-harm (as in the case report mentioned above,[3] for example, or should a patient disclose having taken an overdose of paracetamol with its potential for liver damage). Or, less clearly, in the absence of physical injury, whether they had the capacity to decide whether to accept psychiatric treatment aimed at preventing the acts of self-harm that were being threatened. This would involve treatment for some aspects of the underlying personality disorder. It was at the time of the study questionable whether the Mental Health Act (MHA) 1983 could be employed to treat a person with a diagnosis of "personality disorder." One way of dealing with this dilemma was a consideration of treatment decision-making capacity; we reasoned that if the patient had capacity, it would provide reassurance that involuntary treatment would be unjustified ethically and that autonomously made treatment choices should be respected. (Under the MHA 2007, personality disorder is now considered to constitute a "mental disorder," but whether this helps with ethical decision making is a separate issue, especially if impaired decision making is regarded as important).

Consent was not obtained from the two patients for inclusion in a published case report. Therefore many details are not provided. However, a general description of the findings should suffice to support the main conclusions.

Assessment of Capacity

We adopted the MacCAT-T structure for the assessment of capacity.[4] Four elements were examined: (1) "Understanding," the patient's ability to understand the nature of the disorder and of the benefits and risks associated with treatment; (2) "appreciation," the ability of the patient to appreciate that the disorder is one that the patient has and that the treatment would be of possible benefit to the patient; (3) the "ability to reason" with the information, to generate consequences of having or not having the treatment and to think about their influence on everyday activities; and (4) the ability to "make a choice." These elements parallel the criteria in the Mental Capacity Act (MCA) 2005.[5]

Both patients who were assessed in detail were highly aroused or distressed on presentation to the clinic. Their ideas of self-harm were taken seriously by staff, seriously enough for compulsory admission to hospital to be entertained, initially at least. In both cases the patients said they saw no alternative to suicide. They saw treatment as useless. The criteria for a diagnosis of a depressive illness were not met.

Results of the Capacity Assessments

It was soon apparent that the meaning to be attributed to the concept of personality disorder was of crucial importance when thinking about treatment decision-making capacity. Despite its designation as a "mental disorder" under the MHA 2007, the conceptual status of personality disorder as a "mental disorder" is controversial. For example, Charland has argued that the description of personality disorder is couched in moral terms.[6] This is most evident in "antisocial personality disorder," in which the criteria for diagnosis are essentially a set of socially disapproved behaviors. However, I do not wish to enter into a debate on what kind of "disorder" personality disorder represents. People with personality disorder may present to health care services in states of distress or posing health risks and it is generally accepted that services should provide help.[7] If capacity is to be assessed in this group of patients in a medical setting, then presumably personality disorder must be construed in some way as an "illness" or mental or medical "disorder," the nature of which needs to be discussed with the patient so that his or her understanding and appreciation of the "disorder" can be tested. How is this "disorder" or "mental health problem" to be explained to the patient?

The diagnosis of personality disorder is very different to, say, that of a fracture of the femur or diabetes, or indeed to the "standard" mental disorders such as schizophrenia or bipolar disorder. A straightforward description in terms of symptoms and signs, causes, and relatively clear-cut diagnostic criteria is not possible. Personality disorder is defined as an enduring pattern of maladaptive traits, displayed in a wide range of situations, which results in harms to the person or to others. Justification of the diagnosis requires a relatively detailed account of the patient's life history, looking at personality traits and their interactions with events or situations in which those traits led to personal or social harms or difficulties for the patient or others. Indeed, what needs to be shared with the patient is in essence a "formulation" or narrative that makes comprehensible the predicament that has brought him or her to the health care service. This exploration of the past and its relationship with the present takes quite a long time. It also requires a considerable degree of labor on the part of both the patient and clinician as they try to construct a meaningful account of the patient's life and difficulties. The process involves a dialogue, in the course of which interpretations of events may need to be revised. In the two cases reviewed in detail, it also required the involvement of a relative or friend who provided an important perspective on the development of the problem, in each case instructive for both the clinician and the patient.

In the two cases here, the clinician and patient eventually substantially agreed on the main points of the formulation of the patient's difficulties.

Next, if the patient "understands" the account, there needs to be a discussion of treatment options so the patient can think about what the outcome might be with or without treatment. Again these do not follow the conventional pattern for the majority of illnesses. In the case of personality disorder, recommendations vary greatly, and they are substantially shaped by the nature of the problems as well as a treatment modality's acceptability to the patient. For the patients we assessed, they included in all cases the options of admission to the hospital (possibly involuntary if a case could be made for a "mental disorder" under the MHA 1983), medication, "talking" treatments of various kinds (including supportive psychotherapy, cognitive behavior therapy, dialectic behavior therapy, family therapy, group therapy), and social interventions (including changes to accommodation, financial advice, lifestyle changes, including drug and alcohol misuse, social relations, work). For an assessment of capacity, the patient requires information about these interventions, including the advantages and disadvantages of each put in a way that could be reasonably expected to make sense from their point of view. Connections need to be made between the description of what comprises the personality disorder and the rationale for treatment choices. Again communicating the information to enable decision making is very time-consuming.

Now, decision making having been "enabled," the patient can be asked questions directed to assessing "appreciation" and "reasoning" (or in MCA terms, "using" and "weighing" the information) leading to a choice. Consequences for his or her life goals and choices need to be generated by the patient in weighing the frequently multiple treatment options. This is complex and again takes a lot of time.

Both patients were judged to have capacity to make treatment decisions at the end of this assessment process. Appropriate treatment options became clearer as the discussion developed. Both decided that inpatient admission was not necessary, and this was agreed by the psychiatrist and nursing team who were satisfied that the decision was soundly based. Both patients accepted referral back to their community mental health team for urgent follow-up when further discussion of treatment options, in both cases probably involving some form of psychotherapy, would be considered. Medication was not prescribed for either, but it was agreed that if their condition should deteriorate before the follow-up, they could return to the emergency clinic at any time.

Discussion

Treatment decision-making capacity could be assessed in these patients with personality disorder along the lines described above and given the assumptions stated. The assessment was clearly different to what is usual in health care, reflecting the unusual, if not problematical, conceptual status of personality disorder as a "mental disorder"; it is certainly considerably more complex, but it was, in the end, meaningful.

However, while the assessment in these cases progressed fairly smoothly, it is clear that significant difficulties may arise in other instances. How a threshold for treatment decision-making capacity in such patients can be set is a potential concern. For example, what level of "understanding" or "appreciation" should be expected? How substantive does an agreement between the clinician and the patient on the "formulation" of the problems need to be? Whereas in the two cases discussed above there were no real disagreements, this may not always, or even generally, be the case. There is no simple answer. It is important to bear in mind a temptation for the clinician to raise the threshold when there is disagreement and when there are significant risks. Specifying the threshold in personality disorder is significantly more difficult than in patients with, say, schizophrenia or depression. In the end there may remain an element of indeterminacy if different interpretations can each be reasonably supported by the history of events and behaviors. In such cases one might conclude that it is not possible, in principle, to assess capacity; or that the patient's account, although not the one preferred by the clinician, is an adequate one, and sufficient to demonstrate that the patient has capacity. A study of further cases would establish how significant this issue might prove. The moralized nature of some forms of personality disorder entails a further problem.[6] For example, if a person with an "antisocial personality disorder" were to accept the clinician's formulation of the problem, this could be construed as requiring an admission to engagement in socially disapproved behaviors and an understanding that a course of "treatment" would be aimed at correcting such conduct. This is difficult to reconcile with most people's views of "mental illness" or "mental disorder" and is more in keeping with rehabilitation in the criminal justice system. On the other hand, it could be argued that a failure by someone with an "antisocial personality disorder" to "appreciate" that his or her conduct is unacceptable to society or unlawful would raise a question about his or her mental "capacity," in some sense at least.

At the time the patients were seen, the MCA 2005 had not yet been implemented. However, if one were to view these patients through the lens of the MCA, it is likely that people with a personality disorder might at times, when in states of turmoil, for example, exhibit a "disturbance in the functioning of the mind or brain," making the MCA relevant. It is also noteworthy that the nature and content of the assessments force one to pay full regard to sections 1(3) ("A person is not to be treated as unable to make a decision unless all practicable steps to help him to do so have been taken without success") and 3(2) ("A person is not to be regarded as unable to understand the information relevant to a decision if he is able to understand an explanation of it given to him in a way that is appropriate to his circumstances [using simple language, visual aids or any other means]").

Two further points with a bearing on practical issues can be highlighted:

1. The assessment of capacity along these lines was time-consuming. It could not be completed in a single interview; in each case rest breaks were required, and time was also spent contacting relatives or friends who could help with the formulation. Informants may also be able to help with offers of support that may influence treatment choices—for example, an offer to stay with the patient for a few days could avert the need for admission to the hospital. Capacity assessments during future crisis presentations by these patients might be more quickly assessed, but they will presumably still require a detailed examination of the interaction of personality with recent circumstances and of possible treatment interventions. A diagnostic assessment of patients like these can be lengthy, but the necessary engagement in the type of dialogue described above with its constant creation of "hypotheses," clarifications, and revisions requires substantially more time.

2. Probably as a product of the time spent with the patient and the nature of the discussion, it became evident that the assessment had become an "intervention"—and in each case we judged it to be a therapeutic intervention. The patients, who had many previous contacts with mental health services, had probably never previously experienced the kind of conversation they were now engaged in. An unusual degree of detail about the patient's life and, perhaps more notably, about the clinician's thinking was shared. The patients seemed to find this dialogue helpful. An important outcome in these cases was that the capacity assessment ceased to be the sole or even the main focus of the interview. What would constitute the best intervention in the light of the patient's difficulties came to dominate the discussion.

Although both patients were eventually judged to have capacity, we do not know what proportion of all persons presenting in this way do or do not have capacity in the sense described here. One study suggests only a small proportion lack capacity.[8] The findings raise a significant health service question. How far is it possible to provide a health care setting (short of an inpatient admission, which we generally wish to avoid) that offers the space and time for the prolonged assessment process to take place, together with the containment sufficient to ensure the person's safety in the meantime? Most emergency departments are probably unsuitable. The psychiatric emergency clinic in which our patients were seen and which provided the right kind of environment is now closed. Providing an assessment of people with a personality disorder along the lines described above presents a considerable challenge. When the environment precludes such an assessment, an involuntary admission to hospital becomes more likely, or, if the patient is allowed to leave the emergency room, the staff may be left very anxious about the wisdom of their decision.

References

1. Department of Health & Report of the Expert Committee. (1999). *(Richardson Report): Review of the Mental Health Act.* London: Department of Health.

2. Dawson, J., & Szmukler, G. (2006). Fusion of mental health and incapacity legislation. *British Journal of Psychiatry, 188,* 504–509.

3. Winburn, E., & Mullen, R. (2008). Personality disorder and competence to refuse treatment. *Journal of Medical Ethics, 34,* 715–716.

4. Grisso, T., Appelbaum, P. S., & Hill-Fotouhi, C. (1997). The MacCAT-T: A clinical tool to assess patients' capacities to make treatment decisions. *Psychiatric Services (Washington, D.C.), 48,* 1415–1419.

5. Mental Capacity Act 2005. (2005). London: Stationery Office.

6. Charland, L. C. (2006). Moral nature of DSM-IV cluster B personality disorders. *Journal of Personality Disorders, 20,* 116–125.

7. Bolton, D. (2007). *What is mental disorder? An essay in philosophy, science and values.* Oxford: Oxford University Press.

8. Owen, G. S., Richardson, G., David, A. S., et al. (2008). Mental capacity to make decisions on treatment in people admitted to psychiatric hospitals: cross sectional study. *BMJ (Clinical Research Ed.), 337,* 448.

III

Violence, Trauma, and Treatment

Sadly, violence is the new normal. The twenty-four-hour news cycle often includes coverage of the unremitting violence of mass shootings, child rape at the hands of men in authority, and inner-city gang violence. It is well known that violence and trauma are both a cause and an effect of mental illness. We must be careful not to oversimplify this connection. More often it is the mentally ill who are or have been the victims of violence; they are usually not the perpetrators as is so often depicted in the popular press and media. And as victims of violence, mentally ill persons and their families experience a form of helplessness and suffering that finds its roots in both stigma and social antipathy. Victims of violence are often blamed for their various plights: chronic physical and mental maladies, substance abuse, and homelessness.

The articles in part III address the philosophical and ethical dimensions of first recognizing and then attending to persons who have suffered from traumas resulting from war, the toxic stress of violent inner-city life, and rape. After starting with a conceptual discussion of post-traumatic stress disorder (PTSD), we shift to a qualitative report on the self-perpetuating nature of violence as experienced by young urban black men. Finally, we present a review on the systemic hurdles that rape victims face as they attempt to access medical, legal, and mental health help.

Drawing on work in the philosophy of medicine, two clinician-scholars from a Veterans Affairs hospital, James Beshai and Richard Tushup, provide a phenomenological account of complexities of treating war veterans with PTSD. They discuss the hidden pain of PTSD, the problem of self-disclosure, and the ways in which individual ontologies—the worldviews that patient and clinician hold—may misalign to create confusion in diagnosis, treatment, and recovery. Clinicians also will be challenged by those with PTSD who present them with discordant ethical views about the sanctity of human life—on the one hand, the life of an enemy is expendable, while on the other hand, a buddy's life is sacred. Such dissonance forces clinicians to come to grips with their own views about the sanctity of human life and dignity, as the authors argue that both the diagnosis and treatment of PTSD hinge not on scientific criteria but on subjective value judgments about these deeper concepts. Although Beshai and Tushup focus squarely on PTSD among veterans, their insights will prove valuable across the vast contexts wherein the disorder exists.

We turn then to the streets of US cities where another form of warfare continues unabated: interpersonal violence among persons of color. John Rich and David Stone present qualitative accounts that illustrate how self-respect and the perception of one's peers ultimately drive young urban black men to act violently. There is a perverse logic to the violence that at first blush appears random and irrational. At its base, it is a logical response to a loosely hierarchical social structure that rewards a violent response to personal slights. This rationale for violence is self-amplifying as a response to chronic stress, marginalization from mainstream society, poverty, and discrimination. As this vicious cycle generates pathology after pathology, it challenges clinicians to understand the context from which their traumatized victim-offenders present.

Rebecca Campbell provides an account of the serious difficulties that rape victims face—the minority of whom seek assistance after the assault from legal, medical, and mental health care providers. Campbell explains that the victimization that women seeking this help experience may become a "second rape" as insensitive treatment by medical and legal professionals further dehumanizes and traumatizes them. Campbell describes how sexual assault nurse examiner (SANE) programs provide a model of an ethically informed, victim-centered medical-legal recourse. Because mental health care options for victims are often difficult to access and treatment lags have a significant impact on the psychological well-being of victims, Campbell suggests that mental health care first-aid approaches be more widely deployed.

Campbell's article reiterates an overall theme of this part: that violence begets violence and trauma begets trauma. Mental health care providers share an ethical obligation to both understand and work to arrest this cycle.

9

Sanctity of Human Life in War: Ethics and Post-traumatic Stress Disorder

James A. Beshai and Richard J. Tushup

Perhaps only those willing to wrestle with human anguish and unanswered moral and ethical questions, raised by those who have been splattered by the blood of war and lived to tell of it, unequivocally accept the existential reality of combat-related post-traumatic stress disorder (PTSD). This medical disorder acquired identification first in the Civil War as a "soldier's heart" and as "shell shock" in World War I. World War II and Korea gave us "combat fatigue." There were attempts to dismiss this disorder as a disease related to combat situations as an artificial construct that is politically motivated (Foucault, 1970, 1975). A few veterans report they view it as a "coward's rationalization" to earn benefits. There is a constellation of symptoms that appear in some military veterans as a result of "enduring or witnessing an event that involved actual or threatened death or serious injury, or a threat to the physical integrity of self or others" (American Psychiatric Association, 2000, p. 209). A list of criteria for the diagnosis of PTSD appeared in the *Diagnostic and Statistical Manual of Mental Disorders* (DSM) DSM-III in 1980.

This article focuses on the ethical aspects in diagnosis and treatment of combat-related PTSD. It first addresses the normative function of medical classification in diagnosis and treatment of this disorder and then raises issues with this diagnosis and treatment in view of ethical issues, especially with regard to the moral responsibility of the veteran toward society and toward his own conscience when facing a violation of what many view as the sanctity of human life. Pellegrino and Thomasma (1981, p. 100) make a strong case for the influence of Greek philosophy on ethically sound medical practice and how the Hippocratic oath entails a need for a practical professional ontology to promote health and healing.

This ethical issue over the sanctity of human life is entwined with another political issue: whether the decision to go to war serves the common good in the end. Simply looking at PTSD as a treatable disorder such as diabetes or heart disease falls short of uncovering its uncanny nature of haunting the sensibility of the individual for years afterward.

The specific role a person played in a particular set of events also has relevance and speaks to the ethical integrity of the military officers who give the orders in combat, health care workers treating the people who carried out the combat or who assisted the mission, and even the examiners, usually in the Department of Veterans Affairs, who conduct a compensation and pension examination of the veteran for the government. To stimulate consideration of the ethics and morality of war as something that need not remain in unmentionable obscurity because health care workers show discomfort in dealing with patriotic issues is the aim of this article. Malingering in PTSD was discussed by Burkett (1984, as cited by DeViva & Bloem, 2003) for the individual veteran, not for society.

Normative Functions in Diagnosis and Treatment

McNally's review (2003) of PTSD suggests this medical diagnosis is unique: the only one that relates to a public historical event of a near-death experience that can be verified by reference to military files. It is not based on an identifiable biological or neuropsychological locus in the brain or a recognized neuroscientific process. There have been several neuroscientific attempts (e.g., Blanchard, Kolb, Pallmeyer, & Gerardi, 1982) to identify a specific locus in the brain or a group of neurotransmitters that distinguish those with PTSD from those without, but so far these findings remain unconfirmed. Pellegrino and Thomasma (1981) argued that "the neurosystem is not an organ but an embodiment of the mind and body" (p. 103). Clinicians who engage in diagnosis or treatment of veterans with a medical illness like PTSD face two sets of ethical tasks.

The first issue facing the clinician-examiner is how to translate the well-researched, but abstract, A, B, C, D criteria of PTSD into personal clinical accounts, and vice versa. This issue has been addressed by Pellegrino and Thomasma (1981), Spicker (1976), Straus, Natanson, and Ey (1969), and others. The examiner needs to translate an item like "efforts to avoid thoughts, feelings, or conversations associated with the trauma" into historical events such as "refusing to tell his wife why he singles out a Vietnamese neighbor to help rather than other neighbors." For example, one patient would not tell his wife that he had killed a

Vietnamese woman, first because he had repressed it and second because he did not realize there was any connection between killing her and taking care of a poor Vietnamese immigrant. It took a year of therapy for this veteran to see the connection and to convince both the veteran and his wife that the motive was guilt rather than lust. The conundrum a clinician faces in translating the DSM discipline is manifest here: if the veteran avoids talking about it, how could the examiner know that such a connection exists, and how could that serve as "persistent avoidance of stimuli associated with the trauma"? Every item of the twelve subtitles of criteria C and D can lead to false positives or false negatives in diagnosis. Examiners and therapists need to be aware of these concerns.

The applications of absolute criteria to subjective feelings of "near death," "avoidance," or "high arousal," which are not observable empirically, pose logical dilemmas and need to be relativized or rendered into commonalities in diagnosis. This has to be done even though there is a clinical admission of the specificity and uniqueness of each human experience. A trauma is an experience of a living and changing body. The attribution of etiology requires knowledge and the application of scientific association before moving into therapy and prognosis. But if health is a foundational value, an ethic of medicine must simultaneously consider both individual and social good because both are rooted in the living body.

A value screen is cast on the diagnostic process in which each veteran is a case in an abstract classification, but this particular case must be the correct one for the PTSD classification. The examiner must also provide explanations of the existence of causes and conditions of disease. In the above example, one considers shooting an innocent Vietnamese woman in cold blood because the soldier mistook her for a Vietcong is an ethical issue for the veteran because it violates his sense of the sanctity of human life. According to Pellegrino and Thomasma (1981), "No unitary explanation or logical method can encompass the several different reasoning modes and several kinds of evidence acceptable in responding to the different kinds of questions the clinician must answer" (p. 121).

The Pellegrino and Thomasma (1981) review of positivistic theories in medicine advocates that the ontology of the "lived body" or "wisdom of the body" provides "a bionomic order which is logically prior to individual experience" (p. 117). A veteran presents an organization of reality by his experience of war as a living body. "A living body protoselects health as a desirable goal and considers it obtainable under optimum conditions." Conditions are not optimum during war, and he must consider the value of health and life for every human life not just his own. Health is a value of living bodies if value is defined as that which is judged both obtainable and desirable, that is, a common good. A diagnosis of PTSD is a common good if both the veteran and the examiner are aware of their own practical ontology and how they value not just loss of life but also loss of optimum health as a result of the trauma of war.

During the course of an evaluation for the presence of PTSD, an interviewer conducts a session to match the veteran's account with formal DSM-IV criteria. Given the ethical considerations cited above, it is important to realize that there are at least three unwritten problems in the process of arriving at a diagnosis. (1) The examiner must translate a personal experience with a given practical ontology into an abstract criterion like (A) near death, (B) frequent recurring and distressing flash-backs and nightmares, or (C) avoidance of "stimuli associated with the trauma." (2) The examiner must explain what goes on in this dialogue between him and the veteran. The examiner must engage himself in an inner dialogue of whether the textual material presented by the patient is understood as matching the requirements for a diagnosis. Questions are asked by the examiner to detect presence or absence of verbal and nonverbal signs of traumatic experience with well-defined statements of characteristics. (3) The examiner must have a good grasp of the veteran's ontology and in what manner it may be similar to or different from the examiner's. From this delicate nonverbal, experiential review of the two ontologies, the examiner concludes whether there is a trauma. The compensation and pension examiner makes an assessment of the intensity of the trauma in terms of mild, moderate, and severe. Unlike measuring pain on a ten-point scale, the judgment of the examiner must involve some awareness of a "practical ontology" not disclosed. Pellegrino and Thomasma (1981) drew attention to an understanding of the "implicit" philosophy of life held by the examiner and the veteran in encounters of this sort.

An example of lack of awareness of the other's ontology might be given should a veteran say that in the course of his combat, he killed hundreds of "gooks" or "terrorists." He might feel guilty and disclose or not feel guilty and take pride in serving his country as a decorated combat veteran. Some of the veteran's inner experience may well be accessible to the examiner as a sense of pride, but there may also be a sense of shame for having violated what the individual's ontology would consider as "the sanctity of human life." One veteran might say that he was very good at killing the enemy and find it compatible with his personal ontology, and another just the opposite. He might report this with a sign of "dis-ease" (Straus, 1966) or some cognitive dissonance. What a veteran discloses may or may not tell the truth about what was perceived as the horrific experience of "kill or get killed." This differential in response to the trauma of war may be attributed to the veteran's "practical ontology," and it is not resolved by relying on objective validity scales.

When examiners make a diagnosis of PTSD, they also make a value judgment on behalf of the veteran and interpret this human experience in the light of their own experience. The clinical judgment made may be correct even if the veteran disagrees and takes issue with the diagnosis. Of course, not all diagnostic decisions are valid even though every good decision must be correct to be valid. The examiner is not likely to live peacefully with his decision to deny a veteran a diagnosis of PTSD if that veteran commits suicide as a result of what he perceives as a rejection or lack of understanding of what he went through in war. If criterion A is denied, veterans often tell the examiner "I'd like to see you go through what I went through and tell me if that is traumatic or not."

Ethical Issues: The Individual

The examiner enters into rapport with the veteran with his own implicit views about war and its vicissitudes imparted by society but cast in an undisclosed ontology. Neither the doctor nor the patient knows the basis for their moral judgment. A professional relation is maintained if each refrains from making a judgment of where the other stands on the sanctity of human life. At the same time it is not possible to assess PTSD or treat it without some disclosure of where each one stands on the issue of the sanctity of human life. It is in this nexus that differences in ontological beliefs between therapist and veteran are likely to influence the course of therapy. While the professional training of every therapist includes an awareness of ethical issues in one form or other, it is not so much the amount of knowledge the medical professional may have as it is the belief system that is upheld that makes the difference. In a compensation and pension examination and in therapy, this self-awareness and self-disclosure of one's own position on the sanctity of human life in health and disease, war and peace, enters in and affects the course of diagnosis or therapy.

Nowhere is this sanctity more apparent than it is in medicine with issues like euthanasia, abortion, and end of life. According to Pellegrino and Thomasma (1981), "medicine is a distinctive ethical and moral activity entrusted with the human relationship of healing. One person in need of healing seeks out another who professes to have the knowledge and wisdom to assist in healing" (p. 11). "The ethical component of medicine enters as one moves beyond medicine into a philosophy of medicine which attends in part, to examining judgments about which right decisions were good" (p. 157). In other words, clinical judgments in diagnosis and therapy are both medical and inherently moral. Discussions of both good and bad clinical judgments are not solely dependent on the implementation of scientific rigor and procedure.

Increasingly the interface of psychiatry with ethics seems to agree that a therapist "needs an ontological conception of man which can give order and intelligibility to the objective search of medical science. The pursuit of health, virtue, and common good are inherent in the role of the healing arts and need to be articulated in training" (Pellegrino & Thomasma, 1981) far more than a simple review of how to not run afoul of the law or the Health Insurance Portability and Accountability Act of 1966. Ethical rules and regulations do not become automatically prescriptive unless they are tied to the moral goal of attaining what is good and wholesome for the Other. For a veteran the Other may be the government at large, and while the veteran may be able to disclose his ontology, the government who declared war and sent a veteran into harm's way never declares its ontology. This discrepancy may explain the suspicion that PTSD veterans harbor toward the government. The veteran's motives may be unethical in malingering, but the motives for war are always assumed to be ethical.

Straus makes a phenomenological distinction between "dis-ease" and "disease" where the former is an experience of disruption while disease is a somewhat scientific classification in a manual or DSM which can be discerned, measured, and treated. Certain signs of disease are described and coded accurately in nomenclature, but there is always the additional becoming of the body as a dynamic, sensing, actively lived body. Post-traumatic stress disorder may well be a valid medical classification, but it is also related to a violation of the sanctity of human life. It is entangled with shame, guilt, survival, honor, bravery, and so on. It is not just a dysfunction in locus coeruleus (Gray, 1987) or a group of transmitters. It is a clinical sign of a disruption of lived time in the lived body. It calls for an interpretation of one's ontology and one's relation with the Other in war and peace alike.

Ethical Issues: Society

The therapist enters into three relations: one with the patient, another with disease, and a third with society. The sociocultural and political implications of PTSD are evoked in the third, and it is necessary to concede the relation or rapport with the patient, to the scientific knowledge of the disease as it is summed up in the A, B, C, D criteria of PTSD in DSM-IV. But as Foucault (1970, 1975) stated, there is a tendency to neglect the first two and focus on the third. The individual experience of "shame" or "guilt" at killing the enemy is treated by medication and by informing the veteran that he was serving "a higher purpose" of defending his country. Killing the enemy, a soldier is instructed in boot camp, does not violate the sanctity of life.

Although the object of medicine is essentially seen as curing disease and caring for the patient, there are several ontological themes implicit in social orientation that need to be addressed. Assuming medical knowledge and craft are value laden implies a pragmatic use of science. Doctors must make ethical decisions based on distinctions and priorities between soldiers and civilians. Medical decisions are made on who is likely to live and who is not. Access to treatment determines who is likely to survive and who is not. Ethical judgment is often based on the consequences of action. Treatment of PTSD has ethical consequences in terms of the breakup of marriage, addiction, and suicide. For example, a critical concept such as "normal" engages the examiner or therapist in a discussion of political, social, scientific, and cultural values. A soldier is usually inclined to defend his buddies and ignore "collateral damage." But on a human level, the death of an enemy civilian is also a loss of life. A soldier inherently knows and feels that the sanctity of human life is compromised when he shoots first. A veteran who barricades his house and shoots a neighbor who trespasses his "perimeter" is treated by society as a criminal. How can the veteran reconcile his military ethics with his civilian ethics? How do we treat the category of "normal" in these different circumstances?

After presenting an anatomy of clinical judgment, Pellegrino and Thomasma (1981) stated that "the right action—the best one for a given patient—is not always synonymous with the logically or scientifically deduced action. The amount and kind of information needed to secure a diagnosis may be quite different from that needed for decisive action" (p. 132). Decisive action sometimes involves the counter position of what is good scientifically, what the therapist thinks is good, and what the veteran will accept as good. Scientific, personal, and professional values intersect but can be in conflict.

Such conflicts can be resolved on an interpersonal level by consideration of personal disclosure of where one stands on the sanctity of human life.

Considerations of Personal Ontology and Politics

Rules of prudence such as those cited by Pellegrino and Thomasma (1981) do not provide a recipe for diagnosis, but they may help the health care provider think through the moral problems presented here. There seems to be more variability among PTSD symptoms than among a well-established medical diagnosis like diabetes. Combat may take the form of one individual killing another or using a modern weapon to kill several, but it is a group activity designed to achieve control or power over the enemy. Soldiers who kill one or many Vietnamese in the name of self-defense or providing "freedom and democracy" do not think that they are committing crime at the time, but each one feels differently about the sanctity of human life. In a group each soldier surrenders his free will to his sergeant or to the officer in charge. Prior to induction, recruits need to be told that they are making a moral decision by accepting to surrender their willpower to someone else. The number of casualties and the impact of massive bombing, nuclear or otherwise, is a commander's ethical responsibility. It too cannot be taken lightly as just "collateral damage" and is an ethical dilemma that has to be addressed by the people of a nation. The soldier's brain, no matter what military training he receives, is bound to fail to process the perception of combat adequately. It may be processed as trance logic or as misinformation or as repression depending on personal beliefs to explain PTSD (Beshai, 2004).

Psychiatrists and psychologists may be less interested in philosophy and ontology than they are about curing or caring for the veteran. Research in phenomenology such as that of Straus (1966) and Foucault (1970, 1975) shows that being human is primary, and its fundamental goal is "care," not "power." Care comes closer to the meaning of a personal ontology than power released in every combat.

The medical community cannot create a diagnostic category that distinguishes between normal and abnormal reactions to combat and then stop there, as if all that matters now is how valid and reliable the criteria of PTSD are. With more definitions and more case study, there is bound to be improvement in the accuracy of diagnosis. But the classification of normal and abnormal is a value judgment, and the assumption that there is no such value judgment with regard to PTSD remains fictitious. A medical examiner shirks his ethical responsibility if he stops at that level. It has not yet been demonstrated that those who show constant reexperiencing of the war and who avoid any attempt to deal with it are necessarily patients with PTSD. Nor is it clearly known why some have this disorder and some do not; each answer generates its own set of questions and implications. Personal ethical responsibility cannot be ignored by assuming that the scientific investigation is over. The medical profession and science in general have always had safeguards for such ethical failures, and Pellegrino and Thomasma (1981) make a valuable contribution by drawing attention to the sanctity of life in war and peace.

The existential question facing the young and society is telling the truth about human cost. A society needs to make a moral decision with full disclosure about the social construction of the sanctity of human life. The facts of war are often masked from the young who suffer the most from it. It "is our moral duty toward those we ask to serve on our behalf, and it is our own self-interest as well. Unhealed combat trauma blights not only the life of the veteran but the life of the family and community. . . . It can substantially weaken the society as a whole" (Shay, 1994, p. 195). Post-traumatic stress disorder can cause lifelong disabling psychiatric symptoms and can ruin the ethical and moral fiber of society. "Unhealed combat trauma diminishes democratic participation and can become a threat to democratic political institutions. It originates in violation of trust and destroys the capacity for trust" (Shay, 1994, p. 195).

Providing DSM criteria of PTSD is a first step in a diagnosis and needs to be supplemented with a full and honest disclosure of the human cost of war not only in terms of personal trauma but also in terms of "anomie" for society. This dual disclosure for individual and society provides better coping in the diagnosis and therapy of PTSD than the current focus on sophisticated procedures to do away with the ontological meaning of trauma. This is what may be surmised from Neimeyer and Raskin (2000).

References

American Psychiatric Association. (2000). *Diagnostic and statistical manual of mental disorders* (4th ed., rev.). Washington, DC: Author.

Beshai, J. A. (2004). Toward a phenomenology of trance logic in posttraumatic stress disorder. *Psychological Reports, 94,* 649–654.

Blanchard, E. R., Kolb, L. C., Pallmeyer, T. P., & Gerardi, R. J. (1982). A psychophysiological study of posttraumatic stress disorder in Vietnam veterans. *Psychiatric Quarterly, 54,* 220–229.

DeViva, J. C., & Bloem, W. D. (2003). Symptom exaggeration and compensation seeking among veterans with posttraumatic stress disorder. *Journal of Traumatic Stress, 16,* 503–507.

Foucault, M. (1970). *The order of things: An archaeology of human science.* London: Tavistock.

Foucault, M. (1975). *The birth of the clinic: An archaeology of medical perception.* New York: Random House.

Gray, J. A. (1987). *Fear and stress* (2nd ed.). Cambridge, UK: Cambridge University Press.

McNally, R. J. (2003). Progress and controversy in the study of posttraumatic stress disorder. *Annual Review of Psychology, 54,* 229–252.

Neimeyer, R., & Raskin, J. (2000). *Constructions of disorder: Meaning-making frameworks of psychotherapy.* Washington, DC: American Psychological Association.

Pellegrino, E. D., & Thomasma, D. C. (1981). *A philosophical basis of medical practice.* New York: Oxford University Press.

Shay, J. (1994). *Achilles in Vietnam.* New York: Simon & Schuster.

Spicker, S. (1976). The lived body as catalytic agent. In H. T. Engelhardt Jr. & S. F. Spicker (Eds.), *Evaluation and explanation in the biomedical sciences.* Vol. 1. *Philosophy and medicine* (pp. 181–204). Dordrecht, Holland: Reidel.

Straus, E. W. (1966). *Phenomenological psychology* (E. Eng, Trans.). New York: Basic Books.

Straus, E. W., Natanson, M., & Ey, H. (1969). *Psychiatry and philosophy.* New York: Springer-Verlag.

10

The Experience of Violent Injury for Young African American Men: The Meaning of Being a "Sucker"

John A. Rich and David A. Stone

"If you're living in the inner city, you wouldn't want to be called a sucker cause everybody will take advantage of you. That's why half the people get shot, stabbed these days, trying to defend themselves and not be a sucker."
—shooting victim, age 23

The problem of interpersonal violence continues to grow in the United States. Every day in the United States, on average, sixty-five people die from, and six thousand people are physically injured by, interpersonal violence.[1] Homicide is the leading cause of death for African Americans fifteen to thirty-four years old and the third leading cause of death for all persons fifteen to twenty-four years old. In 1989, the lifetime probability of an African American male being murdered was 1 in 27, while for a white male it was 1 in 205.[2] Homicide rates, however, are only a small part of this tragic picture. According to the National Crime Survey, the ratio of nonfatal violent assaults to homicides exceeds 100:1.[3] Injury due to interpersonal violence disproportionately affects persons of color. Annually in the United States, some 450,000 African Americans and Latinos suffer nonfatal violent injuries.[4] Persons who are violently injured are at high risk of being injured again and of experiencing the comorbidities of substance abuse and unemployment.[5,6] Sims and associates, in a retrospective study of current victims of violence in Detroit in 1989, found that 44 percent of patients suffered a recurrent injury over a five-year period.[5] Over that same period, there was a 20 percent mortality in the retrospective cohort. The prevalence of substance abuse in patients with recurrent violence was 67 percent, as was the rate of unemployment. The authors conclude that violence is a chronic disease with a significant mortality. The study probably underestimates the incidence of violence because it ascertained only episodes that resulted in hospitalization. Goins, Thompson, and Simpkins studied retrospectively and prospectively admissions for abdominal trauma and found recurrence rates to be 48 percent and 47 percent, respectively.[6] Violent injury is, by all accounts, an important, recurrent, and growing problem.

Efforts to detail the incidence and prevalence of violence have been useful, but they do not provide insight into the process of violent injury for victims, including what places individuals at risk of recurrent violent injury. Open-ended interviews and rigorous qualitative analysis are useful in studying processes that may be unfamiliar to researchers because they allow the participants in the study to identify salient issues. These methods allow the generation of hypotheses that are firmly grounded in experiences of the individuals affected. Qualitative methods have been used extensively to study physicians' attitudes about domestic violence,[7] doctor-patient communication,[8] the illness experience for patients with AIDS,[9] and the experience of infant death for families in the inner city.[10]

The purpose of this study is to understand the experience of violent injury from the patient's perspective and to identify important concepts through the analysis of their detailed narratives about the events leading to injury. Here we describe one predominant theme—being a "sucker"— and suggest implications for the prevention of recurrent injury in victims of interpersonal violence.

Methods

Study Site

Boston City Hospital (BCH) is a 350-bed, urban municipal hospital in Boston, Massachusetts. BCH serves patients from the surrounding neighborhoods of Roxbury, Dorchester, and Mattapan, which together comprise 90 percent of the city's minority population. BCH is a regional trauma center, and in 1993 BCH's emergency room and inpatient services treated 298 persons between the ages of 15 and 29 who were victims of interpersonal violence. Of these patients 74 percent were African American and 80 percent were males. BCH treats more than two-thirds of the trauma patients in the city of Boston and therefore is the most appropriate site for a hospital-based exploratory study of violent injury.

Participants

A convenience sample of patients was assembled by sampling patients recruited between August 1992 and August 1994. Inclusion criteria for the study were as follows: African American male between the ages of eighteen and twenty-five; admitted to surgical service with a gunshot or stab wound inflicted by another person; sufficiently medically stable to participate in a sixty-minute interview; and not under police custody. Potential participants satisfying the above criteria were identified in consultation with the head nurse on the surgical ward. Potential participants were approached by one of the authors (J.R.), who explained the purpose of the study and gave them an information sheet about the study. Participants were asked for verbal consent only and informed that the interviews would be taped and transcribed for analysis. The study protocol was approved by the Human Studies Committee at the Trustees of Health and Hospitals for the City of Boston. A total of twenty-seven patients were approached; four refused participation, and five were unable to be scheduled or were discharged before the interview could be conducted. Ten of the participants were interviewed in the hospital, six returned within two months of discharge for the interview, and two were interviewed in their homes within a month of discharge. Each participant received twenty-five dollars.

Data Collection

An open-ended interview guide was developed from the authors' discussions with previous patients and clinical experience. The guide was used to provide structure to the interview and to ensure that the same topics were covered in all interviews, but participants were permitted to elaborate freely on the issues most important to them. Participants were asked to describe the circumstances of their injuries, including the events leading up to the trauma. Probe questions were used to add detail to their narratives. In addition, participants were asked to talk about their plans for avoiding future injury and how they felt the injury would affect future life plans. Demographic information was obtained at the end of the interview. Interviews lasted between forty-five and ninety minutes. One author (J.R.), a physician and health services researcher with training in qualitative methods, conducted thirteen of the interviews; three others were conducted by a trained research assistant and two by a trained mental health worker whose focus is violent injury among children.

Analysis

Interviews were audiotaped and transcribed using standard rules of transcription. All identifiers and names were removed from the final transcripts, and they were reviewed by one of the authors (JR) for accuracy. The transcripts were analyzed using multiple close readings, and recurrent themes were identified. Similar themes noted across interview texts were assembled and analyzed together. The process was facilitated by use of HyperRESEARCH, a software program that organizes textual data.[11] The authors used HyperRESEARCH to identify passages of interview texts and label them as representing specific themes. The program then permitted the authors to examine themes across all of the interviews. Themes were identified by each author independently. The authors then met in a consensus conference, and those themes that were identified by both authors were developed for further analysis. Analysis of interview data commenced after the first interview and was carried out concurrent with subsequent data collection. This approach allowed themes that appeared in early interviews to be explored in greater detail in later ones.

Results

We interviewed eighteen young men who were hospitalized for gunshot wounds or stab wounds on the surgical service at BCH between August 1992 and August 1994. All participants were African American males. Ages ranged from nineteen to twenty-four; educational levels ranged from tenth grade to first year of college. Eleven participants (61 percent) reported that they had been arrested in the past, and four (22 percent) had been incarcerated for more than one month. Two (11 percent) acknowledged carrying a weapon at the time of their injuries; four (22 percent) acknowledged that they had carried weapons in the past but had stopped because of parole. One young man had begun to carry a weapon after his injury. All said they used alcohol, and nine (50 percent) reported regular use of marijuana. None of the participants belonged to any organization such as a church, civic club, or community program.

Being a "Sucker"

Fourteen of the eighteen young men talked about what it means to be a "sucker." The term, which is applied to an individual who fails to fight back or retaliate when he is challenged, disrespected, or hurt, appears to be central to the way many of these young men understand a common type of violent encounter. In what follows, we will examine more closely how "being a sucker" makes sense to these young men and explore the implications of the phenomenon for approaches to violence prevention.

Several participants spontaneously talked about what it means to be a sucker. A twenty-three-year-old man, who was shot in the shoulder by someone who was shooting at an acquaintance, provided this definition:

Table 10.1
Attributes of a "Sucker" versus a "Tough Guy"

"Sucker"	"Tough Guy"
Does nothing, sits there and takes it	Does whatever he has to do
Lets the problem ride	Has to do something
Lets others get the best of him	Stands up for what's right
Disrespected	Gets respect
Unrecognized	Gets a reputation ("rep")
Nobody	Somebody
No dignity	Looked up to

A sucker. A sucker is a person that, if someone does something to them, says something to them, they don't retaliate. You know, they just sit there and take it. Nobody want to be called—if you living in the inner city you wouldn't want to be called a sucker, cause everybody will take advantage of you. That's why half the people get shot, stabbed these days—trying to defend themselves and not be a sucker.

In similar discussions, the young men in the study used a variety of phrases as shown in Table 10.1. The notion of being a sucker is contrasted by the attributes of a "tough guy." The desire to avoid being seen as a sucker is driven by two major concerns. First, if you are a sucker, people will "disrespect you and take advantage of you," and second, you will lose your status in the community and be viewed as a "nobody."

Being Disrespected and Taken Advantage Of
The young men indicated that once you are recognized within your community as one who fails to "stand up for what's yours," others will disrespect you and take what you have. A nineteen-year-old man who described being shot after being caught in the midst of a gun battle explained what being a sucker means for him if he is confronted by someone he doesn't know:

Like if someone walks up on you and starts pushing you, he's pretty much sayin', I don't respect you. Who are you? What are you gonna do? If you ain't doing nothing, he's gonna keep punkin' you, keep callin' you a sucker, showin' you no respect the whole time. . . . I got to get my respect. Cause if I don't go for mine, he's gonna try and take advantage of me and take what I got.

A twenty-five-year-old man who was stabbed by two men trying to rob him also ties being a sucker to the notion of standing up for what he thinks is right and what belongs to him:

A sucker means a person who's not going to stand up for what they feel is right basically. A sucker is a person who will get disrespected. It depends on what the principle is—you know, if you don't stand up for what's yours, you know what I'm saying . . .

A twenty-year-old man shot for an unknown reason by two men who confronted him at his job as a used car salesman gives a similar definition of sucker:

A sucker means that you gonna allow people to walk over you. That's a sucker, a person that lets the same thing happen over and over again and ain't trying to do nothing about standing up for what's yours.

These young men experience their environment as a hostile place and perceive that if they are seen as weak by their peers, they will be targeted for even more victimization. This is evident in the references to being taken advantage of. Closely linked to this fear of victimization is the notion of respect. Respect is clearly something that one must obtain by one's actions, and their comments imply that it is a privilege not routinely afforded young men in the hostile world in which they live. Respect then is earned by projecting an image of toughness. In this way, young men are able to "stand up for what is theirs."

Despite the need to appear tough, the young men also expressed a level of ambivalence about having to respond in this way. They said that they don't want to engage in this type of behavior, but that it is expected and dictated by their peers. A twenty-three-year-old man, deeply involved in a gang, who was shot in retaliation for having shot at another young man, talked about the pressure to act tough: "Cause it's not just me that wants to, but the pressure, peer pressure, you know what I mean? By everybody looking at you, you supposed to be a tough guy." A nineteen-year-old victim expressed his own uncertainty: "If they want to pick up their dukes and beat and scuffle with you, you just go for yours. You just be like, ah damn, you don't want to, but yet, in the back of your mind, you just got to."

The violent response necessary to avoid being a sucker is self-preserving to the extent that it serves notice to others that you do not stand for victimization. The concern of these young men also lies with the surrounding community and peer group. Further, it is in the eyes of one's peers that one becomes known as a sucker. The response is expected by peers, and failure to respond may lead to disapproval from friends. A nineteen-year-old man talked about how his friends respond if he doesn't react: "Well they think you're a punk. They don't be wantin' to hang around with you and shit cause, you see, they know you're not gonna do nothing."

Loss of Status

Young men who react aggressively when confronted not only protect themselves from future injury but also gain some status among their peers, and this in turn bolsters their sense of self-respect. They indicate that status in the community is tied to being able to stand up for oneself. Often one's status in the community is gained by having a reputation for toughness (a "rep"). Having a "rep" bolsters one's own sense of self-respect and self-esteem because it makes you a "somebody." When asked what it means to be a sucker, a twenty-five-year-old stabbing victim summed it up this way: "I feel that a sucker is a person who just don't respect himself basically." An eighteen-year-old talked about the impact of his injury upon his reputation: "I got me a little reputation on the side. I can't have no little stab wound bring me down." The twenty-three-year-old victim of retaliation went further to characterize a sucker as a nobody:

It's like, you get your rep and your dignity around your way man. It's like, it means so much to you. And to be a sucker, to be nobody, understand, to be nobody man—you known what I mean? You might want to be somebody in the community. You might want to be the tough guy. To be a sucker is to be looked down on, you know what I mean? I mean, by everybody looking at you, you supposed to be a tough guy or what we call in the ghetto "a dog." You supposed to be a dog, you know what I mean, a trooper. And you gonna let somebody disrespect you? You a sucker, man, you a nobody. Yesterday you was a dog, today you a sucker. Yesterday you were somebody, today you're a nobody. So nobody wants to be nobody, everybody wants to be somebody. That's why they sell drugs and stuff. They get the gold. They get the car. They somebody. Now they respect you. Everybody looks at you. They get attention. Once you get disrespected, you're nobody now, you're a sucker. Point blank, you know. You're a sucker now and nobody, you know.

The young man quoted here relates community status and self-respect to more than being tough. He also relates selling drugs, owning a car, and wearing gold to being a somebody. He equates external appearances (being tough) or material possessions with his status among his peers and thus his sense of self-respect. The association between status, self-respect, and concrete actions or possessions is important to understand. These young men may have few opportunities to engage in constructive activities to gain a sense of status in their communities, so they use toughness and aggressiveness instead. The implication is that for these young men, finding positive ways to bolster status and self-respect would be productive.

Discussion

Violent behavior among young men often is viewed as senseless and without any underlying cause or logic. Sometimes it is viewed as simply an uncontrolled response to anger, often in the setting of drugs and weapons. The findings in this study indicate that there is an underlying logic to some violence, which stems from the context in which these young men live from day to day and the way in which it shapes their thinking. The problem of recurrent violence among young men of color in the inner city has been particularly difficult to explain. Various demographic factors such as income, age, and ethnicity have been cited as being associated with violent injury, as well as with the likelihood of committing a violent act against someone else.[2] Yet none of these factors provides an explanation for the phenomenon of recurrent violence.

Rosenberg and Mercy reviewed sociological approaches to understanding assaultive violence and identified four major approaches.[12] The *cultural approach* suggests violence is a learned behavior that becomes shared among members of a subgroup or community. Violent norms or behaviors then may be passed from generation to generation. The *structural approach* points to social forces that deprive members of a community from realizing important goals. This deprivation then leads to destructive behaviors in an attempt to deal with lack of opportunity, poverty, discrimination, and so on. The *interactionist approach* suggests violence arises out of a series of responses or "moves" that a person undertakes when his or her safety is threatened. As an offender and victim enter into conflict, the interaction escalates to violent injury. The *economic approach* proposes that the choice to engage in violence is based on rational considerations, particularly whether the benefits of violence outweigh the risks. These various approaches are not viewed as mutually exclusive but represent a range of overlapping possibilities.

The sucker notion is consistent with each of the above frameworks. The sucker notion is a shared understanding among the young men in this study, regardless of whether they themselves have acted on it. In this sense, it is learned by young men through the experiences and stories of their peers. However, it is clear that the sucker notion arises as a result of the perception that the environment in which these young men live is hostile. They feel vulnerable because of structural forces such as crime, lack of opportunity for constructive activity, and the proliferation of firearms. The sucker notion dictates a series of actions and responses when two individuals are in conflict. The interaction is sanctioned and further inflamed by the members of the community who are observing it. These moves may become ingrained responses to conflict. Finally, in a very real sense, these young men are weighing the risks and benefits of violence and deciding that not retaliating has a clear cost: more victimization by those who view you as weak. In this regard, the economic approach may provide some explanation for the sucker phenomenon.

The sucker phenomenon described here offers a different perspective from past research. First, it reflects a belief that the surrounding community or peer group is hostile and ready to take advantage of someone who appears weak. Second, and more important, it reflects a perception that failure to respond violently to a challenge may be more dangerous than striking back. These young men believe that if you appear weak, others will try to victimize you. However, if you show yourself to be strong (by retaliating), then you are perceived as strong and you will be safe.

The notion of sucker is meaningful in contrast to its opposite. If a young man is a "tough guy," peers respect him. If a young man can project an image of strength, he may be able to avoid victimization. The highest value is placed on individuals who defend themselves swiftly, even if by doing so, they place themselves in danger. These men believe that it is better to stand up for yourself and get hurt than not to defend yourself. The impetus for self defense comes largely from the context in which these young men live. Because they feel that being seen as a sucker makes them a target for more extreme victimization (in the form of either physical injury or robbery), they adopt this protective, though violent, posture.

Young men who are hospitalized may feel compelled to prove they are not suckers after they leave the hospital. By so doing, they may arm themselves or expose themselves to dangerous situations, and this may lead to recurrent injury.

Being a sucker is also meaningful with regard to status. Status in the community is tied to one's ability to stand up for oneself in contrast to being a sucker. For these young men, their sense of status is often tied to their ability to "be a man" and defend themselves. Status is also tied to material possessions such as gold and cars. Therefore anyone who threatens to take these material possessions also threatens the young man's sense of self respect. Elijah Anderson, in his studies of young people in inner-city Philadelphia, has noted the tenuous position of self-esteem under these circumstances. He writes:

To run away [from a fight] would likely leave one's self esteem in tatters. Hence people often feel constrained not only to stand up and at least attempt to resist during an assault but also to "pay back"—to seek revenge—after a successful assault on their person. This may include getting a weapon or even getting relatives involved. Their very identity and self respect, their honor is often intricately tied up in the way they perform on the streets during and after such encounters.[13]

Many of these young men recognize the danger in the sucker notion and express ambivalence about it. Still many feel trapped and forced to respond because they feel the benefits of retaliation outweigh those of compromise. Although participants in this case series were from the Boston area, we believe that the phenomenon may be widespread among young men in urban areas, though it may go by a different name.

The results presented here suggest that interpersonal violence is a social phenomenon and not simply the behavior of two individuals. Furthermore, the results suggest that our attempts to stem violence must be broad and must focus not only on the behavior of individuals but also on the perceptions of their peers and realities that prevail within their communities. The young men interviewed for this study live predominantly in impoverished inner-city neighborhoods. Their belief that their neighborhoods are unsafe and replete with weapons is accurate. Their perceptions are the product of the context in which they live. We cannot expect to simply change their perceptions without simultaneously addressing the dangers in their communities.

A previously described young man, injured in retaliation for gang-related violence, said:

It's not gang, it's not drugs or money. Anybody believe that, they getting that from the media thing, you know what I mean, what they show on TV. They pumping everybody up with that. Everybody hears about the shooting, they say drugs and money, drugs and money. I sit back and laugh, cause they get suckered in by that. If they deal with the mentality of the person, that's when they'll be able to deal with the problem. If they can't do that, that's why it continues and gonna be like it is, you know what I mean.

By "mentality" this young man is referring to the meaningful confluence of life circumstances and cultural practices that allows for the possibility of being a sucker in the first place, which then demands retaliation and continues the cycle. As described earlier, this mentality includes the need for material possessions and physical toughness to construct an outward identity and an inward sense of self-esteem. The young man also indicts those of us who too easily accept ("get suckered in by") the popular media explanations of violence that focus on African American males as a homogeneous group involved in crime-related violence. He argues rather for an understanding of the mentality of the person as the only strategy for decreasing violence in the inner city.

As providers we must take up this challenge to "deal with the mentality of the person." We must work to better understand that the life circumstances of our patients who are at risk for violence are meaningful and exist within a culture of practices that permit certain actions (even violent action) to make sense and certain other actions (such as compromise or retreat) not to make sense. Only when we endeavor to understand these practices and the horizons of meaning that they make possible will we begin to propose interventions that will be accepted by young men facing real danger and real choices, and produce positive results. The public health approach must reach beyond the usual confines of hospital clinic and neighborhood health center and collaborate with law enforcement, correctional institutions, educational institutions, economic development and community agencies, and churches to address the conditions that create perceptions of danger.

We would go further to suggest that young African American men who have been injured or involved in violent episodes should be trained and encouraged to serve as agents of change. Young men who understand the pressures of the social phenomenon of violence and who have suffered because of it may be best equipped to recognize the dangers inherent in it. They may also be uniquely qualified to help their peers to develop reasonable and safe responses to confrontation, taking into account the social environment in which they live. Programs that seek to develop young male victims of violence to help to change the community perceptions that lead to violence may be necessary to deal with phenomena such as the sucker notion. In addition, young men who successfully avoid violent encounters while living in the inner city should also be used as resources for developing violence prevention strategies. Furthermore, health care providers must attempt to deal with the larger life issues facing young men who have been injured by referring them to existing supportive programs and agencies for educational and economic development.

The issues identified here are important because they inform the design and potential effectiveness of interventions aimed at decreasing violent injuries. Further research is necessary to refine the sucker notion and incorporate it into survey research and program evaluation. This research will allow the incorporation of the sucker notion into interventions aimed at decreasing interpersonal violence.

Limitations

The results were derived from participants in a single setting: young African American men in Boston who were shot or stabbed and required hospitalization. They were not selected randomly or consecutively. Responses are not necessarily generalizable to other populations in other situations or settings but rather reflect the concerns and beliefs of the young men at this point in their lives. It is possible that the concerns we have uncovered here are widespread among young men in the inner city, and broader studies using surveys and wider sampling techniques would be necessary to confirm this.

References

1. Centers for Disease Control. (1986). *Homicide surveillance: High risk racial and ethnic groups—blacks and Hispanics, 1970–1983*. Bethesda, MD: Centers for Disease Control.

2. National Research Council. (1993). Perspectives on violence. In A. J. Reiss & J. A. Roth (Eds.), *Understanding and Preventing Violence* (pp. 101–181). Washington, DC: National Academy Press.

3. *Criminal Victimization in the United States, 1991*. (1992). Washington, DC: National Center for Health Statistics, National Vital Statistics System, and U.S. Department of Justice.

4. Centers for Disease Control. (1990). Homicide among young black males— United States, 1978–1987. *MMWR, 39*, 869–873.

5. Sims, D. W., Bivins, B. A., Obeid, F. N., Horst, H. M., Sorenson, V. J., & Fath, J. J. (1989). Urban trauma: A chronic recurrent disease. *Trauma, 29*, 940–947.

6. Goins, W. A., Thompson, J., & Simpkins, C. (1992). Recurrent intentional injury. *Journal of the National Medical Association, 84*, 431–435.

7. Sugg, N. K., & Inui, T. (1992). Primary care physicians' response to domestic violence: Opening Pandora's box. *Journal of the American Medical Association, 267*, 3157–3160.

8. Mishler, E. G., Clark, J. A., Ingelfinger, J., & Simon, M. P. (1989). The language of attentive patient care: A comparison of two medical interviews. *Journal of General Internal Medicine, 4*, 325–335.

9. Viney, L. L., & Bousfield, L. (1991). Narrative analysis: A method of psychosocial research for AIDS-affected people. *Social Science and Medicine, 32*, 757–765.

10. McCloskey, L., Power, K., Cruz, A., & Plough, A. (1993). *The social and clinical face of infant mortality: New understandings from qualitative approaches*.

Paper presented at the Third Primary Care Conference of the Agency for Health Care Policy and Research, Atlanta, GA.

11. Hesse-Biber, S., Kinder, T. S., Dupuis, P. R., & Tornabene, E. (1991–1993). HyperRESEARCH. Randolph, MA: Researchware.

12. Rosenberg, M. L., & Mercy, J. A. (1991). Assaultive violence. In M. L. Rosenberg & M. A. Fenley (Eds.), *Violence in America: A Public Health Approach* (pp. 15–50). New York: Oxford University Press.

13. Anderson, E. (1994). The code of the streets. *Atlantic Monthly, 273,* 80–94.

11

The Psychological Impact of Rape Victims' Experiences with the Legal, Medical, and Mental Health Systems

Rebecca Campbell

Sexual violence is a pervasive social problem: National epidemiological data indicate that 17 percent to 25 percent of women are raped in their adult lifetimes (Fisher, Cullen, & Turner, 2000; Koss, Gidycz, & Wisniewski, 1987; Tjaden & Thoennes, 1998). Rape is one of the most severe of all traumas, causing multiple, long-term negative outcomes, such as post-traumatic stress disorder (PTSD), depression, substance abuse, suicidality, repeated sexual victimization, and chronic physical health problems (Kilpatrick & Acierno, 2003; Koss, Bailey, Yuan, Herrera, & Lichter, 2003).[1] Rape victims have extensive postassault needs and may turn to multiple social systems for assistance. Approximately 26 percent to 40 percent of victims report the assault to the police and pursue prosecution through the criminal justice system, 27 percent to 40 percent seek medical care and medical forensic examinations, and 16 percent to 60 percent obtain mental health services (Campbell, Wasco, Ahrens, Sefl, & Barnes, 2001; Ullman, 1996a, 1996b, 2007; Ullman & Filipas, 2001a). When victims reach out for help, they place a great deal of trust in the legal, medical, and mental health systems as they risk disbelief, blame, and refusals of help. How these system interactions unfold can have profound implications for victims' recovery. If victims are able to receive the services they need and are treated in an empathic, supportive manner, then social systems can help facilitate recovery. Conversely, if victims do not receive needed services and are treated insensitively, then system personnel can magnify victims' feelings of powerlessness, shame, and guilt. Postassault help seeking can become a "second rape," a secondary victimization to the initial trauma (Campbell & Raja, 1999; Campbell et al., 2001).

Victims' postassault help-seeking experiences are not uniformly bad or retraumatizing (Campbell et al., 2001; Ullman, 1996a, 1996b; Ullman & Filipas, 2001a). But there is reason—many reasons, actually—to be concerned about what happens to victims when they seek community help. Although some victims have positive experiences, secondary victimization is a widespread problem that happens, in varying degrees, to most survivors who seek postassault care. Who gets services, and how they get them, reflects privilege and discrimination. Ethnic minority and/or low-socioeconomic-status (SES) women, for instance, are more likely to have difficulty obtaining help (Martin, 2005). Furthermore, our social systems do not treat all rapes equally. Persistent, stubborn myths remain about what constitutes "real rape"—stranger assaults committed with a weapon, resulting in visible physical injuries to victims (Estrich, 1987). Social systems respond to these assaults with the highest attention. Yet prevalence studies consistently demonstrate that nonstranger rape is far more typical (approximately 80 percent are committed by someone known to the victim) and that assailants use a variety of tactics—not just weapons—to gain control over their victims (Koss et al., 1987, 2007). Our social systems are least likely to respond to the most common kinds of assaults.

At a time of tremendous vulnerability and need, rape victims turn to their communities for help and risk further hurt. The trauma of rape extends far beyond the actual assault, and intervention strategies must address the difficulties rape survivors encounter when seeking community help. Although prevention efforts to eliminate rape are clearly needed, it is also important to consider how we can prevent further trauma among those already victimized. A growing literature is emerging on postassault help seeking and its impact on victims' mental health outcomes. The purpose of this article is to review the extant research on rape victims' experiences with legal, medical, and mental health systems and how those interactions affect survivors' psychological well-being.[2] The contributions of rape crisis centers, community-based agencies that work as advocate intermediaries between victims and social systems, are examined throughout. In response to growing concerns about the community response to rape, new interventions and programs have emerged that seek to improve services and prevent secondary victimization. These innovative alternatives are also reviewed to explore strategies for creating more consistently positive, postassault help seeking experiences for all rape victims.

The Legal System

Victims' Help-Seeking Experiences

Rape prosecution is a complex, multistage process, and few cases make it all the way through the criminal justice system (Bouffard, 2000). Most victims' first contact will be with a patrol officer, which will be the first of numerous times victims will be asked to describe the assault. Typically a detective is then assigned to investigate and decide whether the case should be referred to the prosecutor. Detectives have considerable discretion in conducting investigations, and what happens during this process can be quite upsetting for victims. Many victims report that law enforcement personnel actively discouraged them from reporting (Campbell, 2005, 2006; Campbell & Raja, 2005; Filipas & Ullman, 2001; Ullman, 1996b). Police may graphically portray the personal costs involved for victims should they pursue prosecution, such as repeated trips to court or humiliating cross-examination (Kerstetter & Van Winkle, 1990; Madigan & Gamble, 1991). Detectives issue warnings of impending prosecution not to assailants, but to victims, threatening them that they will be charged if at some point in the investigation doubt emerges about the accuracy of their claims (Logan, Evans, Stevenson, & Jordan, 2005). Victims are questioned about elements of the crime (e.g., penetrations, use of force, or other control tactics) over and over again to check for consistency in their accounts, which can be emotionally unsettling and, given that trauma can impede concentration and memory (Halligan, Michael, Clark, & Ehlers, 2003), cognitively challenging as well. Many victims report that this questioning strays into issues such as what they were wearing, their prior sexual history, and whether they responded sexually to the assault (Campbell, 2005, 2006; Campbell & Raja, 2005; Campbell et al., 2001). Victims rate these questions as particularly traumatic (Campbell & Raja, 2005), and their legal relevance is minimal at best because all states have rape shield laws that limit information about the victims from being discussed in court, should the case reach that far (Flowe, Ebbesen, & Putcha-Bhagavatula, 2007). In spite of rape shield laws, law enforcement personnel confirm that these are typical investigational practices (Campbell, 2005). The police investigation is designed to weed out cases, and to that end, it is very effective: Most reported rapes never progress past this stage. Approximately 56 percent to 82 percent of all reported rape cases are dropped (i.e., not referred to prosecutors) by law enforcement (67 percent on average; Bouffard, 2000; Crandall & Helitzer, 2003; Frazier & Haney, 1996).

If a case progresses past the investigation stage, prosecutors often conduct their own interviews with the victims prior to deciding whether to file criminal charges (Martin & Powell, 1994). Again, what happens in this process is largely unknown, but Frohmann's (1997a, 1997b) ethnographic research revealed that prosecutors require victims to go through the details of the rape again multiple times. If prosecutors are disinclined to charge the case, then they engage in a lengthy exploration of any discrepancies in victims' accounts and press victims for explanations and proof. If prosecutors are inclined to press charges, they cover much of this same ground but try to coach victims, grooming them for how to respond to and withstand such questioning. Either way, victims go through a punishing process of reliving the assaults and defending their characters (Koss & Achilles, 2008). More cases drop out of the legal system at this stage: on average, approximately 44 percent of the cases referred by law enforcement to prosecutors for further consideration are dismissed by the prosecutors, and about half on average (56 percent) move forward (Frazier & Haney, 1996; Spohn, Beichner, & Davis-Frenzel, 2001).

For the cases that are accepted for prosecution, victims must prepare for a series of court hearings (e.g., preliminary hearings, trials, plea hearings, sentencing). Research is limited on these end-stage processes, perhaps because they are relatively rare occurrences. Through extensive recruitment efforts, Konradi (2007) interviewed forty-seven victims whose cases made it to trial or plea bargaining. Approximately one-third of these women felt inadequately prepared by the prosecutors: Although they had been questioned repeatedly, they were given very little information about the procedural process and felt thrown into the hearings with little understanding of what to expect. Most victims did receive extensive preparation, but it was grueling: reading and rereading police reports, practicing how to tell what happened in the rape, simulating cross-examination, and figuring out how to dress, speak, show emotion, or not show emotion in court. If a case makes it this far, more often than not, it results in a guilty verdict or a guilty plea bargain. Of prosecuted cases, 76 percent to 97 percent end with guilty verdicts or pleas (88 percent on average; Frazier & Haney, 1996; Spohn et al., 2001). These cases were carefully selected, and these victims were tested and then groomed, so that what went forward through the system had good odds for conviction.

But overall, case attrition is staggering: for every one hundred rape cases reported to law enforcement, on average thirty-three would be referred to prosecutors, sixteen would be charged and moved into the court system, twelve would end in a successful conviction, and seven would end in a prison sentence (Bouffard, 2000; Crandall & Helitzer, 2003; Frazier & Haney, 1996; Spohn et al., 2001). Successful prosecution is not random: it is more likely for those from privileged backgrounds and those who experienced assaults that fit stereotypic notions of what constitutes rape. Younger women, ethnic minority women, and women of lower SES are more likely to have their cases rejected by the criminal justice system (Campbell et al., 2001; Frohmann, 1997a, 1997b; Spears & Spohn, 1997; Spohn et al., 2001; cf. Frazier & Haney, 1996). Cases of stranger rape (where the suspect was eventually identified) and those that occurred with the use of a weapon and/or resulted in physical injuries to victims are more likely to be prosecuted (Campbell et al., 2001; Frazier & Haney, 1996; Kerstetter, 1990; Martin & Powell, 1994; Spears & Spohn, 1997; Spohn et al., 2001). Alcohol and drug use by the victim significantly increases the likelihood that a case will be dropped (Campbell et al., 2001; Frohmann, 1997a, 1997b; Spears & Spohn, 1997; cf. Frazier & Haney, 1996).

These data suggest that the odds of a case being prosecuted are not good, and the treatment victims receive from legal system personnel along the way is not much better. Across multiple samples, 43 percent to 52 percent of victims who had contact with the legal system rated their experience as unhelpful and/or hurtful (Campbell et al., 2001; Golding, Siegel, Sorenson, Burnam, & Stein, 1989; Filipas & Ullman, 2001; Monroe et al., 2005; Ullman, 1996b). In qualitative focus group research, survivors described their contact with the legal system as a dehumanizing experience of being interrogated, intimidated, and blamed. Several women mentioned that they would not have reported if they had known what the experience would be like (Logan et al., 2005). Even victims who had the opportunity to go to trial described the experience as frustrating, embarrassing, and distressing, but they also took tremendous pride in their ability to exert some control in the process and to tell what happened to them (Konradi, 2007).

These experiences of secondary victimization take a toll on victims' mental health. In self-report characterizations of their psychological health, rape survivors indicated that as a result of their contact with legal system personnel, they felt bad about themselves (87 percent), depressed (71 percent), violated (89 percent), distrustful of others (53 percent), and reluctant to seek further help (80 percent) (Campbell, 2005; Campbell & Raja, 2005). The harm of secondary victimization is also evident on objective measures of PTSD symptomatology. Ullman and colleagues found that contact with formal help systems, including the police, was more likely to result in negative social reactions, which were associated with increased PTSD symptomatology (Filipas & Ullman, 2001; Starzynski, Ullman, Filipas, & Townsend, 2005; Ullman & Filipas, 2001a, 2001b).

In a series of studies dealing directly with victim/police contact, Campbell and colleagues found that low legal action (i.e., the case did not progress or was dropped) was associated with increased PTSD symptomatology, and high secondary victimization was also associated with increased PTSD (Campbell et al., 2001; Campbell & Raja, 2005). In tests of complex interactions, Campbell, Barnes, et al. (1999) identified that it was the victims of nonstranger rape whose cases were not prosecuted and who were subjected to high levels of secondary victimization who had the highest PTSD of all—worse than those who chose not to report to the legal system at all. It is interesting that when victims who did *not* report to the police were asked why they did not pursue prosecution, they specifically stated that they were worried about the risk of further harm and distress; their decision was a self-protective choice to guard their fragile emotional health (Patterson, Greeson, & Campbell, 2008).

Alternatives and Innovations: Restoring Survivors

Rape is a felony crime, and the take-home message should not be that prosecution is a futile, psychologically damaging endeavor. What can be done to change the legal system's response to rape victims? Since the beginning of the antirape movement in the 1970s, rape crisis centers have led multiple successful efforts for legal reform (e.g., repealing marital exemption laws, enacting rape shield laws; see Matthews, 1994). But there is the law as written and the law in practice—and changing the latter has required the daily dedication of rape victim advocates. Most rape crisis centers have legal advocacy programs whereby trained paraprofessional advocates help victims navigate their contacts with the criminal justice system (see Campbell & Martin, 2001, for a review). Advocates explain the legal process to victims and inform them of their rights, and in many communities, advocates can be present for the police and prosecution interviews as well as accompany victims to court. The advocates' job is to watch, witness, and advocate on behalf of victims to improve case processing and prevent secondary victimization.

Few studies have examined the effectiveness of rape victim advocates, but the limited studies on this topic are promising. Survivors consistently rate advocates as supportive and informative (Campbell et al., 2001; Golding et al., 1989; Wasco et al., 2004). Wasco, Campbell, Barnes, and Ahrens (1999) found that survivors who worked with advocates had significantly lower PTSD scores than those who had legal system involvement without the help of advocates. Pursuing this issue further, I (Campbell, 2006) used a naturalistic quasi-experimental design to compare the experiences with police of victims who had a rape crisis center victim advocate available to them and those who did not. Rape survivors who had the assistance of an advocate were significantly more likely to have police actually take a report and were less likely to be treated negatively by law enforcement (e.g., less likely to be discouraged from reporting, less likely to be questioned about their sexual histories). These victims also had significantly less emotional distress after their contact with the legal system. Rape victim advocates continue to provide support and advocacy through the later stages of trials or plea bargains (Martin, 2005), and the victims in Konradi's (2007) qualitative study noted that advocates provided useful information about their rights, helped them prepare for making their victim impact statements at the offenders' sentencing hearings, and supported them by attending the hearings. However, not all communities have rape crisis centers, so many victims do not have the option of working with an advocate (Campbell & Martin, 2001).

Although rape crisis centers have been instrumental in changing the legal culture of rape prosecution, many victims have little faith that justice is possible (Logan et al., 2005; Patterson et al., 2008). Sarason's (1972) theory of alternative settings suggests that interventions that step outside existing systems may be more effective: creating something altogether different is often more successful than tinkering with existing settings. In that vein, restorative justice programs for sexual assault victims have emerged as a promising alternative to traditional justice systems (Koss, 2006).[3] Restorative justice programs operate outside the criminal justice system but are often developed by community-wide teams that include victims/survivors, rape crisis center advocates, and representatives from the legal, medical, and mental health systems. These programs work from the fundamental position that the needs of the victims, as well as their significant others, friends, family, and all others who were hurt by the rape, are paramount and that offenders need to accept responsibility for that harm and make amends (Koss, 2006; Koss & Achilles, 2008). The philosophy and operation of restorative justice programs are multidisciplinary in nature (see Koss, 2006, for a review), but psychology and allied professions have been clearly influential, as these interventions strive to create an empowering experience for survivors, prevent psychological distress, and promote social support from the survivors' families and communities (Koss, Bachar, Hopkins, & Carlson, 2004).

In the context of sexual assault, restorative justice programs often use conferencing methods, whereby the victim, the offender, and their families agree to prepare for a meeting, at which time the offender will publicly take responsibility for the assault. Detailed procedures are developed to prevent secondary victimization in the conference and to provide a respectful environment (see RESTORE, 2006). At the conferences, specially trained facilitators cue offenders to make a statement accepting responsibility for their actions, and then the victims (and others) have the opportunity to describe how they have been affected by the assault. The offenders then have to verbally acknowledge that they have heard what has been said about the harm caused by their actions. A redress plan is then developed that outlines how the offenders will repair the harm and make amends. In the United States, only one operational restorative justice program for sexual assault exists, codeveloped by Koss and multiple stakeholders in Pima County, Arizona (see Koss et al., 2004). Victims who initially report to the criminal justice system are offered the opportunity to participate in the RESTORE program if their cases meet eligibility criteria (the offender is eighteen years old or older, is a first-time offender, is accused of raping someone known to him, or is charged with a misdemeanor sex offense; RESTORE, 2006). Evaluation of RESTORE is in progress, but preliminary findings suggest that offenders who successfully completed the program exhibited positive changes in their understanding of the harm they had caused to the victim and others (Koss & Achilles, 2008).

The Medical System

Victims' Help-Seeking Experiences

Rape victims have extensive postassault medical needs, including injury detection and care, medical forensic examination, screening and treatment for sexually transmitted infections (STIs), and pregnancy testing and emergency contraception. Although most victims are not physically injured to the point of needing emergency care (Ledray, 1996), traditionally, police, rape crisis centers, and social service agencies have advised victims to seek treatment in hospital emergency departments for a medical forensic exam (Martin, 2005). The survivor's body is a crime scene, and due to the invasive nature of rape, a medical professional, rather than a crime scene technician, is needed to collect the evidence. The "rape exam" or "rape kit" usually involves plucking head and pubic hairs; collecting loose hairs by combing the head and pubis; swabbing the vagina, rectum, and/or mouth to collect semen, blood, or saliva; and obtaining fingernail scrapings in the event the victim scratched the assailant. Blood samples may also be collected for DNA, toxicology, and ethanol testing (Martin, 2005).

Victims often experience long waits in hospital emergency departments because rape is rarely an emergent health threat, and during this wait, victims are not allowed to eat, drink, or urinate so as not to destroy physical evidence of the assault (Littel, 2001; Taylor, 2002). When victims are finally seen, they get a cursory explanation of what will occur, and it often comes as a shock that they have to have a pelvic exam immediately after such an egregious, invasive violation of their bodies (Martin, 2005; Parrot, 1991). Many victims describe the medical care they receive as cold, impersonal, and detached (Campbell, 2005, 2006; Campbell & Raja, 2005). Furthermore, the exams and evidence collection procedures are often performed incorrectly (Martin, 2005; Sievers, Murphy, & Miller, 2003). Most hospital emergency department personnel lack training in rape forensic exams, and those with training usually do not perform exams frequently enough to maintain proficiency (Littel, 2001; Plichta, Vandecar-Burdin, Odor, Reams, & Zhang, 2006).

Forensic evidence collection is often the focus of hospital emergency department care, but rape survivors have other medical needs, such as information on the risk of STIs/HIV and prophylaxis (preventive medications to treat any STIs that may have been contracted through the assault). The Centers for Disease Control and Prevention (2002) and the American Medical Association (1995) recommend that all sexual assault victims receive STI prophylaxis and HIV prophylaxis on a case-by-case basis after risk assessment. Yet analyses of hospital records have shown that only 34 percent of sexual assault patients are treated for STIs (Amey & Bishai, 2002). However, data from victims suggest much higher rates of STI prophylaxis: 57 percent to 69 percent of sexual assault patients reported that they received antibiotics during their hospital emergency department care (Campbell, 2005, 2006; Campbell et al., 2001; National Center for Victims of Crime & National Crime Victims Research and Treatment Center, 1992). But not all victims are equally likely to receive STI-related medical services. Victims of nonstranger rape are significantly less likely to receive information on STIs/HIV or STI prophylaxis (Campbell & Bybee, 1997; Campbell et al., 2001), even though knowing one's assailant does not mitigate one's risk. In addition, one study found that Caucasian women were significantly more likely to get information on HIV than were ethnic minority women (Campbell et al., 2001).

Postassault pregnancy services are also inconsistently provided to rape victims. Only 40 percent to 49 percent of victims receive information about the risk of pregnancy (Campbell et al., 2001; National Center for Victims of Crime & National Crime Victims Research Center, 1992). The American Medical Association (1995) and the American College of Obstetricians and Gynecologists (1998) recommend emergency contraception for victims at risk for pregnancy, but only 21 percent to 43 percent of sexual assault victims who need emergency contraception actually receive it (Amey & Bishai, 2002; Campbell, 2005, 2006; Campbell & Bybee, 1997; Campbell et al., 2001). To date, no studies have found systematic differences in the provision of emergency contraception as a function of victim or assault characteristics, but hospitals affiliated with the Catholic church are significantly less likely to provide emergency contraception (Campbell & Bybee, 1997; Smugar, Spina, & Merz, 2000).

In the process of administering the forensic exam, STI services, and pregnancy-related care, doctors and nurses ask victims many of the same kinds of questions as do legal personnel regarding their prior sexual histories, sexual responses during the assault, what they were wearing, and what they did to "cause" the assault. Medical professionals may view these questions as necessary and appropriate, but rape survivors find them upsetting (Campbell & Raja, 2005). Comparative studies suggest that victims encounter significantly fewer victim-blaming questions and statements from medical system personnel than from legal personnel (Campbell, 2005, 2006; Campbell & Raja, 2005; Campbell, Barnes, et al., 1999), but this questioning still has a demonstrable negative impact on victims' mental health. Campbell (2005) found that as a result of their contact with emergency department doctors and nurses, most rape survivors stated that they felt bad about themselves (81 percent), depressed (88 percent), violated (94 percent), distrustful of others (74 percent), and reluctant to seek further help (80 percent; see also Campbell & Raja, 2005). Only 5 percent of victims in Ullman's (1996b) study rated physicians as a helpful source of support, and negative responses from formal systems, including the medical system, significantly exacerbated victims' PTSD symptomatology (Filipas & Ullman, 2001; Starzynski et al., 2005; Ullman & Filipas, 2001a, 2001b). Victims who did not receive basic medical services rated their experiences with the medical system as more hurtful, which has been associated with higher PTSD levels (Campbell & Raja, 2005; Campbell et al., 2001). Specifically, nonstranger rape victims who received minimal medical services but encountered high secondary victimization appeared to be the most at risk: These women had significantly higher levels of PTSD symptoms than victims who did not seek medical services at all (Campbell, Barnes, et al., 1999).

Alternatives and Innovations: A SANE Approach

The conclusion cannot be that victims should not seek postassault medical care. Forensic evidence may be crucial for a successful legal case (Frazier & Haney, 1996; Spohn et al., 2001), but even more important is the fact that there are significant long-term health consequences for untreated injuries and STIs/HIV (Aral, 2001). Rape crisis centers have been instrumental in improving postassault medical care, including leading efforts to create standardized rape kits and providing medical advocates on a 24/7 basis to help victims in hospital emergency departments (Martin, 2005). Unfortunately, not all hospitals work with rape crisis centers, which may compromise victim care. In a quasi-experimental study, I (Campbell, 2006) compared victims' medical forensic exam experiences in two urban hospitals that were highly similar (e.g., number of victims served per year, patient sociodemographic characteristics) except that one had a policy of paging rape crisis center advocates to assist victims, and the other did not work with advocates. Victims who had the assistance of an advocate were significantly more likely to receive comprehensive medical care and were less likely to experience secondary victimization. Although these differences cannot be solely attributed to the efforts of the rape crisis center advocates, this study suggests that victims may benefit from some assistance in navigating the chaos of hospital emergency departments.

Alternatively, it may be more effective to change the postassault medical care delivery system entirely, which was the founding premise of Sexual Assault Nurse Examiner (SANE) programs. SANE programs were created by the nursing profession in the 1970s and rapidly grew in numbers during the 1990s (Ledray, 1999; Littel, 2001; U.S. Department of Justice, 2004). These programs were designed to circumvent many of the problems of traditional hospital emergency department care by having specially trained nurses, rather than doctors, provide 24/7 crisis intervention and medical care to sexual assault victims in either hospital emergency department or community clinic settings (Campbell, Patterson, & Lichty, 2005). Influenced by psychiatric and community mental health nursing, as well as clinical psychology, SANE programs place strong emphasis on treating victims with dignity and respect in order to decrease postassault psychological distress (Ledray, 1992, 1999; Taylor, 2002). Many SANE programs work with their local rape crisis centers so that victim advocates can be present for the exam to provide emotional support, which combines the potential benefits of both service programs (Littel, 2001; Taylor, 2002).

The medical forensic exams and the evidence collection kits provided by SANE programs are more thorough than those victims receive in traditional emergency department care. Most SANE programs utilize specialized forensic equipment (e.g., a colposcope), which allows for the detection of microlacerations, bruises, and other injuries (Ledray, 1999). Even though the exam is more lengthy, *how* it is performed is qualitatively different. SANE programs provide a full explanation of the process *before* the exam begins and then continue to describe what they find throughout the exam, giving patients the opportunity to reinstate some control over their bodies by participating when appropriate (e.g., combing their own hair). In an evaluation of a midwestern SANE program, victims gave strong positive feedback about their exam experiences: all patients indicated that they were fully informed about the process and that the nurses took their needs and concerns seriously and allowed them to stop or pause the exam if needed (Campbell, Patterson, Adams, Diegel, & Coats, 2008). This patient-centered care also seems to help victims' psychological well-being, as survivors reported feeling supported, safe, respected, believed, and well-cared for by their SANE nurses (see also Ericksen et al., 2002).

With respect to STI/HIV and emergency contraception care, national surveys of SANE programs find service provision rates of 90 percent or higher (Campbell et al., 2006; Ciancone, Wilson, Collette, & Gerson, 2000). As with traditional emergency department medical care, SANE programs affiliated with Catholic hospitals are significantly less likely to conduct pregnancy testing or offer emergency contraception (but they do so at higher rates than non-SANE, Catholic-affiliated emergency departments; Campbell et al., 2006). In a quasi-experimental longitudinal study, Crandall and Helitzer (2003) compared medical service provision rates two years before to four years after the implementation of a hospital-based SANE program and found significant increases in STI prophylaxis care (from 89 percent to 97 percent) and emergency contraception (from 66 percent to 87 percent).

In addition to beneficial effects on victims' health, SANE programs may be instrumental in increasing legal prosecution of reported cases. Multiple case studies suggest that SANE programs increase prosecution, particularly plea bargains, because when confronted with the forensic evidence collected by the SANE programs, assailants will plead guilty (often to a lesser charge) rather than face trial (see Littel, 2001). When cases do go to trial, the SANE programs' expert witness testimony can help obtain convictions (see Ledray, 1999). Quasi-experimental pre-post designs have found that police referral and prosecution rates have increased significantly after the implementation of SANE programs (Campbell, Patterson, & Bybee, 2007; Crandall & Helitzer, 2003). Key informant interviews suggest this happens because SANE programs help centralize what is often disjointed, fragmented care for victims, which improves working relationships between the legal and medical systems. The development and launch of SANE programs are often accompanied by formal and informal cross-agency trainings to improve communication, collaboration, and coordination. These trainings typically emphasize strategies for establishing rapport with victims, which may prevent secondary victimization and increase victims' engagement in the prosecution process (Campbell et al., 2007; Crandall & Helitzer, 2003). Although more research on SANE programs is clearly needed, it appears that changing postassault victim care practices in one social system can have positive ripple effects in other systems as well.

The Mental Health System

Victims' Help-Seeking Experiences
The mental health effects of rape have been extensively studied, yet it is still difficult to convey just how devastating rape is to victims' emotional well-being (Campbell, 2002). Many women experience this trauma as a fundamental betrayal of their sense of self, identity, judgment, and safety (Janoff-Bulman, 1992; Koss et al., 1994; Moor, 2007). Between 31 percent and 65 percent of rape survivors develop PTSD, and 38 percent to 43 percent meet diagnostic criteria for major depression (for reviews, see Kilpatrick & Acierno, 2003; Kilpatrick, Amstadter, Resnick, & Ruggiero, 2007; Koss et al., 2003). These sequelae are largely due to the trauma of the rape itself, but as noted previously, negative responses from the legal and medical systems exacerbate victims' distress. Clearly, victims may *need* mental health services, but there has been comparatively less research on what services they actually receive and whether that care improved their psychological health. Victims may obtain mental health services in myriad ways (e.g., treatment outcome research, community clinics/private practice, specialty agencies such as rape crisis centers), and their experiences vary considerably as a function of treatment setting.

First, some victims receive mental health services by participating as research subjects in randomized control trial (RCT) treatment outcome studies (e.g., Foa, Rothbaum, Riggs, & Murdock, 1991; Krakow et al.,

2001; Resick et al., 2008; Resick, Nishith, Weaver, Astin, & Feuer, 2002). This option is available only to rape survivors who live in communities where such research is being conducted and who fit eligibility criteria. However, this kind of research is not intended to provide large-scale services; the goal is to establish empirically supported treatments (ESTs) that can then be disseminated for wider-scale benefit (American Psychological Association, 1995; American Psychological Association Presidential Task Force on Evidence-Based Practice, 2006). Indeed, the results of these trials suggest that cognitive-behavioral therapies, such as cognitive processing therapy and prolonged exposure, are effective in alleviating PTSD symptoms (Foa, Keane, & Friedman, 2000; Russell & Davis, 2007). The victims who participate in these trials receive high-quality treatment and benefit tremendously, but this is not the experience of the typical rape victim seeking postassault mental health services (Koss et al., 2003).

A second, and more typical, way victims receive postassault mental health services is through community-based care provided by psychologists, psychiatrists, or social workers in private or public clinic settings. More victims receive mental health services in these settings than in treatment outcome studies, but these settings are still highly underutilized and have serious accessibility limitations. Most victims who seek traditional mental health services, for example, are Caucasian (Campbell et al., 2001; Golding et al., 1989; Starzynski, Ullman, Townsend, Long, & Long, 2007; Ullman & Brecklin, 2002). Ethnic minority women are more likely to turn to informal sources of support (e.g., friends and family; Wyatt, 1992) and may not necessarily place the same value on formal psychotherapy (Bletzer & Koss, 2006). Victims without health insurance are also significantly less likely to obtain mental health services (Koss et al., 2003; Starzynski et al., 2007).

When victims do receive community-based mental health services, it is unclear whether practitioners are consistently using empirically supported treatments. Two statewide random sample studies of practitioners suggest it is unlikely. Campbell, Raja, and Grining's (1999) survey of licensed mental health professionals in a midwestern state found that most (52 percent) reported using cognitive-behavioral methods with victims of violence (including, but not limited to sexual assault victims), but almost all practitioners stated that they rarely use a single approach and intentionally combine multiple therapeutic orientations and treatments. Sprang, Craig, and Clark's (2008) study of mental health practitioners in a southern state also found high use of cognitive-behavioral interventions with trauma victims (including but not limited to sexual assault survivors), but again, these were not in exclusive use. Exposure therapy, a cognitive-behavioral therapy approach with strong empirical support (Foa et al., 2000), was rarely cited as a preferred treatment (see Ruscio & Holohan, 2006). These studies suggest that cognitive-behavioral therapy approaches are often used by community practitioners, but without in-depth data on how the services were implemented, it would be a stretch to conclude that most victims receive empirically supported care in traditional, community-based mental health services. As is often the case in the efficacy-effectiveness-dissemination research cycle, it can take quite a while for evidence-based practice to become standard care (Huppert, Fabbro, & Barlow, 2006; Kazdin, 2008; Ruscio & Holohan, 2006; Sprang et al., 2008; Westen, Novotny, & Thompson-Brenner, 2004).

Few studies have examined if and how victims benefit from community-based mental health services. In general, victims tend to rate their experiences with mental health professionals positively and to characterize their help as useful and supportive (Campbell et al., 2001; Ullman, 1996a, 1996b). Whether positive satisfaction results in demonstrable mental health benefit is largely unknown, although Campbell, Barnes, et al. (1999) found that community-based mental health services were particularly helpful for victims who had had negative experiences with the legal and/or medical systems. Victims who encountered substantial difficulty obtaining needed services and experienced high secondary victimization from the legal and medical systems had high PTSD symptomatology, but among this high-risk group of survivors, those who had been able to obtain mental health services had significantly lower PTSD, which suggests that there may have been some benefit from receiving such services. In this same sample, however, 25 percent of women who received postassault mental health services rated this contact as hurtful (with 19 percent characterizing it as severely hurtful; Campbell et al., 2001). Indeed, some mental health practitioners have expressed concern about whether their own profession works effectively with sexual assault victims: 58 percent of practitioners in a statewide study felt that mental health providers engage in practices that would be harmful to victims and questioned the degree to which victims benefit from services (Campbell & Raja, 1999).

A third setting in which victims may obtain mental health services is specialized violence-against-women agencies, such as rape crisis centers and domestic violence shelter programs. Rape crisis centers help victims negotiate their contact with the legal and medical systems, and they also provide individual and group counseling (Campbell & Martin, 2001). These agencies are perhaps the most visible and accessible source for mental health services for rape victims (Koss et al., 2003), as they provide counseling free of charge and do not require health insurance. As with traditional mental health services, there is still evidence of racial differences in service utilization, as Caucasian women are significantly more likely to utilize rape crisis center services than are ethnic minority women (Campbell et al., 2001; Martin, 2005; Wgliski & Barthel, 2004).

Little is known about the therapeutic orientations and treatment approaches used in rape crisis centers, but current data indicate a strong feminist and/or empowerment theoretical orientation (e.g., shared goal setting, focus on gender inequalities, identification of rape as not only a personal problem but a social problem too; Edmond, 2006; Goodman & Epstein, 2008; Howard, Riger, Campbell, & Wasco, 2003; Ullman & Townsend, 2008; Wasco et al., 2004). In a national survey of rape crisis centers and domestic violence shelters,[4] approximately 70 percent of the agencies reported using cognitive-behavioral methods—in combination with other methods (e.g., client centered and feminist; Edmond, 2006). With respect to counseling outcomes, Wasco et al. (2004) and Howard et al. (2003) compared self-reported PTSD symptoms pre- and postcounseling among victims receiving rape crisis center counseling services and found significant reductions in distress levels and self-blame over time and increases in social support, self efficacy, and sense of control. Because these studies did not examine the content of services or include comparison groups, it is unclear whether these observed improvements are attributable to the services provided.

Alternatives and Innovations: Mental Health Services Sooner and Better

Victims have extensive postassault mental health needs, and several researcher-practitioners have called for increased use of empirically supported treatments in rape crisis centers and other community-based mental health services settings (Edmond, 2006; Russell & Davis, 2007; Sprang et al., 2008). Future work in this arena can benefit from the large, multidisciplinary literature on the adoption of evidence-based practice in community settings. Miller and Shinn's (2005) extensive review of the science-practice gap across multiple social issues highlights several challenges that may be particularly relevant for improving mental health services for rape victims (see also Kazdin, 2008). Making providers aware of evidence-based practice and/or empirically supported treatments is a necessary first step (Sprang et al., 2008), but knowledge is rarely sufficient for innovation adoption (Miller & Shinn, 2005). Changing existing practice requires that individuals and organizations have the training, expertise, and funding to adopt the innovation. Training may be a particularly salient resource because most mental health professionals do not receive adequate instruction on working with victims (Goodman & Epstein, 2008; Campbell, Raja, & Grining, 1999; Ullman, 2007). In response to this situation, several national/federal research agendas on interpersonal violence have called for more training of mental health workers (Koss, 2008). Ullman (2007) argued that such training must focus on teaching professionals how to inquire in a sensitive manner about women's histories of victimization; survivors may be reluctant, and understandably so, to disclose abuse, and yet the underlying reason for their distress may be a history of victimization. As Resick (2004) aptly noted, "Treatment needs to focus on processing the core traumas, not just on symptoms" (p. 1292). Training is an important first step in ensuring that mental health professionals are responding appropriately to the needs of victimized women.

But Miller and Shinn (2005) found that even with adequate training and resources, practitioners can be resistant to evidence-based practice if they perceive that the innovation is incongruent with their values. In the context of mental health services for rape victims, this seems quite possible given that rape crisis centers' roots stem from the antirape social movement, which is a markedly different historical context from that of the mental health profession. The limited empirical data on rape crisis centers' mental health services suggest a strong valuing of feminist, empowerment-focused approaches (Edmond, 2006; Wasco et al., 2004), which could be perceived as incongruent with therapeutic approaches that do not emphasize the broader social context of rape (Goodman & Epstein, 2008). Similarly, non–rape-crisis-center-affiliated mental health practitioners specifically favor integrating multiple therapeutic orientations and approaches (Campbell, Raja, et al., 1999; Sprang et al., 2008), which could be viewed as antithetical to the adoption of manualized interventions. Kazdin (2008) noted that mental health practitioners' skepticism of evidence-based practice may run even deeper. Participant samples and treatment success are often narrowly defined in efficacy research, leaving clinicians to question whether such treatments can create meaningful improvement in clients' everyday life functioning. Research on clinical decision making is clearly warranted to understand how rape crisis center counselors' and other community-based mental health providers' beliefs and values shape their choice and implementation of treatment approaches.

Miller and Shinn's (2005) analysis also invites critical examination of the presumptive advantage of empirically supported treatments. There is a well-documented "pro-innovation bias" in the social sciences: the notion that evidence-based practice and/or empirically supported treatments are widely considered to have benefits over indigenous practices that have not been studied and indeed may prove effective if studied (Mayer & Davidson, 2000; Rogers, 1995). Miller and Shinn (2005) advocated for more research that seeks to understand what is being offered in community settings, to identify indigenous strategies that are effective, and to capture local knowledge and expertise, because closing the research-practice gap requires partnerships with the "agencies, organizations, and associations that are the lifeblood of the community" (p. 179). In that vein, translational research projects with rape crisis centers and other community-based mental health services are needed to evaluate current services, assess the need for adoption of empirically supported treatments, and disseminate effective clinical practice (see National Institute of Mental Health, 2004, 2006).

A more fundamental innovation for improving mental health services for rape victims is reconceptualizing the role of mental health professionals in postassault care. When victims obtain mental health services, it is usually after the fact. Psychologists and allied professionals are largely absent in the immediate, postassault community response to rape, which is unfortunate because during this vulnerable time, victims encounter substantial secondary victimization from the legal and medical systems. Bringing trained mental health professionals in earlier could make a significant difference in victims' well-being, and a promising, empirically informed model of early intervention is psychological first aid. Based on years of research on crisis intervention techniques, psychological first aid was developed for working with victims of disasters, violence, and other traumas in their immediate aftermath (Everly & Flynn, 2005; Parker, Everly, Barnett, & Links, 2006; Ruzek et al., 2007). The goal of psychological first aid is to accelerate recovery and promote mental health through eight core goals and actions: (1) initiate contact in a nonintrusive, compassionate, helpful manner; (2) enhance safety and provide physical and emotional comfort; (3) calm and orient emotionally distraught survivors; (4) identify immediate needs and concerns and gather information; (5) offer practical help to address immediate needs and concerns; (6) reduce distress by connecting to primary support persons; (7) provide individuals with information about stress reactions and coping; and (8) link individuals to services and inform them about services they may need in the future (Ruzek et al., 2007).

Ruzek and colleagues (2007) examined how and why these eight principles of psychological first aid can curb posttrauma distress. Focusing on psychological and physical safety can interrupt the biological mechanisms of posttrauma stress reactions (see Bryant, 2006) and can challenge cognitive beliefs about perceived dangerousness (see Foa & Rothbaum, 1998). Grounding techniques that focus individuals on the relative safety of the present time can also be effective in interrupting processes that begin to link nonthreatening persons, places, and things to the original trauma event (see Resick & Schnicke, 1992). Trying to calm victims can significantly decrease the likelihood that their immediate anxiety will generalize to other situations (see Bryant, 2006) and can reduce high arousal levels, which, if prolonged, can lead to acute stress disorder (and later PTSD) as well as significant somatic symptoms (see Harvey, Bryant, & Tarrier, 2003). Mobilizing resources to respond to victims' immediate needs and linking them to services in the community have been found to reduce distress and increase long-term quality of life (see Sullivan & Bybee, 1999). Providing information about effective coping strategies can foster self-efficacy, which can help victims set realistic expectations for the long-term recovery process (see Benight & Harper, 2002). Strengthening social support and coping can help with practical and material resource needs but also provides additional outlets for emotional processing of the traumatic events (see Norris, Friedman, & Watson, 2002). Each of the individual components of psychological first aid has good empirical support, but there has been limited research on how the *combined* set of intervention strategies can curb posttrauma distress (Ruzek et al., 2007). However, a recent meta-analysis of multistrategy crisis intervention methods for medical patients found that these techniques can significantly mitigate PTSD, depression, and anxiety symptoms (Stapleton, Lating, Kirkhart, & Everly, 2006). Future research is needed to examine how the full complement of psychological first aid components can prevent distress among diverse groups of trauma survivors.

Given these promising findings regarding the effectiveness of psychological first aid, it is worth considering how this intervention could be used to assist rape survivors in the immediate postassault aftermath. Psychological first aid was purposively designed for simple, practical administration wherever trauma survivors are, including hospitals, shelters, and police departments (National Child Traumatic Stress Network and National Center for PTSD, 2006). Psychological first aid can be performed by mental health professionals, but another role for psychologists and allied professionals is to provide training to public health workers and other first responders so that they can also offer psychological first aid (Parker, Barnett, Everly, & Links, 2006). Mental health professionals could work with hospital emergency departments, SANE programs, and police departments—either as providers of psychological first aid or as training consultants. Similarly, because the medical and legal advocacy provided by rape crisis centers includes crisis intervention, mental health professionals could partner with these centers to ensure that advocates are trained in all psychological first aid core competencies.

Conclusion

Rape victims encounter significant difficulties obtaining help from the legal, medical, and mental health systems, and what help they do receive can leave them feeling blamed, doubted, and revictimized. As a result, survivors' postrape distress may be due not only to the rape itself but also to how they are treated by social systems after the assault. The community response to rape is not haphazard: certain victims and certain kinds of assaults are more likely to receive systemic attention. Ethnic minority and/or low-SES victims and those raped by someone they know are at particularly high risk for having difficult postassault help-seeking experiences. Some victims are virtually missing in the research on this issue and indeed may be missing in our social systems as well. What happens to immigrant victims; to survivors living in rural areas; to lesbian, bisexual, and transgendered victims; and to survivors with disabilities is largely unknown, but given that privilege and discrimination so strongly influence system response, there is more than enough reason to be concerned about highly marginalized and vulnerable victims.

This review has highlighted the experiences of victims who sought help from formal social systems and the difficulties they encountered. But one must remember that many victims, indeed most, do not seek help from the legal, medical, and mental health systems. When these survivors are asked why they do not, they say that they are concerned about whether they would even get help and that they are worried about being treated poorly. Unfortunately, empirical research suggests that this apprehension is probably warranted. At the same time, for some victims, social system contact is beneficial and healing. The challenge, then, is to address the underlying problems in our social systems so that good care is more consistently provided to all victims, who have survived all kinds of assaults. We need interventions and programs that victims will trust and that will help them through the healing process.

Several promising innovations have emerged to improve the community response to rape. For the legal system, SANE programs seem to be making a positive difference in prosecution rates, but the criminal justice system remains inherently adversarial—as it was designed and intended to be. Restorative justice programs offer a way to "restore survivors" (Koss, 2006) by creating an alternative setting that focuses on victims' needs to speak of the assault and to be heard and recognized. Offenders are held accountable for their actions and must make amends. This is what many survivors say they want, and it can be done without a grueling, drawn-out court battle (Koss & Achilles, 2008). Although legal issues still garner a great deal of attention from researchers, practitioners, and policymakers, the medical and mental health needs of victims are also paramount. A founding goal of SANE programs was to provide more comprehensive medical care and to do so in a way that addressed victims' emotional needs for respect, privacy, and control. Emerging data suggest that these programs are successful in these aims, but there is still a need for more focus on victims' mental health needs. Developing central roles for psychologists and allied professionals in the immediate postassault community response to rape could be instrumental in preventing secondary victimization and preventing further distress. Psychological first aid provides one approach for creating linkages between the mental health community, victims, and other social system personnel. Collaborative, multisystem innovations, informed by social science research, are changing the community response to rape. The trauma associated with negative postassault help seeking can be prevented, and our communities can be more effective in helping survivors heal from rape.

Notes

1. First, to clarify the meaning of key terms used in this article (adapted from Koss & Achilles, 2008), *rape* refers to an unwanted act of oral, vaginal, or anal penetration committed by the use of force, the threat of force, or when the recipient of the unwanted penetration is incapacitated; *sexual assault* refers to a broader range of contact and noncontact sexual offenses, up to and including

rape. The focus of this review is rape, but because sexual assault can include rape, selected research on sexual assault was also included when appropriate. Second, the terms *victim* and *survivor* are used interchangeably in this article. The term *survivor* conveys the strength of those who have been raped; the term *victim* reflects the criminal nature of this act.

2. There is a parallel literature on victims' experiences disclosing to informal sources of support (e.g., family and friends) and the resulting impact on survivors' psychological health. The focus of this article is formal systems (legal, medical, and mental health systems and rape crisis centers), but see Ullman (1999, 2000) for reviews on informal support.

3. Sexual Assault Nurse Examiner (SANE) programs, which were developed within the medical system, may also have positive effects on the legal system. These programs are reviewed later in this article.

4. Domestic violence shelters are included in studies of community-based mental health services for rape/sexual assault victims because some communities do not have free-standing rape crisis centers and instead have combined sexual assault/ domestic violence programs (Campbell, Baker, & Mazurek, 1998; National Sexual Violence Resource Center, 2006). Domestic violence programs are also included in such research because irrespective of their organizational linkages to rape crisis centers, these agencies provide counseling services to victims of marital rape/intimate partner rape (Howard et al., 2003).

References

American College of Obstetricians and Gynecologists. (1998). Sexual assault (ACOG educational bulletin). *International Journal of Gynaecology and Obstetrics*, *60*, 297–304.

American Medical Association. (1995). *Strategies for the treatment and prevention of sexual assault*. Chicago, IL: Author.

American Psychological Association. (1995). *Template for developing guidelines: Interventions for mental disorders and psychosocial aspects of physical disorders*. Washington, DC: Author.

American Psychological Association Presidential Task Force on Evidence-Based Practice. (2006). Evidence-based practice in psychology. *American Psychologist*, *61*, 271–285.

Amey, A. L., & Bishai, D. (2002). Measuring the quality of medical care for women who experience sexual assault with data from the National Hospital Ambulatory Medical Care Survey. *Annals of Emergency Medicine*, *39*, 631–638.

Aral, S. O. (2001). Sexually transmitted diseases: Magnitude, determinants, and consequences. *International Journal of STD and AIDS*, *12*, 211–215.

Benight, C. C., & Harper, M. L. (2002). Coping self-efficacy perceptions as a mediator between acute stress response and long-term distress following natural disasters. *Journal of Traumatic Stress*, *15*, 177–186.

Bletzer, K. V., & Koss, M. P. (2006). After rape among three populations in the Southwest: A time for mourning, a time for recovery. *Violence against Women, 12,* 5–29.

Bouffard, J. (2000). Predicting type of sexual assault case closure from victim, suspect and case characteristics. *Journal of Criminal Justice, 28,* 527–542.

Bryant, R. A. (2006). Cognitive behavior therapy: Implications from advances in neuroscience. In N. Kato, M. Kawata, & R. K. Pitman (Eds.), *PTSD: Brain mechanisms and clinical implications* (pp. 255–270). Toyko: Springer.

Campbell, R. (2002). *Emotionally involved: The impact of researching rape.* New York: Routledge.

Campbell, R. (2005). What really happened? A validation study of rape survivors' help-seeking experiences with the legal and medical systems. *Violence and Victims, 20,* 55–68.

Campbell, R. (2006). Rape survivors' experiences with the legal and medical systems: Do rape victim advocates make a difference? *Violence against Women, 12,* 1–16.

Campbell, R., Baker, C. K., & Mazurek, T. (1998). Remaining radical? Organizational predictors of rape crisis centers' social change initiatives. *American Journal of Community Psychology, 26,* 465–491.

Campbell, R., Barnes, H. E., Ahrens, C. E., Wasco, S. M., Zaragoza-Diesfeld, Y., & Sefl, T. (1999). Community services for rape survivors: Enhancing psychological well-being or increasing trauma? *Journal of Consulting and Clinical Psychology, 67,* 847–858.

Campbell, R., & Bybee, D. (1997). Emergency medical services for rape victims: Detecting the cracks in service delivery. *Women's Health (Hillsdale, N.J.), 3,* 75–101.

Campbell, R., & Martin, P. Y. (2001). Services for sexual assault survivors: The role of rape crisis centers. In C. Renzetti, J. Edleson, & R. Bergen (Eds.), *Sourcebook on violence against women* (pp. 227–241). Thousand Oaks, CA: Sage.

Campbell, R., Patterson, D., Adams, A. E., Diegel, R., & Coats, S. (2008). A participatory evaluation project to measure SANE nursing practice and adult sexual assault patients' psychological well-being. *Journal of Forensic Nursing, 4,* 19–28.

Campbell, R., Patterson, D., & Bybee, D. (2007, October). *Prosecution rates for adult sexual assault cases: A ten year analysis before and after the implementation of a SANE program.* Paper presented at the International Forensic Nursing Scientific Assembly, Salt Lake City, UT.

Campbell, R., Patterson, D., & Lichty, L. F. (2005). The effectiveness of sexual assault nurse examiner (SANE) programs: A review of psychological, medical, legal, and community outcomes. *Trauma, Violence, and Abuse: A Review Journal, 6,* 313–329.

Campbell, R., & Raja, S. (1999). The secondary victimization of rape victims: Insights from mental health professionals who treat survivors of violence. *Violence and Victims, 14,* 261–275.

Campbell, R., & Raja, S. (2005). The sexual assault and secondary victimization of female veterans: Help-seeking experiences in military and civilian social systems. *Psychology of Women Quarterly, 29*, 97–106.

Campbell, R., Raja, S., & Grining, P. L. (1999). Training mental health professionals on violence against women. *Journal of Interpersonal Violence, 14*, 1003–1013.

Campbell, R., Townsend, S. M., Long, S. M., Kinnison, K. E., Pulley, E. M., Adames, S. B., et al. (2006). Responding to sexual assault victims' medical and emotional needs: A national study of the services provided by SANE programs. *Research in Nursing and Health, 29*, 384–398.

Campbell, R., Wasco, S. M., Ahrens, C. E., Sefl, T., & Barnes, H. E. (2001). Preventing the "second rape": Rape survivors' experiences with community service providers. *Journal of Interpersonal Violence, 16*, 1239–1259.

Centers for Disease Control and Prevention. (2002). Sexual assault and STDs— Adults and adolescents. *Morbidity and Mortality Weekly Report, 51*(RR-6), 69–71.

Ciancone, A., Wilson, C., Collette, R., & Gerson, L. W. (2000). Sexual Assault Nurse Examiner programs in the United States. *Annals of Emergency Medicine, 35*, 353–357.

Crandall, C., & Helitzer, D. (2003). *Impact evaluation of a Sexual Assault Nurse Examiner (SANE) program* (Document No. 203276). Washington, DC: National Institute of Justice.

Edmond, T. (2006, February). *Theoretical and intervention preferences of service providers addressing violence against women: A national survey.* Paper presented at the Council on Social Work Education Conference, Chicago, IL.

Ericksen, J., Dudley, C., McIntosh, G., Ritch, L., Shumay, S., & Simpson, M. (2002). Clients' experiences with a specialized sexual assault service. *Journal of Emergency Nursing, 28*, 86–90.

Estrich, S. (1987). *Real rape: How the legal system victimizes women who say no.* Cambridge, MA: Harvard University Press.

Everly, G. S., & Flynn, B. W. (2005). Principles and practice of acute psychological first aid. In G. S. Everly & C. L. Parker (Eds.), *Mental health aspects of mass disasters: Public health preparedness and response* (pp. 79–89). Baltimore, MD: Johns Hopkins Center for Public Health Preparedness.

Filipas, H. H., & Ullman, S. E. (2001). Social reactions to sexual assault victims from various support sources. *Violence and Victims, 16*, 673–692.

Fisher, B. A., Cullen, F. T., & Turner, M. G. (2000). *The sexual victimization of college women* (NCJ 182369). Washington, DC: U.S. Department of Justice, Office of Justice Programs.

Flowe, H. D., Ebbesen, E. B., & Putcha-Bhagavatula, A. (2007). Rape shield laws and sexual behavior evidence: Effects of consent level and women's sexual history on rape allegations. *Law and Human Behavior, 31*, 159–175.

Foa, E. B., Keane, T. M., & Friedman, M. J. (Eds.). (2000). *Effective treatments for PTSD: Practice guidelines from the International Society for Traumatic Stress Studies.* New York: Guilford Press.

Foa, E. B., & Rothbaum, B. O. (1998). *Treating the trauma of rape: Cognitive-behavioral therapy for PTSD.* New York: Guilford Press.

Foa, E. B., Rothbaum, B. O., Riggs, D. S., & Murdock, T. B. (1991). Treatment of posttraumatic stress disorder in rape victims: A comparison between cognitive-behavioral procedures and counseling. *Journal of Consulting and Clinical Psychology, 59,* 715–723.

Frazier, P., & Haney, B. (1996). Sexual assault cases in the legal system: Police, prosecutor and victim perspectives. *Law and Human Behavior, 20,* 607–628.

Frohmann, L. (1997a). Complaint-filing interviews and the constitution of organizational structure: Understanding the limitations of rape reform. *Hastings Women's Law Journal, 8,* 365–399.

Frohmann, L. (1997b). Discrediting victims' allegations of sexual assault: Prosecutorial accounts of case rejections. *Social Problems, 38,* 213–226.

Golding, J. M., Siegel, J. M., Sorenson, S. B., Burnam, M. A., & Stein, J. A. (1989). Social support sources following sexual assault. *Journal of Community Psychology, 17,* 92–107.

Goodman, L. A., & Epstein, D. (2008). *Listening to battered women: A survivor-centered approach to advocacy, mental health, and justice.* Washington, DC: American Psychological Association.

Halligan, S. L., Michael, T., Clark, D. M., & Ehlers, A. (2003). Posttraumatic stress disorder following assault: The role of cognitive processing, trauma memory, and appraisals. *Journal of Consulting and Clinical Psychology, 71,* 419–431.

Harvey, A. G., Bryant, R. A., & Tarrier, N. (2003). Cognitive behavior therapy for posttraumatic stress disorder. *Clinical Psychology Review, 23,* 501–522.

Howard, A., Riger, S., Campbell, R., & Wasco, S. M. (2003). Counseling services for battered women: A comparison of outcomes for physical and sexual abuse survivors. *Journal of Interpersonal Violence, 18,* 717–734.

Huppert, J. D., Fabbro, A., & Barlow, D. H. (2006). Evidence-based practice and psychological treatments. In C. D. Goodheart, A. E. Kazdin, & R. J. Sternberg (Eds.), *Evidence-based psychotherapy: Where practice and research meet* (pp. 131–152). Washington, DC: American Psychological Association.

Janoff-Bulman, R. (1992). *Shattered assumptions: Towards a new psychology of trauma.* New York: Free Press.

Kazdin, A. E. (2008). Evidence-based treatment and practice: New opportunities to bridge clinical research and practice, enhance the knowledge base, and improve patient care. *American Psychologist, 63,* 146–159.

Kerstetter, W. (1990). Gateway to justice: Police and prosecutor response to sexual assault against women. *Journal of Criminal Law and Criminology, 81,* 267–313.

Kerstetter, W., & Van Winkle, B. (1990). Who decides? A study of the complainant's decision to prosecute in rape cases. *Criminal Justice and Behavior, 17,* 268–283.

Kilpatrick, D. G., & Acierno, R. (2003). Mental health needs of crime victims: Epidemiology and outcomes. *Journal of Traumatic Stress, 16*, 119–132.

Kilpatrick, D. G., Amstadter, A. B., Resnick, H. S., & Ruggiero, K. J. (2007). Rape-related PTSD: Issues and interventions. *Psychiatric Times, 24*, 50–58.

Konradi, A. (2007). *Taking the stand: Rape survivors and the prosecution of rapists.* Westport, CT: Praeger.

Koss, M. P. (2006). Restoring rape survivors: Justice, advocacy, and a call to action. *Annals of the New York Academy of Sciences, 1087*, 206–234.

Koss, M. P. (2008, February). *Interpersonal violence agendas: Past and future.* Paper presented at the American Psychological Association Summit on Violence and Abuse in Relationships, Bethesda, MD.

Koss, M. P., Abbey, A., Campbell, R., Cook, S., Norris, J., Testa, M., et al. (2007). Revising the SES: A collaborative process to improve assessment of sexual aggression and victimization. *Psychology of Women Quarterly, 31*, 357–370.

Koss, M., & Achilles, M. (2008). *Restorative justice responses to sexual assault.* Retrieved March 3, 2008, from http://www.vawnet.org/category/Main_Doc .php?docid=1231.

Koss, M. P., Bachar, K. J., Hopkins, C. Q., & Carlson, C. (2004). Expanding a community's justice response to sex crimes through advocacy, prosecutorial, and public health collaboration. *Journal of Interpersonal Violence, 19*, 1435–1463.

Koss, M. P., Bailey, J. A., Yuan, N. P., Herrera, V. M., & Lichter, E. L. (2003). Depression and PTSD in survivors of male violence: Research and training initiatives to facilitate recovery. *Psychology of Women Quarterly, 27*, 130–142.

Koss, M. P., Gidycz, C. A., & Wisniewski, N. (1987). The scope of rape: Incidence and prevalence of sexual aggression and victimization in a national sample of higher education students. *Journal of Consulting and Clinical Psychology, 55*, 162–170.

Koss, M. P., Goodman, L. A., Browne, A., Fitzgerald, L. F., Keita, G. P., & Russo, N. F. (1994). *No safe haven: Male violence against women at home, at work, and in the community.* Washington, DC: American Psychological Association.

Krakow, B., Hollifield, M., Johnston, L., Koss, M., Schrader, R., Warner, T. D., et al. (2001). Imagery rehearsal therapy for chronic nightmares in sexual assault survivors with posttraumatic stress disorder: A randomized control trial. *Journal of the American Medical Association, 296*, 537–545.

Ledray, L. (1992). The sexual assault nurse clinician: A fifteen-year experience in Minneapolis. *Journal of Emergency Nursing, 18*, 217–222.

Ledray, L. (1996). The sexual assault resource service: A new model of care. *Minnesota Medicine, 79*, 43–45.

Ledray, L. E. (1999). *Sexual assault nurse examiner (SANE) development & operations guide.* Washington, DC: Office for Victims of Crime, U.S. Department of Justice.

Littel, K. (2001). Sexual assault nurse examiner programs: Improving the community response to sexual assault victims. *Office for Victims of Crime Bulletin, 4*, 1–19.

Logan, T., Evans, L., Stevenson, E., & Jordan, C. E. (2005). Barriers to services for rural and urban survivors of rape. *Journal of Interpersonal Violence, 20,* 591–616.

Madigan, L., & Gamble, N. (1991). *The second rape: Society's continued betrayal of the victim.* New York: Lexington Books.

Martin, P. Y. (2005). *Rape work: Victims, gender, and emotions in organization and community context.* New York: Routledge.

Martin, P. Y., & Powell, R. M. (1994). Accounting for the "second assault": Legal organizations' framing of rape victims. *Law and Social Inquiry, 19,* 853–890.

Matthews, N. A. (1994). *Confronting rape: The feminist anti-rape movement and the state.* New York: Routledge.

Mayer, J. P., & Davidson, W. S. (2000). Dissemination of innovation as social change. In J. Rappaport & E. Seidman (Eds.), *Handbook of community psychology* (pp. 421–438). New York: Plenum Press.

Miller, R. L., & Shinn, M. (2005). Learning from communities: Overcoming difficulties in dissemination of prevention and promotion efforts. *American Journal of Community Psychology, 35,* 169–183.

Monroe, L. M., Kinney, L. M., Weist, M. D., Dafeamekpor, D. S., Dantzler, J., & Reynolds, M. W. (2005). The experience of sexual assault: Findings from a state-wide victim needs assessment. *Journal of Interpersonal Violence, 20,* 767–777.

Moor, A. (2007). When recounting the traumatic memories is not enough: Treating persistent self-devaluation associated with rape and victim-blaming myths. *Women and Therapy, 30,* 19–33.

National Center for Victims of Crime and National Crime Victims Research and Treatment Center. (1992). *Rape in America: A report to the nation.* Arlington, VA: National Center for Victims of Crime.

National Child Traumatic Stress Network and National Center for PTSD. (2006). *Psychological first aid: Field operations guide* (2nd ed.). Retrieved March 3, 2008, from http://www.nctsn.org/content/psychological-first-aid.

National Institute of Mental Health. (2004). *Bridging science and service: A report by the National Advisory Mental Health Council's Clinical Treatment and Services Research Workgroup.* Bethesda, MD: Author.

National Institute of Mental Health. (2006). *The road ahead: Research partnerships to transform services: A report by the National Advisory Mental Health Council's Workgroup on Services and Clinical Epidemiology Research.* Bethesda, MD: Author.

National Sexual Violence Resource Center. (2006). *Directory of sexual assault centers in the United States.* Enola, PA: Author.

Norris, F. H., Friedman, M. J., & Watson, P. J. (2002). 60,000 disaster victims speak: Part II. Summary and implications of the disaster mental health research. *Psychiatry, 65,* 240–260.

Parker, C. L., Barnett, D. J., Everly, G. S., & Links, J. M. (2006). Expanding disaster mental health response: A conceptual training framework for public health professionals. *International Journal of Emergency Mental Health*, 8, 101–110.

Parker, C. L., Everly, G. S., Barnett, D. J., & Links, J. M. (2006). Establishing evidence-informed core intervention competencies in psychological first aid for public health personnel. *International Journal of Emergency Mental Health*, 8, 83–92.

Parrot, A. (1991). Medical community response to acquaintance rape—Recommendations. In A. Parrot & L. Bechhofer (Eds.), *Acquaintance rape: The hidden crime* (pp. 304–316). New York: Wiley.

Patterson, D., Greeson, M. R., & Campbell, R. (2008). *Protect thyself: Understanding rape survivors' decisions not to seek help from social systems*. Manuscript submitted for publication.

Plichta, S. B., Vandecar-Burdin, T., Odor, R. K., Reams, S., & Zhang, Y. (2006). The emergency department and victims of sexual violence: An assessment of preparedness to help. *Journal of Health and Human Services Administration*, 29, 285–308.

Resick, P. A. (2004). A suggested research agenda on treatment-outcome research for female victims of violence. *Journal of Interpersonal Violence*, 19, 1290–1295.

Resick, P. A., Galovski, T. E., Uhlmansiek, M., Scher, C. D., Clum, G. A., & Young-Xu, Y. (2008). A randomized control trial to dismantle components of cognitive processing therapy for posttraumatic stress disorder in female victims of interpersonal violence. *Journal of Consulting and Clinical Psychology*, 76, 243–258.

Resick, P. A., Nishith, P., Weaver, T. L., Astin, M. C., & Feuer, C. A. (2002). A comparison of cognitive-processing therapy with prolonged exposure and a waiting condition for the treatment of chronic posttraumatic stress disorder in female rape victims. *Journal of Consulting and Clinical Psychology*, 70, 867–879.

Resick, P. A., & Schnicke, M. K. (1992). Cognitive processing therapy for sexual assault victims. *Journal of Consulting and Clinical Psychology*, 60, 748–756.

RESTORE. (2006). *Overview manual*. Retrieved March 3, 2008, from http://www.restorativejustice.org/articlesdb/articles/7182.

Rogers, E. M. (1995). *Diffusion of innovations* (4th ed.). New York: Free Press.

Ruscio, A. M., & Holohan, D. R. (2006). Applying empirically supported treatments to complex cases: Ethical, empirical, and practical considerations. *Clinical Psychology: Science and Practice*, 13, 146–162.

Russell, P. L., & Davis, C. (2007). Twenty-five years of empirical research on treatment following sexual assault. *Best Practices in Mental Health*, 3, 21–37.

Ruzek, J. I., Brymer, M. J., Jacobs, A. K., Layne, C. M., Vernberg, E. M., & Watson, P. J. (2007). Psychological first aid. *Journal of Mental Health Counseling*, 29, 17–49.

Sarason, S. B. (1972). *The creation of settings and the future societies.* San Francisco: Jossey-Bass.

Sievers, V., Murphy, S., & Miller, J. (2003). Sexual assault evidence collection more accurate when completed by sexual assault nurse examiners: Colorado's experience. *Journal of Emergency Nursing, 29,* 511–514.

Smugar, S. S., Spina, B. J., & Merz, J. F. (2000). Informed consent for emergency contraception: Variability in hospital care of rape victims. *American Journal of Public Health, 90,* 1372–1376.

Spears, J., & Spohn, C. (1997). The effect of evidence factors and victim characteristics on prosecutors' charging decisions in sexual assault cases. *Justice Quarterly, 14,* 501–524.

Spohn, C., Beichner, D., & Davis-Frenzel, E. (2001). Prosecutorial justifications for sexual assault case rejection: Guarding the "gateway to justice." *Social Problems, 48,* 206–235.

Sprang, G., Craig, C., & Clark, J. (2008). Factors impacting trauma treatment practice patterns: The convergence/divergence of science and practice. *Journal of Anxiety Disorders, 22,* 162–174.

Stapleton, A., Lating, J., Kirkhart, M., & Everly, G. S. (2006). Effects of medical crisis intervention on anxiety, depression, and posttraumatic stress symptoms: A meta-analysis. *Psychiatric Quarterly, 77,* 231–238.

Starzynski, L. L., Ullman, S. E., Filipas, H. H., & Townsend, S. M. (2005). Correlates of women's sexual assault disclosure to informal and formal support sources. *Violence and Victims, 20,* 417–432.

Starzynski, L. L., Ullman, S. E., Townsend, S. M., Long, D. M., & Long, S. M. (2007). What factors predict women's disclosure of sexual assault to mental health professionals? *Journal of Community Psychology, 35,* 619–638.

Sullivan, C. M., & Bybee, D. (1999). Reducing violence using community-based advocacy for women with abusive partners. *Journal of Consulting and Clinical Psychology, 67,* 43–53.

Taylor, W. K. (2002). Collecting evidence for sexual assault: The role of the sexual assault nurse examiner (SANE). *International Journal of Gynaecology and Obstetrics, 78,* S91–S94.

Tjaden, P., & Thoennes, N. (1998). *Full report of the prevalence, incidence, and consequences of violence against women: Findings from the National Violence against Women Survey.* Washington, DC: National Institute of Justice.

Ullman, S. E. (1996a). Correlates and consequences of adult sexual assault disclosure. *Journal of Interpersonal Violence, 11,* 554–571.

Ullman, S. E. (1996b). Do social reactions to sexual assault victims vary by support provider? *Violence and Victims, 11,* 143–156.

Ullman, S. E. (1999). Social support and recovery from sexual assault: A review. *Aggression and Violent Behavior, 4,* 343–358.

Ullman, S. E. (2000). Psychometric characteristics of the Social Reactions Questionnaire: A measure of reactions to sexual assault victims. *Psychology of Women Quarterly, 24,* 169–183.

Ullman, S. E. (2007). Mental health services seeking in sexual assault victims. *Women and Therapy, 30,* 61–84.

Ullman, S. E., & Brecklin, L. R. (2002). Sexual assault history, PTSD, and mental health service seeking in a national sample of women. *Journal of Community Psychology, 30,* 261–279.

Ullman, S. E., & Filipas, H. H. (2001a). Correlates of formal and informal support seeking in sexual assault victims. *Journal of Interpersonal Violence, 16,* 1028–1047.

Ullman, S. E., & Filipas, H. H. (2001b). Predictors of PTSD symptom severity and social reactions in sexual assault victims. *Journal of Traumatic Stress, 14,* 369–389.

Ullman, S. E., & Townsend, S. M. (2008). What is an empowerment approach to working with sexual assault survivors? *Journal of Community Psychology, 36,* 1–14.

U.S. Department of Justice. (2004). *A national protocol for sexual assault medical forensic examinations: Adults/adolescents.* Washington, DC: Author.

Wasco, S. M., Campbell, R., Barnes, H., & Ahrens, C. E. (1999, June). *Rape crisis centers: Shaping survivors' experiences with community systems following sexual assault.* Paper presented at the Biennial Conference on Community Research and Action, New Haven, CT.

Wasco, S. M., Campbell, R., Howard, A., Mason, G., Schewe, P., Staggs, S., et al. (2004). A statewide evaluation of services provided to rape survivors. *Journal of Interpersonal Violence, 19,* 252–263.

Westen, D., Novotny, C. M., & Thompson-Brenner, H. (2004). The empirical status of empirically supported psychotherapies: Assumptions, findings, and reporting in controlled clinical trials. *Psychological Bulletin, 130,* 631–663.

Wgliski, A., & Barthel, A. K. (2004). Cultural differences in reporting of sexual assault to sexual assault agencies in the United States. *Sexual Assault Report, 7*(84), 92–93.

Wyatt, G. E. (1992). The sociocultural context of African American and White American women's rape. *Journal of Social Issues, 48,* 77–91.

IV

Addiction

The following four contributions on addiction wrestle with one of the toughest challenges those in mental health care face. Addiction is not only devastating for those in its grasp, but addiction to alcohol and drugs also exacts a staggering toll on families, friends, coworkers, and societies. The costs of addiction extend to the crime associated with some addictive behavior; attempts to prevent access to addictive substances such as heroin, cocaine, or prescription pain medications; and the cost of dealing with the physical and mental toll that addiction takes.

Craig Reinerman begins by reminding us that the addiction model is a double-edged sword. Lumping behavior such as regular heroin use into the addiction category is a humane strategy for granting access to treatment and other services, but also a justification for punitive policies against those who choose to use and those who choose to sell drugs.

The triumph of addiction as disease is well illustrated by the history of alcohol use and abuse. Reinerman reminds us that for centuries, very heavy drinking was an accepted part of ordinary life. Those who abused alcohol were thought of as loving drink too much to choose to give it up. It was the rise of industrialized societies that greatly valued sobriety and tried to encourage self-control in all areas of life that drove drinking into the emerging disease model of addiction.

Using the discourse of disease has had progressive effects insofar as it has helped trigger a shift in which drug use is now seen as "properly belonging in the realm of public health rather than criminal law." However, it also means that the powerful can use medicine to declare war on citizens who ingest substances that lead to behavior that the culture disvalues.

Thomas Szasz, in his widely read and debated article, follows the admission of the cultural dimension of addiction with an argument that addiction is entirely a creation of those in power in any given society.

Drug abuse may be undesirable, but it is not the provenance of medicine to fix it. It is the task of those involved in ethics, education, and religion to try and discourage behavior they find offensive or perverse. Unless you are a child abusing substances or you harm others by your behavior, Szasz maintains that medicine and even the state should not interfere with your choices as to what you ingest, smoke, or use for stimulation.

Prominent researchers Charles O'Brien and Thomas McLellan do not agree. They believe that research has begun to reveal both the underlying biological risk factors that lead to addiction and how it is that addictive stimuli and substances can coerce and compel behavior in those who are addicts. They note that addiction is not an acute illness but rather a chronic condition. As such its control or cure is contingent on many factors including patient compliance. Seen in this light, addiction is a struggle to manage for mental health care providers, but no more so than trying to achieve improvement with respect to arthritis, diabetes, hypertension, allergies, and many other chronic illnesses.

Laura Weiss Roberts and Kim Bullock pick up on the theme of addiction as chronic illness by noting that it is a challenge to care for the noncompliant patient and by offering advice about how best to proceed ethically with these difficult patients. Addicts are often poor, disenfranchised, and isolated, which leads their caretakers' duties and obligations to try and engage families, friends, social networks, peer counselors, and local resources. They see addiction as socially constructed and, as such, a set of problems that require social responses.

Nonetheless, more and more studies are revealing biological risk factors in our genes or our brains for addiction. At the same time, more and more behaviors are being brought forward for possible classification as addiction, including uncontrolled overeating, gambling, promiscuity, and online gaming. It is likely that attention to the biological bases of such behavior will reveal evidence of difference. Whether that evidence is enough to shift these behaviors toward a medical rather than a moral framework remains to be seen.

12

Addiction as Accomplishment: The Discursive Construction of Disease

Craig Reinarman

"An ideology is reluctant to believe that it was ever born, since to do so is to acknowledge that it can die. . . . It would prefer to think of itself as without parentage, sprung parthenogenetically from its own seed. It is equally embarrassed by the presence of sibling ideologies, since these mark out its own finite frontiers and so delimit its sway. To view an ideology from the outside is to recognize its limits."
—Terry Eagleton (1991:58)

In the United States and many other Western industrialized societies at the start of the twenty-first century, "addiction" is said to be a "disease." Virtually everyone in the treatment industry embraces the notion that "addiction" is a "disease," as do nearly all people who understand themselves to be "in recovery" from it. Officials of the U.S. National Institute of Drug Abuse have adopted the claim that "addiction is a brain disease" as a kind of mantra (e.g., Enos, 2004; Leshner, 1997, 2001; Volkow, 2003). Even the drug policy reform movement, which advocates decriminalization of drugs, invokes the disease concept of addiction when advocating treatment in lieu of prison for drug offenders (see, e.g., Bertram, Blachman, Sharp & Andreas, 1996:233–241). The disease concept of addiction is now so widely believed, so taken for granted in public discourse about drug problems, it is difficult to imagine that it was not always part of the basic perceptual schema of human knowledge.

Yet addiction-as-disease did not emerge from the natural accumulation of scientific discoveries; its ubiquity is a different species of social accomplishment. The disease concept was invented under historically and culturally specific conditions, promulgated by particular actors and institutions, and internalized and reproduced by means of certain discursive practices. This article begins by briefly reviewing some of the questions that have been raised about whether it is a discrete empirical entity with an identifiable etiology. The core of the article then traces the social construction and cultural dissemination of addiction-as-disease to show how it achieved its status as the dominant framework for understanding drug problems. The concluding discussion attempts to situate the lived experience of problematic drug use within this construction and notes the double-edged character of this discourse of disease: a humane strategy for gaining access to treatment and other services, but at the same time a justification for punitive drug policies.

Heretical Doubts about Entitivity and Etiology

Addiction-as-disease is not as discrete or as readily identifiable an entity as many people believe it is. One of the principal reasons for this is that the user behaviors presumed to constitute it are protean, forged in interaction with features of users' environments. What are taken as empirical indicators of an underlying disease of addiction consist of a broad range of behaviors that are interpreted as "symptoms" only under some circumstances. They can be aggregated to fit under the heading of "addiction" only by means of some degree of epistemic force. As Room (1983) and others have shown in the case of alcoholism, these symptoms can be better described empirically and grasped theoretically if they are not conceptualized as constituent elements of a discrete disease entity, but instead disaggregated and understood as drinking practices and problems.

The etiology of addiction-as-disease has also been difficult to nail down. For most of the nineteenth century, it was widely believed that alcohol was inherently addicting and therefore that anyone who drank it would become addicted. We now know that most drinkers and drug users do not become addicts, so the pharmacological properties of the psychoactive substances cannot be the proximate cause of addiction-as-disease in the sense that tubercle bacillus is the cause of tuberculosis. This means that if addiction can be said to be a disease, it must be a person-specific disease, one that some people get but most do not (Levine, 1978). Yet despite decades of research, the biological basis for addiction-as-disease remains elusive. Addiction researchers thus far have been unable to identify either a gene as the source or an organ as the site of the core pathology of addiction in affected individuals.

In recent years, the brain is typically cited as the organ in which addiction-as-disease is said to reside, but this is not yet clear. Neuroscientists have done promising new research using magnetic resonance imaging (MRI) to show how the brain's so-called pleasure center or reward circuitry reacts and even makes longer-term adaptations to psychoactive substances (see Volkow, 2003, for a useful overview). While such studies confirm that there is a biological component in what is called addiction, they have yielded an embarrassment of riches. The trend in neuropharmacological research is toward the "common pathway" hypothesis (e.g., Nestler & Malenka, 2004). Changes in brain function along this pathway occur with the use of a wide variety of very different drugs, licit and illicit, but also for many adrenaline-inducing and other pleasurable or merely satisfying activities involving no drugs at all. These activities include gambling (e.g., Blakeslee, 2002; Goleman, 1989); acts of cooperation, trust, and generosity (e.g., Angier, 2002); maternal support (e.g., Moles, Kieffer & D'Amato, 2004); talk therapy (e.g., Brody et al., 2001); and even looking at beautiful faces (e.g., Aharon et al., 2001). Indeed, Dr. Roy Wise, a NIDA addiction researcher, notes that people will like and thus tend to repeat "anything you can do that turns on these dopamine neurons" (Kolata, 2002).

That the brain is centrally involved in drug use behaviors is not in question; whether this new neuroscience research has identified a specific locus of addiction-as-disease in the brain is another matter. At present, it is not clear if there is a site of pathology in the brain that distinguishes repetitive drug taking from, say, sex, sailing, symphonies, and other activities people learn to repeat because they provide pleasure. For purposes of understanding how addiction-as-disease achieved its hegemonic status, however, such questions have little relevance, for the disease concept preceded this brain research by decades and took hold for reasons unrelated to neuroscience.

Numerous alcohol and drug scholars voiced the blasphemy of doubt about addiction-as-disease well before the new brain research. As early as 1962, for example, Seeley noted that "the statement that 'alcoholism is a disease' is most misleading, since it conceals that a step in public policy is being recommended, not a scientific discovery announced" (1962:587). He supported strongly the notion that drinkers who needed help should have it, but he balked when this sort of compassion made its case by masquerading as science. Zinberg's study of controlled heroin users, *Drug, Set, and Setting* (1984), demonstrated that "loss of control," which many consider the sine qua non of addiction-as-disease, was not the inevitable outcome of regular use but rather contingent upon social and psychological variables (see also Hanson, Beschner, Walters & Bovelle, 1985; Prebble & Casey, 1969; and Waldorf, 1973, all of whom make parallel points about heroin users). Similarly, in *Heavy Drinking:*

The Myth of Alcoholism as Disease (1988), Fingarette shows that neither tolerance nor withdrawal, the two most traditional and basic criteria for addiction, are actually manifest in many so-called alcoholics. He advanced instead the notion of heavy drinking as a "way of life"—an often unhealthy and problematic way of life, to be sure, but not technically a disease state. In *Diseasing of America* (1989) and several other books, Peele documents numerous empirical inadequacies in the disease concept of addiction and delineates the interests behind its promulgation.

Questions of entitivity and etiology aside, Davies' *The Myth of Addiction* (1992) employs attribution theory to show that people choose to interpret habitual drug taking as an addictive disease that is beyond the control of the user not because this interpretation best fits the observable facts, but because it is a view that serves useful purposes for users themselves and for society in general. Addiction-as-disease functions, for example, as an excuse for bad behavior, a means of absolving blame, an explanation of otherwise "irrational" behavior, and as legitimation for punishment and/or treatment (see also Davies, 1997, on drug discourse). The giving of accounts for actions is a behavior in its own right, independent of the actions they purport to explain (Mills, 1940). For example, Room has observed that "we are living at a historic moment when the rate of alcohol dependence as a cognitive and existential experience is rising, although the rate of alcohol consumption and of heavy drinking is falling" (1991:154).

Numerous critiques of addiction-as-disease have been published in *Addiction Research and Theory* (see, e.g., volume 5, number 1, 1997). One of the broadest and most sharply posed was by Cohen (2000). He argues that addiction-as-disease is essentially a religious notion in that it functions to manage our fears about how firmly we are in control of our behaviors and destinies—a myth-like social construction of no greater scientific validity than the pre-Galilean cosmology of flat-earthers. Once the Protestant Reformation and market capitalism gave rise to the notion of "the autonomous individual" in the West somewhere around the seventeenth century, Cohen suggests, we began to see the development of its opposite—a modern sort of devil that takes the form of people who are thought to have lost the capacity for the self-regulation, independence, and entrepreneurial activity, which were considered the essence of the autonomous individual.

While these and many other scholars have raised profound questions about the ontological status of addiction-as-disease, this does not appear to have slowed its march. In what follows, I address the more modest question of how addiction-as-disease came to be so widely adopted for so many different problems. *Specifically, by what historical, institutional, and interactional processes was the concept of addictive disease rendered culturally available such that it could become the dominant framework for understanding drug problems?*

Addiction as a Historical Accomplishment

As Room has argued, "addiction" is "a set of ideas which have a history and a cultural location" (2004:221). In his famous painting of 1559, *The Fight between Carnival and Lent,* Peter Breugel depicts an agrarian village in preindustrial Europe in full celebration. Feasting, drinking, and even drunkenness are seen everywhere, as was the case with numerous peasant holidays that were traditionally passed in varying degrees of intoxicated revelry. Drinking was a common part of everyday life, engaged in by most people, with the exception of the few monk-like figures from ascetic Protestant sects who, in the painting, can be seen in dark robes solemnly stepping toward the church while their fellow villagers frolic in drink-crazed abandon. Breugel gives us a liminal moment, a glimpse of an historic shift—the beginning of the problematization of intoxication at the dawn of Western modernity (see Burke, 1978). The ancient bacchanalian drinking traditions that persisted from at least classical antiquity through the Middle Ages began to be contested by ascetic Protestantism and early capitalism, each of which helped create the modern Western "individual" and at the same time demanded the renunciation of pleasure for the sake of piety and productivity. As Levine (1978), Cohen (2000), and Room (2004) all note, it was in this historical and cultural context that the notion that a substance might "cause" one to "lose" self-control became thinkable.

Levine's classic article, "The Discovery of Addiction" (1978), documents the emergence in the Western world of a discursive formation in which the self was understood in a new way, an understanding that began to emerge in the United States only at the end of the eighteenth century. Before this, Levine shows, drunks were assumed to have a will, to have the capacity to make choices; they did not have a disease that robbed them of volition, they just loved drink too much. In the early nineteenth century, industrialization and its attendant mobility were transforming U.S. society—straining family ties and traditional community support networks such that the economic fate of families increasingly depended upon self-control (Room, 2004). The moral enterprise of Dr. Benjamin

Rush and the early temperance crusaders gave a specific form to this spreading concern over self-control: drunks were reconceptualized as people stricken with a *disease of the will* (cf. Valverde, 1998)—a disease that rendered them powerless (prefiguring the first of the twelve steps of Alcoholics Anonymous). In a few decades in the early nineteenth century, the growing temperance movement transformed alcohol from what even leading Puritan preachers had called "the good creature of God" into a "demon destroyer" held to be the direct cause of crime, violence, poverty, divorce, and virtually all other problems in America.

The notion that an intoxicating substance could cripple self-control and thus cause bad behavior that would not otherwise occur is a culturally specific attribution; "not all cultures make this kind of causal connection" (Room, 2004:225; see also Davies, 1992, 1997; MacAndrew & Edgerton, 1969; Peele, 1989). It is a notion that made sense and took hold at a point in history and in those societies in which social life was organized such that individualism had become the taken-for-granted frame of reference. The notion that drinking or drug use can cause the neglect of other activities makes sense in "the context of a culture attuned to the clock, a cultural frame in which time is viewed as a commodity which is used or spent rather than simply experienced" (Room, 2004:226).

A Chronicle of Conceptual Acrobatics

Physicians now claim ownership of addiction-as-disease, but this was not always so. In the latter half of the nineteenth century, the fledgling profession of psychiatry mostly resisted the attribution of disease to habitual drinkers; they were not, it seems, considered desirable patients. Toward the end of the nineteenth century in England, some of the leaders of the British Society for the Scientific Study of Inebriety tried to popularize "inebriety" as a concept covering all the drug-taking phenomena now aggregated under the heading of addiction-as-disease. But through the 1880s "smoking and drug taking" were not classified under "any scientific definition" of inebriety or addiction (Valverde, 1998:51). Indeed, the definition of addiction-as-disease has been regularly reworked—and not in the direction of greater focus and precision as is typically the case with other diseases.[1]

In the early part of the twentieth century, opiate addiction came to be defined as physiological dependence as indicated by tolerance and withdrawal symptoms. But this definition eventually proved too restrictive. For one thing, tolerance and withdrawal are not universal even among regular heroin users (e.g., Blackwell, 1983, 1985; Hanson et al., 1985;

Zinberg, 1984). Moreover, the habitual or problematic use of many other illicit drugs does not necessarily lead to such symptoms. Even among extreme users of a so-called hard drug like crack cocaine, for example, what is called addiction is sociologically contingent rather than physiologically inevitable, as the disease model implies (Morgan & Zimmer, 1997; Reinarman, Waldorf & Murphy, 1994; Reinarman, Waldorf, Murphy & Levine, 1997).

In 1950, a World Health Organization (WHO) committee defined "drug addiction" as a state of chronic or periodic intoxication due to regular use of a drug, including a compulsion to continue, a tendency to increase dose, both psychic and physical dependence, and detrimental effects on the user as well as society. Faced with the recalcitrant fact that lots of illicit drug use did not entail these characteristics, the WHO added a new concept to its armamentarium in 1957: "drug habituation." Drug habituation was defined much the same way as drug addiction but without compulsion, increasing doses, or societal consequences. By the 1960s, WHO's search for some common denominator of addiction led it to drop both these concepts in favor of the looser "drug dependence," defined simply as psychic and/or physical dependence on a drug, the characteristics of which vary by drug type (Christie & Bruun, 1968:66–7). By 1981, the WHO definition of *dependence* was redefined still more loosely as a syndrome in which drug taking is "given a much higher priority than other behaviors that once had a higher value" (Shaffer & Jones, 1989:42). Yet this broader definition leads back to the embarrassment-of-riches problem noted earlier, for it fits virtually any behavior that is substituted for a prior behavior—even behaviors that entail no use of psychoactive substances.

Like their counterparts at WHO, other addiction researchers continued to hunt for a definition malleable enough to encompass both the growing range of illicit drug-taking practices and stubborn empirical anomalies. For example, in 1972, the American Psychiatric Association (APA) shifted away from "addiction" toward a broader concept of "drug abuse," which it defined as the nonmedical use of drugs that alter consciousness in ways that "are considered by social norms and defined by statute [as] inappropriate, undesirable, harmful . . . or culture-alien" (cited in Zinberg, 1984:39). But most of these terms were normative, not scientific, and the definition itself was marked by a revealing circularity: lawmakers justify laws against drug abuse in terms of medical evidence, but here the medical experts framed their definition of drug abuse in terms of laws.

This repeated redrawing of the definitional boundaries of addiction is one reason for the essential elasticity of addiction-as-disease, which is evidenced by the extraordinary range of phenomena to which it has been applied. The disease of addiction is now used to describe not merely the habitual use of alcohol and other drugs but the over- and underconsumption of food, gambling, shopping, credit card use, sex, love, attachment to and need for other people ("co-dependency" [Rice, 1992, 1996]), and even shades into forms of obsessive-compulsive disorder such as pulling out one's hair (tricotillomania), a form of addictive disease for which there are treatment and recovery centers (Reinarman, 1995).

Finally, the currently dominant definition of addiction-as-disease derives from a series of criteria listed in the *Diagnostic and Statistical Manual* (DSM) published by the American Psychiatric Association. To be diagnosed as having what is now termed "dependence," a drug user must meet any three of seven criteria that range from vague and context-dependent behavioral indicators such as using more of a drug than intended to classical tolerance and withdrawal. One commonsense indicator that is also a key DSM-IV criterion is persistent use despite harmful consequences, but this too is problematic. Such harms are not always present in habitual users and even when present are not always attributable to drug use alone. Many of the harms taken as key indicators of addiction are not caused directly by repeated use of a drug; rather they are a function of the *interaction* between the various characteristics of users' psychological sets and those of the social settings of use (e.g., deviant subcultures that arose under and are sustained by prohibitionist policies), the relative social stability or marginalization of the user, as well as dosage, chronicity of use, and other more standard variables, which are themselves influenced by such sets and settings (Zinberg, 1984).

Despite this long history of conceptual acrobatics, the complexities of drug-using behaviors continue to defy rigorous categorization under the heading of addiction-as-disease. After decades of diligent scientific labor, we still await a truly uniform set of symptoms and a distinct site, source, and course of pathology that are necessary and sufficient for the presence of the disease of addiction. In this sense, addiction-as-disease may be a little like the Loch Ness Monster: the indigenous faithful swear they have seen it and know exactly what it looks like, but skeptical outsiders have seen only shadows of something for which they have no more compelling explanation available.

Nonetheless, this definition of addiction-as-disease using the flexible DSM-IV diagnostic criteria has been widely adopted.

Addiction as a Political-Institutional Accomplishment

In the United States, the temperance movement and the early alcohol prohibitionists had claimed throughout the nineteenth and into the twentieth century that the evil was in the bottle (Levine, 1978), that all who touched alcoholic beverages were vulnerable to addiction. By the time the Prohibition amendment was repealed in 1932, however, it had become clear once again that most people drank in moderation and did not become drunks. The temperance crusaders and prohibitionists had lost credibility; a new formulation was needed. In 1935, a new lay organization of former "drunks," Alcoholics Anonymous (AA), took one of the first steps toward the modern version of addiction-as-disease. AA drew a clear "distinction between the alcoholic and the non-alcoholic" in these terms:

If, when you honestly want to, you find you cannot quit entirely, or if when drinking, you have little control over the amount you take, you are probably an alcoholic. If that be the case, you may be suffering from an illness which only a spiritual experience will conquer. (Alcoholics Anonymous, 1976:44)

A key principle in AA was the importance of reaching out and providing support to other alcoholics, which helped spread the disease concept. As noted earlier, the AA model was subsequently adopted by dozens of offshoots, some concerned with other forms of drug use (Narcotics Anonymous, Cocaine Anonymous), others having nothing to do with drugs (Sex and Love Addicts Anonymous, Shopaholics Anonymous).

In 1942, the alcoholism movement was founded by Marty Mann, a public relations executive and former "drunk," and others. By 1944, she joined with Dr. E. M. Jellinek at Yale to create an organization whose purpose was to popularize the disease concept by putting it on a scientific footing. Note the chronology: science was not the source of the concept but a resource for promoting it. This organization later became the National Council on Alcoholism (NCA). Its goal was to create a new "scientific" approach that would allow it to get beyond the old, moralistic "wet" versus "dry" battle lines of the temperance and Prohibition period (Roizen, 1991). While there were a few scientists doing research on alcohol in the 1930s, the bulk of the scientific research that Mann and her allies hoped would be the basis for their new disease concept had not yet been done. Indeed, they hoped the NCA would generate contributions needed to fund that research. The 1942 "manifesto" of the alcoholism movement clearly stated that they sought to "inculcate" into public opinion the idea that alcoholics were "sick," and therefore "not responsible" for their drinking and its consequences, and were thus deserving of medical treatment (Anderson, 1942; Roizen, 1991; Room & Collins, 1983).

As Schneider (1978) among others has shown, AA, the Yale Center for Alcohol Studies, and the National Council on Alcoholism provided the institutional foundation on which the disease concept of alcoholism was constructed. All of them attempted to shape public opinion and public policy to accept the disease concept. By the early 1970s, the movement had succeeded in persuading the U.S. government to spin off from the National Institute of Mental Health an autonomous National Institute of Alcohol Abuse and Alcoholism, which for the first time gave the disease of alcoholism the official imprimatur of the state and a large research funding base. This in turn gave crucial institutional support, political legitimacy, and cultural momentum to the more general concept of addiction-as-disease.

Other institutions have played supporting roles in promulgating the disease concept. Since the 1980s, drug courts have adopted addiction-as-disease as the core rationale for sentencing drug offenders into treatment (on penalty of prison). They have since been joined by the strange bedfellow of the drug policy reform movement, which has found it politically useful to rely, implicitly or explicitly, upon the disease model in order to pass ballot initiatives mandating treatment instead of jail (e.g., in Arizona and California). This endorsement of addiction-as-disease by the leading critics of national drug policy has further broadened its cultural currency.

A final institution warrants brief mention here: the mass media. The countless temperance tales that appeared in pulp fiction form in the nineteenth century depicted drunks as powerless before alcohol. In the early twentieth century, the so-called yellow journalism of the Hearst newspapers included hundreds of ruin-and-redemption stories that exaggerated the evils of drink and drugs. Early films like *The Dividend* and *Man with the Golden Arm* used the same stock depictions. More recently, there have been numerous studies of how the news media have created or abetted various drug scares that construct chemical bogymen of one sort or another, nearly all such scares implying that addiction-as-disease was the inevitable and tragic result of use of the demon drug du jour (e.g., Becker, 1963; Brecher, 1972; Gusfield, 1963; Lindesmith, 1947, 1965; Reeves & Campbell, 1994; Reinarman & Levine, 1989, 1997).

Most recently, the Oscar-winning film *Traffic* took the arguably courageous step of asserting that the drug war has not worked and was unlikely ever to do so. But the director apparently felt that in order to make this controversial point acceptable to mass American audiences, it was necessary to employ a traditional drug scare narrative. In the film, a fictional drug czar's daughter—an upper-middle-class, top-ranked student with all manner of healthy involvements in school, sports, and the community—smokes some cannabis and a few scenes later is a heroin addict having sex with a gun-wielding African American drug dealer. In the film's denouement, she is shown with her father and mother in a Twelve Step meeting reciting the scripted text of recovery: admitting that she is powerless before her addictive disease.

I do not mean to suggest that affluent, accomplished youth with extraordinary life chances *never* find themselves in trouble with drugs, only that such a caricatured depiction inverts the well-known probabilities regarding what sorts of people under what sorts of conditions are most likely to end up in that situation or suffer its worst consequences. Whether news or film, the media tend to frame their addiction stories as if it is a disease that "can happen to anyone." This is true enough as far as it goes, but it ignores all the sociological variables that make such an outcome far less likely for such a privileged person. As Best (1999) shows, the it-can-happen-to-anyone frame is preferred by the media not because it is statistically accurate but because it attracts the broadest interest in the story and thus the largest market share of audience.

Addiction as an Interactional Accomplishment

In his seminal 1953 article, "Becoming a Marijuana User," Becker showed that the marijuana high did not result from the mere mechanical ingestion of the smoke but had to be learned in interaction with experienced users. Much the same may be said for addiction-as-disease. There are at least two processes involved in becoming a person who is afflicted with addiction-as-disease. First, there is what might be called the *pedagogical* process, in which addicts-to-be learn the lexicon of disease and recovery from counselors, therapists, judges, probation and parole officers, treatment providers, and other addicts (see Phillips, 1990; Rapping, 1996; Reinarman, 1995). They are taught to retrospectively reinterpret their lives and behavior in terms of addiction-as-disease.

As Weinberg shows in rich ethnographic detail, those drawn or forced into a treatment setting are typically required to "admit that they suffer from a disease that prevents them from controlling their drug use." Since many are at first reluctant to make such an admission, the initial therapeutic objective becomes "break[ing] down the putative denial that keeps the addicted person . . . unconsciously complicit with his or her disease." And to accomplish this, "a good deal of treatment discourse is taken up with inducing and offering confessions of the depths to which one's disease has forced one to sink" (Weinberg, 2000:611). Rice similarly shows that the group processes of Codependents Anonymous function to induce members to "select [codependency, or the disease of being addicted to other people] as a narrative of their lives to acquire a new and more satisfying sense of identity" (1992:338; see also Rice, 1996). In effect, the accounts that putative "addicts" give of their behaviors are not naturally occurring, objective descriptions of an unambiguous reality. Rather, accounts that get accepted as adequate, that is, those that begin with the admission of "addiction," are produced when the messy details of life histories are organized by the discursive procedures (e.g., typification) applied in social control and therapeutic settings (cf. Zimmerman, 1969).

Second, almost immediately there is the *performative* process, in which addicts tell and retell their newly reconstituted life stories according to the grammatical and syntactical rules of disease discourse that they have come to learn. In so doing, they not only spread the word (e.g., "carry this message to other" addicts) but also help to "save" themselves from relapsing back "into" their "disease."

One can observe these processes in almost any Twelve Step meeting, in most treatment programs, and even on a syndicated cable television show called *The Recovery Network*. In one recent broadcast of *The Recovery Network*, for example, a "recovering addict" explained his savagely bad behavior as "my disease talking." Likewise, a member of the treatment group observed by Weinberg rhetorically distanced himself from his own addicted self and past behavior by means of disease discourse: "When I was out there in my addiction, I fucked over a lot of people" (2000:611).

In this sense, as Davies (1992) suggests, addiction-as-disease is functional for the now-"recovering" addict in that it provides a narrative that allows him or her simultaneously to "own" and yet disown deviant acts committed while addicted. In this manner, they admit the sins of the old addicted self while laying claim to a new self-in-the-making. The etiology implicit in such disease discourse shares certain similarities in logical structure with seventeenth-century theological narratives in which demonic possession was thought to be causal; in disease discourse, addiction is a kind of "secular possession" (Room, 2004:231). In each case, an exogenous force or foreign agent ("the devil," "the disease") is held to be the effective cause of the individual's bad behavior.

It should also be noted that once "in recovery," such "addicts" are often called upon to speak in the community, in schools, and in the media as experts on addiction. Their accounts are afforded respect, legitimacy, and authority because they have "been there."[2] This completes the loop and conceals, like a good magic trick, the actual procedures by which it was accomplished.

What about the Lived Experience of Problematic Drug Use?
The notion that addiction-as-disease is a historically and culturally specific social construction and political accomplishment should not be taken to mean that the lived experience of what is called addiction is therefore somehow less "real," less powerful, or less deserving of attention. The related critiques noted earlier to the effect that the physiological-pharmacological dimension of what is called addiction has been overemphasized and is not the sufficient cause of addiction does not imply that pharmacology and physiology are unimportant parts of the puzzle that is called addiction. Users decide to ingest drugs in part because they are psychoactive, consciousness-altering chemicals that make us feel different in some way (Room & Collins, 1983:v–vi). But again, this material substratum where molecules meet receptor sites cannot by itself explain drug-using behaviors. Regular ingestion may or may not lead to the sorts of habitual or problematic use patterns that diseasists call addiction, and even physiological dependence may or may not lead to desperate "junkie" behavior that is so often taken as a clear indicator of the disease.

What are taken to be physiological-pharmacological effects do not present themselves to users in some raw, precategorical form, without the linguistic encasements provided prior to ingestion by culture. Becker (1967), Weil (1972), Davies (1992), and others have shown that the subjective effects reported by drug users are produced in important part by users' active interpretation of the often ambiguous physiological cues produced by ingestion of a drug. Such interpretations are assembled from the conceptual categories available in culture. The particular features of and the meanings attributed to drug experiences, as well as the behavior thought to follow from them, are culturally specific. For example, MacAndrew and Edgerton's (1969) pioneering cross-cultural research on drunken behavior demonstrated that people come to understand their experience of altered states—and learn how to behave in those states—from their culture. As Peele has argued, the cultural belief that "alcohol has the power to addict a person goes hand in hand with more alcoholism"

(1989:170). Conversely, cultures in which people do not believe drugs can cause the "loss of control" exhibit very little of it. But just because "loss of control" is as much a cultural construct as a physiological fact should not be taken to imply that users' *feelings* of "loss of control" are any less acute.

Most of those who get defined as addicts and come to adopt the addict identity (especially in treatment and/or recovery) find that addiction-as-disease resonates with their experience. This suggests that there is a reasonable cognitive fit between the discourse of disease and their experience of drug use. But such resonance and cognitive fit are matters of culture too, not an external validation of the concept of addiction-as-disease. The question of which came first, phenomenological experience or the cultural-cognitive frameworks available for making sense of it, is, like the proverbial chicken and egg question to which it is cousin, very difficult to disentangle. From birth, human beings are raised inside their culture, and there is no simple way to separate their lived experience from the discursive practices operating in that culture which name it and give it specific shape and valence.

Discussion: Disease as a Double-Edged Sword

In this article, I have tried to sketch some of the processes by which addiction-as-disease was socially constructed and made culturally available as a framework for understanding drinking, drug use, and other behaviors involving self-regulation, and how this framework then gets inscribed upon lived experience. If this disease discourse was only a rhetorical strategy for gaining the right to various services for people who need them, as most proponents of addiction-as-disease claim, then all this might not matter much. But addiction-as-disease has been put to other, arguably less noble uses.

In 1975, British historian E. P. Thompson wrote *Whigs and Hunters*, a book about the origins of the Black Act, a law passed without debate by the English Parliament in the early eighteenth century. This strange law created some fifty new capital offenses, including traditional practices of foresters like hunting, fishing, gathering wood in royal forests, and especially painting one's face black in disguise to be able to get away with these activities. It seems that the ruling Whig government found such agrarian rule breaking to be a form of dissent that threatened the "delicate structure of patronage" on which the legitimacy of the English state then depended (Sutton, 2001:90). Walpole and company needed the support of officers, courtiers, and other newly moneyed types to whom the Crown had given large swaths of the common forests as deer parks and country estates. The Black Act was a harsh overreaction that was vitiated in its administration and thus remained largely ineffectual. But it was intended to serve as a weapon in defense of the Whig regime at a precarious moment in England's transition from feudalism to capitalism. In the cool, clear light of retrospect, it is easier to see that the excessive punitiveness of this law undermined the very legitimacy it was designed to buttress.

How will twentieth-century U.S. drug laws be read a century or two into the new millennium? Since the 1980s, the United State has imprisoned a higher proportion of its citizens than any other nation, and drug offenses have been the largest single category of crimes in what has been the most massive wave of imprisonment in U.S. history. Those who have ended up behind bars for drug offenses are overwhelmingly poor people and people of color. Many leading judges, high officials from closely allied nations, and a growing chorus of international human rights organizations look upon the U.S. drug war and imprisonment wave of 1986–2003 as not only ineffective but inhumane and unjust. And in response to the many cries for reform, the reply in congressional hearings, in medical science conferences, and on television talk shows has been to invoke the dreaded "disease of addiction" as justification.

Addiction-as-disease, then, is something of a double-edged sword. When attached to sympathetic (Betty Ford) or well-connected (Rush Limbaugh) individuals, it becomes part of the larger, positive gestalt surrounding them. But when addiction-as-disease gets attached to less reputable individuals ("street junkies," "ghetto crackheads"), it becomes part of a larger, very negative gestalt. Thus, the disease concept sometimes serves as a humane warrant for the right of access to services, but it also serves, paradoxically, as a key justification for punitive prohibition. It is at least partly on the grounds of avoiding or reducing this dread "disease" that the U.S. government passes and enforces a modern American version of the Black Act, and then pressures other governments and the United Nations to follow their example (Bewley-Taylor, 1999; Levine, 2003).

The discourse of disease may have potentially progressive effects insofar as it has helped trigger a shift of gaze in which drug use comes to be seen as properly belonging in the realm of public health rather than criminal law. But addiction-as-disease has just as often been a discursive weapon wielded by a state that has declared war upon citizens who ingest disapproved substances. It is a weapon that helps to justify—*"for their own good"*—the suspension of the Bill of Rights under what the Supreme Court openly calls "the drug exception" and the mass incarceration of the powerless.

Notes

1. For an insightful analysis of these processes of redefinition, see Woolgar and Pawluch's (1985) discussion of "ontological gerrymandering."

2. Ethan Nadelmann has suggested that the media asking addicts to serve as experts on drug use is rather like asking those who have gone bankrupt to serve as experts on business.

References

Aharon, I., Etcoff, N., Ariely, D., Chabris, C., O'Connor, E., & Breiter, H. C. (2001). Beautiful faces have variable reward value: fMRI and behavioral evidence. *Neuron, 32,* 537–551.

Alcoholics Anonymous. (1976). *Alcoholics Anonymous: The story of how many thousands of men and women have recovered from alcoholism* (3rd ed.). New York: Alcoholics Anonymous World Services.

Anderson, D. (1942). Alcohol and public opinion. *Quarterly Journal of Studies on Alcohol, 3*(3), 376–392.

Angier, N. (2002). Why we're nice: The feel-good factor. *International Herald Tribune,* July 25, 2002, p. 8.

Becker, H. S. (1953). Becoming a marijuana user. *American Journal of Sociology, 59,* 235–242.

Becker, H. S. (1963). *Outsiders: Studies in the sociology of deviance.* New York: Free Press.

Becker, H. S. (1967). History, culture, and subjective experience: An exploration of the social bases of drug-induced experiences. *Journal of Health and Social Behavior, 8,* 162–176.

Bertram, E., Blachman, M., Sharp, K., & Andreas, P. (1996). *Drug war politics: The price of denial.* Berkeley: University of California Press.

Best, J. (1999). *Random violence: How we talk about new crimes and new victims.* Berkeley: University of California Press.

Bewley-Taylor, D. R. (1999). *The United States and international drug control, 1909–1997.* London: Pinter.

Blackwell, J. S. (1983). Drifting, controlling, and overcoming: Opiate users who avoid becoming chronically dependent. *Journal of Drug Issues, 13,* 219–236.

Blackwell, J. S. (1985). Opiate dependence as a psychophysical event: Users' reports of subjective experience. *Contemporary Drug Problems, 12,* 331–350.

Blakeslee, S. (2002). Hijacking the brain circuits with a nickel slot machine. *New York Times,* Feb. 19, 2002, p. D1.

Brecher, E. M. (1972). *Licit and illicit drugs*. Boston, MA: Little, Brown.

Brody, A., et al. (2001). Regional brain metabolic changes in patients with major depression treated with either paroxetine or interpersonal therapy. *Archives of General Psychiatry, 58*, 631–640.

Burke, P. (1978). *Popular culture in early modern Europe*. New York: Harper and Row.

Christie, N., & Bruun, K. (1968). The conceptual framework. In M. Keller & T. C. Coffey (Eds.), *Proceedings of the 28th International Congress on Alcohol and Alcoholism* (Vol. 2, pp. 65–73). Highland Park, NJ: Hillhouse Press.

Cohen, P. (2000). Is the addiction doctor the voodoo priest of Western man? *Addiction Research and Theory, 8*, 589–598.

Davies, J. B. (1992). *The myth of addiction: An application of the psychological theory of attribution to illicit drug use*. Chur, Switzerland: Harwood.

Davies, J. B. (1997). *Drugspeak: The analysis of drug discourse*. Reading, England: Harwood.

Eagleton, T. (1991). *Ideology*. London: Verso.

Enos, G. (2004). The future of addiction services: It's in the science. *Addiction Professional, 2*(6), 17–21.

Fingarette, H. (1988). *Heavy drinking: The myth of alcoholism as a disease*. Berkeley: University of California Press.

Goleman, D. (1989). Biology of brain may hold key for gamblers. *New York Times*, October 5, 1989, p. B1.

Gusfield, J. (1963). *Symbolic crusade: Status politics and the American temperance movement*. Urbana: University of Illinois Press.

Hanson, B., Beschner, G., Walters, J., & Bovelle, E. (Eds.). (1985). *Life with heroin: Voices from the inner city*. Lexington, MA: Health.

Kolata, G. (2002). Runner's high? Endorphins? Fiction, some scientists say. *New York Times*, May 21, 2002, p. D1.

Leshner, A. I. (1997). Addiction is a brain disease, and it matters. *Science, 278*, 45–57.

Leshner, A. I. (2001). Countering abuse and addiction with information audiences can use. *Nida Notes, 16*(4), 4–5.

Levine, H. G. (1978). The discovery of addiction: Changing conceptions of habitual drunkenness in America. *Journal of Studies on Alcohol, 39*, 143–174.

Levine, H. G. (2003). Global drug prohibition: Its uses and crises. *International Journal on Drug Policy, 14*, 145–153.

Lindesmith, A. R. (1947). *Opiate addiction*. Evanston, IL: Principia Publishers.

Lindesmith, A. R. (1965). *The addict and the law*. Bloomington: Indiana University Press.

MacAndrew, C., & Edgerton, R. (1969). *Drunken Comportment*. Chicago, IL: Aldine.

Mills, C. W. (1940). Situated actions and vocabularies of motive. *American Sociological Review, 5*, 904–913.

Moles, A., Kieffer, B. L., & D'Amato, F. R. (2004). Deficit in attachment behavior in mice lacking the mu-opiod receptor gene. *Science, 304*(5679), 1983–1986.

Morgan, J. P., & Zimmer, L. (1997). The social pharmacology of smokeable cocaine. In C. Reinarman & H. G. Levine (Eds.), *Crack in America: Demon drugs and social justice* (pp. 131–170). Berkeley: University of California Press.

Nestler, E. J., & Malenka, R. C. (2004). The addicted brain. *Scientific American, 290*(3), 78–85.

Peele, S. (1989). *Diseasing of America: Addiction treatment out of control.* Lexington, MA: Lexington Books.

Phillips, M. D. (1990). *Breaking the code: Toward a lexicon of recovery.* Paper presented at the Kettil Bruun Society Alcohol Epidemiology Meetings, Budapest.

Prebble, E., & Casey, J. H. (1969). Taking care of business: The heroin user's life on the street. *International Journal of the Addictions, 4,* 1–24.

Rapping, E. (1996). *The culture of recovery.* Boston, MA: Beacon Press.

Reeves, J. L., & Campbell, R. (1994). *Cracked coverage: Television news, the anti-cocaine crusade, and the Reagan legacy.* Durham, NC: Duke University Press.

Reinarman, C. (1995). Twelve-step movements and advanced capitalist culture: On the politics of self-control in postmodernity. In M. Darnovsky, B. Epstein, & R. Flacks (Eds.), *Cultural politics and social movements* (pp. 90–109). Philadelphia, PA: Temple University Press.

Reinarman, C., & Levine, H. G. (1989). Crack in context: Politics and media in the making of a drug scare. *Contemporary Drug Problems, 16,* 535–577.

Reinarman, C., Waldorf, D., & Murphy, S. (1994). Pharmacology is not destiny: The contingent character of cocaine abuse and addiction. *Addiction Research, 2,* 21–36.

Reinarman, C., Waldorf, D., Murphy, S., & Levine, H. G. (1997). The contingent call of the pipe: Bingeing and addiction among heavy cocaine smokers. In C. Reinarman & H. G. Levine (Eds.), *Crack in America: Demon drugs and social justice* (pp. 77–97). Berkeley: University of California Press.

Reinarman, C., & Levine, H. G. (1997). Crack in context: America's latest drug demon. In C. Reinarman & H. G. Levine (Eds.), *Crack in America: Demon drugs and social justice* (pp. 1–17). Berkeley: University of California Press.

Rice, J. S. (1992). Discursive formation, life stories, and the emergence of co-dependency. *Sociological Quarterly, 33,* 337–364.

Rice, J. S. (1996). *A disease of one's own: Psychotherapy, addiction, and the emergence of co-dependency.* New Brunswick, NJ: Transaction Publishers.

Roizen, R. (1991). *The American discovery of alcoholism, 1933–1939.* PhD dissertation, University of California, Berkeley.

Room, R. (1983). Sociological aspects of the disease concept of alcoholism. *Research Advances in Alcohol and Drug Problems, 7,* 47–91.

Room, R. (1991). Cultural changes in drinking and trends in alcohol problems indicators: Recent U.S. experience. In W. Clark & M. Hilton (Eds.), *Alcohol in America: Drinking practices and problems* (pp. 149–162). Albany: State University of New York Press.

Room, R. (2004). The cultural framing of addiction. *Janus Head, 6*(2), 221–234.

Room, R., & Collins, G. (1983). *Alcohol and disinhibition: The nature and meaning of the link* (National Institute of Alcoholism and Alcohol Abuse, Research Monograph 12). Washington, DC: U.S. Department of Health and Human Services.

Schneider, J. (1978). Deviant drinking as disease: Alcoholism as a social accomplishment. *Social Problems, 25*, 361–372.

Seeley, J. R. (1962). Alcoholism is a disease: Implications for social policy. In D. J. Pittman & C. R. Snyder (Eds.), *Society, culture, and drinking patterns* (pp. 586–593). New York: Wiley.

Shaffer, H. J., & Jones, S. B. (1989). *Quitting cocaine: The struggle against impulse*. Lexington, MA: Lexington Books.

Sutton, J. R. (2001). *Law/society*. Thousand Oaks, CA: Sage.

Thompson, E. P. (1975). *Whigs and hunters: The origins of the Black Act*. New York: Pantheon.

Valverde, M. (1998). *Diseases of the will: Alcohol and the dilemmas of freedom*. Cambridge, UK: Cambridge University Press.

Volkow, N. (2003). The addicted brain: Why such poor decisions? *Nida Notes, 18*, 3–4.

Waldorf, D. (1973). *Careers in dope*. Englewood Cliffs, NJ: Prentice Hall.

Weil, A. (1972). *The natural mind*. Boston, MA: Houghton Mifflin.

Weinberg, D. (2000). "Out there": The ecology of addiction in drug abuse treatment discourse. *Social Problems, 47*, 606–621.

Woolgar, S., & Pawluch, D. (1985). Ontological gerrymandering: The anatomy of social problems explanations. *Social Problems, 32*, 214–227.

Zimmerman, D. H. (1969). Fact as practical accomplishment. In S. Wheeler (Ed.), *On record: Files and dossiers in American life* (pp. 319–354). New York: Russell Sage Foundation.

Zinberg, N. E. (1984). *Drug, set, and setting: The basis for controlled intoxicant use*. New Haven, CT: Yale University Press.

13

The Ethics of Addiction

Thomas S. Szasz

Much of my work during the past fifteen years has been devoted to showing that for the most part, psychiatric problems are not medical but moral problems (1–3). Almost nowhere is this now more obvious than in the case of addiction, yet almost nowhere is the moral perspective now more vehemently rejected and the medical perspective more ardently embraced.

Lest we take for granted that we know what "drug addiction" or "drug abuse" is, let me begin with a definition of it.

Webster's Third New International Dictionary (unabridged) defines addiction as "the compulsory uncontrolled use of habit-forming drugs beyond the period of medical need or under conditions harmful to society." This definition imputes lack of self-control to the addict over his taking or not taking a drug, a dubious proposition at best; at the same time, by classifying an act as an addiction according to whether it harms society, it offers a moral definition of an ostensibly medical condition.

Likewise, the currently popular term *drug abuse* places this behavior squarely in the category of ethics, for it is ethics that deals with the right and wrong uses of man's power and possessions.

Clearly, drug addiction and drug abuse cannot be defined without specifying the proper and improper uses of certain pharmacologically active agents. The regular administration of morphine by a physician to a patient dying of cancer is the paradigm of the proper use of a narcotic, whereas even its occasional self-administration by a physically healthy person for the purpose of "pharmacological pleasure" is the paradigm of drug abuse.

I submit that these judgments have nothing whatsoever to do with medicine, pharmacology, or psychiatry. They are moral judgments. Indeed, our present views on addiction are astonishingly similar to some of our former views on sex. Intercourse in marriage with the aim of procreation was the paradigm of the proper use of one's sexual organs, whereas intercourse outside of marriage with the aim of carnal pleasure was the paradigm of their improper use. Moreover, until recently masturbation—or self-abuse as it was called—was professionally declared to be, and popularly accepted as, both the cause and the symptom of a variety of illnesses.

To be sure, it is now virtually impossible to cite a contemporary American (or foreign) medical authority to support the concept of self-abuse. Medical opinion now holds that there is simply no such thing, that whether a person masturbates or not is medically irrelevant, and that engaging in the practice or refraining from it is a matter of personal morals or lifestyle. On the other hand, it is now virtually impossible to cite a contemporary American (or foreign) medical authority to oppose the concept of drug abuse. Medical opinion now holds that drug abuse is a major medical, psychiatric, and public health problem; that drug addiction is a disease similar to diabetes, requiring prolonged (or life-long) and careful medically supervised treatment; and that taking or not taking drugs is primarily, if not solely, a matter of medical concern and responsibility.

The Bases of Our Drug Laws

Like any other social policy, our drug laws may be examined from two entirely different points of view: technical and moral. Our present inclination, however, is either to ignore the moral perspective or to mistake the technical for the moral.

An example of our misplaced overreliance on a technical analysis of the so-called drug problem is the professionalized mendacity about the dangerousness of certain types of drugs. Since most of the propaganda against drug abuse seeks to justify certain repressive policies by appeals to the alleged dangerousness of various drugs, the propagandists often must, in order to enlist significant support, falsify the facts about the true pharmacological properties of the drugs they seek to prohibit. They must do so for two reasons: (1) because there are too many substances in daily use that are just as harmful as, if indeed they are not more harmful than, the substances they want to prohibit, and (2) because they realize that dangerousness alone can *never* be a sufficient justification for prohibiting any drug, substance, or artifact. Thus, the more they ignore the moral dimensions of the problem, the more they must escalate their fraudulent claims about the dangers of drugs.

Clearly, the argument that marijuana—or heroin, or methadone, or morphine—is prohibited because it is addictive or dangerous cannot be supported by facts. For one thing, there are many drugs—from insulin to penicillin—that are neither addictive nor dangerous but are neverthe-less also prohibited: they can be obtained only through a physician's prescription. For another, there are many things—from dynamite to guns—that are much more dangerous than narcotics (especially to others!) but that are not prohibited.

As everyone knows, it is still possible in the United States to walk into a store and walk out with a shotgun. We enjoy this right not because we do not believe that guns are dangerous, but because we believe even more strongly that civil liberties are precious. (It also so happens that historical precedent favors those who want to preserve this right, not those who want to abolish it.) At the same time it is not possible in the United States to walk into a store and walk out with a bottle of barbiturates, codeine, or other drug. We are deprived of this right (which the citizens of some other countries, such as Lebanon, enjoy) because we have come to value medical paternalism more highly than the right to obtain and use drugs without recourse to medical intermediaries.

In short, our so-called drug abuse problem is an integral part of our present social ethic, which accepts "protections" and repressions justified by appeals to health similar to those that medieval societies accepted when they were justified by appeals to faith. The problem of drug abuse (as we now know it) is one of the inevitable consequences of the medical monopoly over drugs, a monopoly whose value is daily acclaimed by science and law, state and church, the professions and the laity. As for-merly the Church regulated man's relations to God, so Medicine now regulates his relations to his body. Deviation from the rules set forth by the Church was then considered heresy and was punished by appropriate theological sanctions, called penance; deviation from the rules set forth by Medicine is now considered drug abuse (or some sort of "mental illness") and is punished by appropriate medical sanctions, called treatment.

The problem of drug abuse will thus be with us so long as we live under medical tutelage. This is not to say that if all access to drugs were free, some people would not medicate themselves in ways that might upset us or harm them. That, of course, is precisely what happened when religious practices became free.

Legitimizing Social Policies

To command adherence, social policy must be respected, and to be respected, it must be considered legitimate. In our society, there are two principal sources of legitimacy: tradition and science.

Time is a supreme ethical arbiter. Whatever a social practice might be, if people engage in it, generation after generation, then that practice becomes accepted not only as necessary but also as good. Slavery is an example.

Many opponents of illegal drugs thus admit that tobacco may be more harmful to health than marijuana; nevertheless, they urge that smoking tobacco should be legal but smoking marijuana should not be, because the former habit is socially accepted while the latter is not. This is a perfectly reasonable argument. But let us understand it for what it is: a plea for legitimizing old and accepted practices and for illegitimizing novel and unaccepted ones. It is a justification that rests on precedence, not on evidence.

The other basis for legitimizing policy, increasingly more important in the modern world, is science. In matters of health—a vast and increasingly elastic category—physicians thus play important roles not only as healers, but also as legitimizers and as illegitimizers. One result is that, regardless of the pharmacological effects of a drug on the person who takes it, if he obtains it through a physician and uses it under medical supervision, that use is ipso facto legitimate and proper, but if he obtains it through nonmedical channels and uses it without medical supervision (and especially if the drug is illegal and the individual uses it solely for the purpose of altering his mental state), then that use is ipso facto illegitimate and improper. In short, being medicated by a doctor is drug use, while self-medication (especially with certain classes of drugs) is drug abuse.

Again, it is perfectly reasonable to insist on such an arrangement. But let us understand it for what it is: a plea for legitimizing what doctors do, because they do it with "good therapeutic" intent, and for illegitimizing what laymen do, because they do it with bad self-abusive ("masturbatory") intent. This justification rests on the principle of professionalism, not of pharmacology. Hence it is that we applaud the systematic medical use of methadone and call it "treatment for heroin addiction," but decry the occasional nonmedical use of marijuana and call it "dangerous drug abuse."

Our present concept of drug abuse thus articulates and symbolizes a fundamental policy of Scientific Medicine: namely, that a layman should not medicate his own body but should place its medical care under the supervision of a duly accredited physician. Before the Reformation, the practice of True Christianity rested on a similar policy: namely, that a layman should not himself commune with God but should place his spiritual care under the supervision of a duly accredited priest.

The self-interests of the Church and of Medicine in such policies are obvious enough. What might be less obvious is the interest of the laity in them: by delegating responsibility for the spiritual and medical welfare of the people to a class of authoritatively accredited specialists, these policies—and the practices they ensure—relieve individuals from assuming the burdens of these responsibilities for themselves. As I see it, then, our present problems with drug use and drug abuse are among the consequences of our pervasive ambivalence about personal autonomy and responsibility.

Luther's chief heresy was to remove the priest as intermediary between man and God, giving the former direct access to the latter. He also demystified the language in which man could henceforth address God, approving for this purpose what until then had significantly been called the "vulgar" tongue. But perhaps it is true that familiarity breeds contempt: Protestantism was not just a new form of Christianity, but the beginning of its end, at least as it had been known until then.

I propose a medical reformation analogous to the Protestant Reformation, specifically a "protest" against the systematic mystification of man's relationship to his body and his professionalized separation from it. The immediate aim of this reform would be to remove the physician as intermediary between man and his body and to give the layman direct access to the language and contents of the pharmacopoeia. It is significant that until recently, physicians wrote prescriptions in Latin and that medical diagnoses and treatments are still couched in a jargon whose chief aim is to awe and mystify the laity. Were man to have unencumbered access to his own body and the means of chemically altering it, it would spell the end of Medicine, at least as we now know it. This is why, with faith in Scientific Medicine so strong, there is little interest in this kind of medical reform: physicians fear the loss of their privileges; laymen, the loss of their protections.

Our present policies with respect to drug use and drug abuse thus constitute a covert plea for legitimizing certain privileges on the part of physicians and for illegitimizing certain practices on the part of everyone else. The upshot is that we act as if we believed that only doctors should be allowed to dispense narcotics, just as we used to believe that only priests should be allowed to dispense absolution.

Fortunately, however, we do not yet live in a technically perfected world. Our technical approach to the "drug problem" has thus led, and will undoubtedly continue to lead, to some curious attempts to combat it.

In one such attempt, the American government is now pressuring Turkey to restrict its farmers from growing poppy (the source of morphine and heroin) (4). If turnabout is fair play, perhaps we should expect the Turkish government to pressure the United States to restrict its farmers from growing corn and wheat. Or should we assume that Muslims have enough self-control to leave alcohol alone, but that Christians need all the controls politicians, policemen, and physicians, both native and foreign, can bring to bear on them to enable them to leave opiates alone?

In another such attempt, the California Civil Liberties Union has recently sued to enforce a paroled heroin addict's "right to methadone maintenance treatment" (5). In this view, the addict has more rights than the nonaddict: for the former, methadone supplied at taxpayer's expense is a "'right"; for the latter, methadone supplied at his own expense is evidence of addiction.

The Right of Self-Medication

I believe that just as we regard freedom of speech and religion as fundamental rights, so should we also regard freedom of self-medication as a fundamental right, and instead of mendaciously opposing or mindlessly promoting illicit drugs, we should, paraphrasing Voltaire, adopt as our position: "I disapprove of what you take, but I will defend to the death your right to take it."

However, like most other rights, the right of self-medication should apply only to adults, and it should not be an unqualified right. Since these qualifications are important it is necessary to specify their precise range.

John Stuart Mill said (approximately) that a person's right to swing his arm ends where his neighbor's nose begins. Likewise, the limiting condition with respect to self-medication should be the inflicting of actual (as against symbolic) harm on others.

Our present practices with respect to alcohol embody and reflect this individualistic ethic. We have the right to buy, possess, and consume alcoholic beverages. Regardless of how offensive drunkenness might be to a person, he cannot interfere with another person's right to become inebriated so long as that person drinks in the privacy of his own home or at some other appropriate location, and so long as the drinker conducts himself in an otherwise law-abiding manner. In short, we have a right to be intoxicated—in private. Public intoxication is considered an offense against others and is therefore a violation of the criminal law.

The right to self-medication should be hedged in by similar limits. "Public intoxication," not only with alcohol but with any other drug, should be an offense punishable by the criminal law. Furthermore, acts that may injure others—such as driving a car—should, when carried out in a drug-intoxicated state, be punished especially strictly and severely. The habitual use of certain drugs, such as alcohol and opiates, may also harm others indirectly by rendering the subject unmotivated for working and thus unemployed. In a society that supports the unemployed, such a person would, as a consequence of his own conduct, place a burden on the shoulders of his working neighbors. How society might best guard itself against this sort of hazard I cannot discuss here. However, it is obvious that prohibiting the use of habit-forming drugs offers no protection against this risk, but only further augments the tax burdens laid upon the productive members of society.

The right to self-medication must thus entail unqualified responsibility for the effects of one's drug-intoxicated behavior on others. Unless we are willing to hold ourselves responsible for our own behavior, and hold others responsible for theirs, the liberty to use drugs (or to engage in other acts) degenerates into a license to hurt others. Herein exactly is the catch: we are exceedingly reluctant to hold people responsible for their misbehavior; this is why we prefer diminishing rights to increasing responsibilities. The former requires only the passing of laws, which can then be more or less freely violated or circumvented, whereas the latter requires prosecuting and punishing offenders, which can be accomplished only by just laws justly enforced. The upshot is that we increasingly substitute tender-hearted tyranny for tough-spirited liberty.

Such then would be the situation of adults, were we to regard the freedom to take drugs as a fundamental right similar to the freedom to read and the freedom to worship. What would be the situation of children? Since many people who are now said to be drug addicts or drug abusers are minors, it is especially important that we think clearly about this aspect of the problem.

Children and Drugs

I *do not* believe, and I *do not* advocate, that children should have a right to ingest, inject, or otherwise use any drug or substance they want. Children do not have the right to drive, drink, vote, marry, make binding contracts, and so on; they acquire these rights at various ages, coming into their full possession at maturity (usually between the ages of eighteen and twenty-one). The right to self-medication should similarly be withheld until maturity.

In this connection, it is well to remember that children lack even such basic freedoms as the opportunity to read what they wish or worship God as they choose, freedoms we consider elementary rights for adult Americans. In these as well as other important respects, children are wholly under the jurisdiction of their parents or guardians. The disastrous fact that many parents fail to exercise proper authority over the conduct of their children does not, in my opinion, justify depriving adults of the right to engage in conduct we deem undesirable for children.

This remedy only further aggravates the situation. For if we consider it proper to prohibit the use of narcotics by adults to prevent their abuse by children, then we would also have to consider it proper to prohibit sexual intercourse, driving automobiles, piloting airplanes—indeed virtually everything!—because these activities too are likely to be abused by children.

In short, I suggest that "dangerous" drugs be treated, more or less, as alcohol is treated now. Other drugs should be as freely available as are items on the shelves of grocery stores. Neither the use of narcotics nor their possession nor their sale to adults should be prohibited, but only their sale to minors. Of course, this would result in the ready availability of all kinds of drugs among minors, though perhaps their availability would be no greater than it is now, but these drugs would be more visible and hence more easily subject to proper controls. This arrangement would place responsibility for the use of all drugs by children where it belongs: on the parents and their children. This is where the major responsibility rests for the use of alcohol. It is a tragic symptom of our refusal to take personal liberty and responsibility seriously that there appears to be no public desire to assume a similar stance toward other "dangerous" drugs.

Consider what would happen if a child should bring a bottle of gin to school and get drunk there. Would the school authorities blame the local liquor stores as pushers? Or would they blame the parents and the child himself? There is liquor in practically every home in America, and yet children rarely bring liquor to school, whereas marijuana, dexedrine, heroin, substances that children do not find in the home and whose very possession is a criminal offense, frequently find their way into the school.

Our attitude toward sexual activity provides another model for our attitude toward drugs. Although we generally discourage children below a certain age from engaging in sexual activities with others (we no longer "guard" them against masturbation), we do not prohibit such activities by law. What we do prohibit by law is the sexual seduction of children by adults. The "pharmacological seduction" of children by adults should be similarly punishable. In other words, adults who give or sell drugs to children should be regarded as offenders. Such a specific and limited prohibition—as against the kinds of generalized prohibitions that we had under the Volstead Act or have now with respect to countless drugs—would be relatively easy to enforce. Moreover, it would probably be rarely violated, for there would be little psychological interest and no economic profit in doing so. On the other hand, the use of drugs by and among children (without the direct participation of adults) should be a matter entirely outside the scope of the criminal law, just as is their engaging in drinking or sexual activities under like circumstances.

There is, of course, a fatal flaw in my proposal. Its adoption would remove minors from the ranks of our most cherished victims. We could no longer spy on them and persecute them in the name of protecting them from committing drug abuse on themselves. Hence, we cannot— indeed we shall not—abandon such therapeutic tyrannizations and treat children as young persons entitled to dignity from us and owing responsibility to us, until we are ready to cease psychiatrically oppressing children "in their own best interests."

The Fundamental Issue

Sooner or later we shall have to confront the basic moral and political issue underlying the problem of addiction (and many other problems, such as sexual activity between consenting adults, pornography, contraception, gambling, and suicide), that is, in a conflict between the individual and the state, where should the former's autonomy end and the latter's right to intervene begin?

The Declaration of Independence speaks of our inalienable right to "life, liberty, and the pursuit of happiness." How are we to interpret this? By asserting that we ought to be free to smoke tobacco but not marijuana? The Constitution and the Bill of Rights are silent on the subject of drugs, implying that the adult citizen has or ought to have the right to medicate his own body as he sees fit.

The nagging questions remain. As American citizens, do we and should we have the right to take narcotics and other drugs? Further, if we take drugs and conduct ourselves as law-abiding citizens, do we and should we have the right to remain unmolested by the government? Finally, if we take drugs and break the law, do we and should we have the right to be treated as persons accused of crime, rather than as patients accused of mental illness?

These are fundamental questions that are conspicuous by their absence from contemporary discussions of problems of drug abuse and drug addiction. In this area, as in so many others, we have allowed a moral problem to be disguised as a medical question and have then engaged in shadow-boxing with metaphoric diseases and medical attempts, ranging from the absurd to the appalling, to combat them.

References

1. Szasz, T. S. (1961). *The myth of mental illness.* New York: Harper & Row.

2. Szasz, T. S. (1970). *Ideology and insanity.* Garden City, NY: Anchor, Doubleday.

3. Szasz, T. S. (1970). *The manufacture of madness.* New York: Harper & Row.

4. Pursuit of the poppy. (1970). *Time,* September 14, 28–30.

5. CLU says addict has right to use methadone. (1970). *American Civil Liberties Union,* July, 5.

14

Myths about the Treatment of Addiction

Charles P. O'Brien and A. Thomas McLellan

Although addictions are chronic disorders, there is a tendency for most physicians and for the general public to perceive them as being acute conditions such as a broken leg or pneumococcal pneumonia. In this context, the acute-care procedure of detoxification has been thought of as appropriate "treatment." When the patient relapses, as most do sooner or later, the treatment is regarded as a failure. However, contrary to commonly held beliefs, addiction does not end when the drug is removed from the body (detoxification) or when the acute post-drug-taking illness dissipates (withdrawal). Rather, the underlying addictive disorder persists, and this persistence produces a tendency to relapse to active drug-taking. Thus, although detoxification as explained by Mattick and Hall can be successful in cleansing the person of drugs and withdrawal symptoms, detoxification does not address the underlying disorder, and thus is not adequate treatment.[1]

As we shall discuss, addictions are similar to other chronic disorders such as arthritis, hypertension, asthma, and diabetes. Addicting drugs produce changes in brain pathways that endure long after the person stops taking them. Further, the associated medical, social, and occupational difficulties that usually develop during the course of addiction do not disappear when the patient is detoxified. These protracted brain changes and the associated personal and social difficulties put the former addict at great risk of relapse. Treatments for addiction therefore should be regarded as being long term, and a "cure" is unlikely from a single course of treatment.

Is Addiction a Voluntary Disorder?

One reason that many physicians and the general public are unsympathetic toward the addict is that addiction is perceived as being self-afflicted: "they brought it on themselves." However, there are numerous involuntary components in the addictive process, even in the early stages. Although the choice to try a drug for the first time is voluntary, whether the drug is taken can be influenced by external factors such as peer pressure, price, and, in particular, availability. In the United States, there is a great deal of cocaine in all areas of the country, and in some regions the availability of heroin is widespread. Nonetheless, it is true that despite ready availability, most people exposed to drugs do not go on to become addicts. Heredity is likely to influence the effects of the initial sampling of the drug, and these effects are in turn likely to be influential in modifying the course of continued use. Individuals for whom the initial psychological responses to the drug are extremely pleasurable may be more likely to repeat the drug taking and some of them will develop an addiction. Some people seem to have an inherited tolerance to alcohol, even without previous exposure.[2] At some point after continued repetition of voluntary drug taking, the drug "user" loses the voluntary ability to control its use. At that point, the "drug misuser" becomes "drug addicted," and there is a compulsive, often overwhelming *involuntary* aspect to continuing drug use and to relapse after a period of abstinence. We do not yet know the mechanisms involved in this change from drug taking to addiction, and we are searching for pharmacological mechanisms to reverse this process.

Comparison to Other Medical Disorders

The view of addiction as a chronic medical disorder puts it in a category with other conditions that show a similar confluence of genetic, biological, behavioral, and environmental factors. There are many examples of chronic illnesses that are generally accepted as requiring life-long treatment. Here, we will focus on only three: adult-onset diabetes, hypertension, and asthma. Like substance-use disorders, the onset of these three diseases is determined by multiple factors, and the contributions of each factor are not yet fully specified. In adult-onset diabetes and some forms of hypertension, genetic factors have a major, though not exclusive, role in the etiology. Parenting practices, stress in the home environment, and other environmental factors are also important in determining whether these diseases actually get expressed, even among individuals who are genetically predisposed. Behavioral factors are also important at the outset in the development of these disorders. The control of diet and weight and the establishment of regular exercise patterns are two important determinants of the onset and severity. Thus, although a diabetic, hypertensive, or asthmatic patient may have been genetically predisposed and may have been raised in a high-risk environment, it is also true that behavioral choices such as the ingestion of high sugar and/or high-cholesterol foods, smoking, and lack of exercise also play a part in the onset and severity of their disorder.

Treatment Results

Almost everyone has a friend or relative who has been through a treatment program for addiction to nicotine, alcohol, or other drugs. Since most of these people have a relapse to drug-taking at some time after the end of treatment, there is a tendency for the general public to believe that addiction treatment is unsuccessful. However, this expectation of a cure after treatment is unrealistic—just as it is for other chronic disorders. The persistent changes produced by addiction are still present and require continued maintenance treatment—either psychosocial or pharmacological or a combination. As with other chronic disorders, the only realistic expectation for the treatment of addiction is patient improvement rather than cure. Consistent with these expectations, studies of abstinence rates at one year after completion of treatment indicate that only 30 to 50 percent of patients have been able to remain completely abstinent throughout that period, although an additional 15 to 30 percent have not resumed compulsive use.[3–6]

Successful treatment leads to substantial improvement in three areas: reduction of alcohol and other drug use, increases in personal health and social functions, and reduction in threats to public health and safety. All these domains can be measured in a graded fashion with a method such as the Addiction Severity Index (ASI).[7] In the ASI, a structured interview determines the need for treatment in seven independent domains. These measurements allow us to see addiction not as an all-or-none disease, but in degrees of severity across all the areas relevant to successful treatment.

Success rates for treatment of addictive disorders vary according to the type of drug and the variables inherent in the population being treated. For example, prognosis is much better in opioid addicts who are professionals, such as physicians or nurses, than in individuals with poor education and no legitimate job prospects, who are addicted to the same or even lesser amounts of opioids obtained on the street and financed by crime. Figure 14.1 compares the ASI profiles of two patients admitted to our treatment program. One was a resident physician who had few personal or professional difficulties except for heavy compulsive cocaine use. The other patient was a pregnant teenager who was admitted while

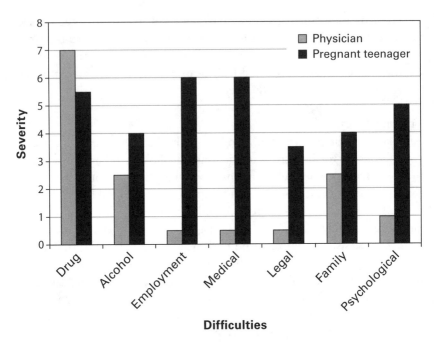

Figure 14.1
Admission severity profiles of two patients admitted for drug misuse

Table 14.1
Success rates for addictive disorders

Disorder	Success rate (percent)*
Alcoholism[8]	50 (40–70)
Opioid dependence[9]	60 (50–80)
Cocaine dependence[10]	55 (50–60)
Nicotine dependence[11]	30 (20–40)

*Follow-up 6 months. Data are median (range).

in premature labor induced by cocaine. The profile shows less drug use in the young woman, but in other areas shown to be important determinants of the outcome of treatment, she has severe problems. The types of treatment needed by these two patients are clearly different. Although the treatment of the physician will be challenging, his prognosis is far better than that of the young woman.

Success rates for the treatment of various addictive disorders are shown in table 14.1. Improvement is defined as a greater than 50 percent reduction on the drug-taking scale of the ASI. Another measure of the success of addiction treatment is the monetary savings that it produces. That addiction treatment is cost-effective has been shown in many studies in North America. For example, in one study in California, the benefits of alcohol and other drug treatment outweighed the cost of treatment by four- to twelve-fold depending on the type of drug and the type of treatment.

There has been progress in the development of medications for the treatment of nicotine, opioid, and alcohol addictions. For heroin addicts, *maintenance* treatment with a long-acting opioid such as methadone, l-α-acetylmethadol (LAAM), or buprenorphine can also be regarded as a success. The patient may be abstinent from illegal drugs and capable of functioning normally in society while requiring daily doses of an orally administered opioid medication—in very much the same way that dia-betic patients are maintained by injections of insulin and hypertensive patients are maintained on beta-blockers to sustain symptom improve-ments. Contrary to popular belief, patients properly maintained on meth-adone do not seem "drugged." They can function well, even in occupations requiring quick reflexes and motor skills, such as driving a subway train or motor vehicle. Of course not all patients on methadone can achieve high levels of function. Many street heroin addicts, such as the young cocaine-dependent woman in figure 14.1, have multiple additional psy-chosocial difficulties, are poorly educated, and misuse many drugs. In such cases, intensive psychosocial supports are necessary in addition to methadone; even then, the prognosis is limited by the patient's ability to learn skills for legitimate employment.

Nicotine is the addicting drug that has the poorest success rate (table 14.1). That these success rates are for individuals who came to a special-ized clinic for the treatment of their addiction implies that the patients tried to stop or control drug use on their own but have been unable to do so. Of those who present for treatment for nicotine dependence, only about 20 to 30 percent have not resumed smoking by the end of twelve months.

Treatment Compliance
Studies of treatment response have uniformly shown that patients who comply with the recommended regimen of education, counseling, and medication that characterizes most contemporary forms of treatment, have typically favorable outcomes during treatment and longer-lasting post-treatment benefits.[5,13-16] Thus, it is discouraging for many practitio-ners that so many drug-dependent patients do not comply with the recommended course of treatment and subsequently resume substance use. Factors such as low socioeconomic status, comorbid psychiatric

conditions, and lack of family or social supports for continuing abstinence are among the most important variables associated with lack of treatment compliance, and ultimately to relapse after treatment.[17–19]

Patient compliance is also especially important in determining the effectiveness of medications in the treatment of substance dependence. Although the general area of pharmacotherapy for drug addiction is still developing, in opioid and alcohol dependence there are several well-tested medications that are potent and effective in completely eliminating the target problems of substance use. Disulfiram has proven efficacy in preventing the resumption of alcohol use among detoxified patients. Alcoholics resist taking disulfiram because they become ill if they take a drink while receiving this medication; thus compliance is very poor.[20]

Naltrexone is an opioid antagonist that prevents relapse to opioid use by blocking opioid receptors; it is a nonaddicting medication that makes it impossible to return to opioid use, but it has little acceptance among heroin addicts who simply do not comply with this treatment. Naltrexone is also helpful in the treatment of alcoholism. Animal and human studies have shown that the reward produced by alcohol involves the endogenous opioid system. After patients are detoxified from alcohol, naltrexone reduces craving and blocks some of the rewarding effects of alcohol if the patient begins to drink again.[22,23] Although compliance is substantially better for naltrexone in the treatment of alcoholism than in opioid addiction, efforts to improve compliance are pivotal in the treatment of alcoholism. Continuing clinical research in this area is focused on the development of longer-acting forms of these medications and behavioral strategies to increase patient compliance.

The diseases of hypertension, diabetes, and asthma are also chronic disorders that require continuing care for most, if not all, of a patient's life. At the same time, these disorders are not necessarily unremitting or unalterably lethal, provided that the treatment regimen of medication, diet, and behavioral change is followed. This last point requires emphasis. As with the treatment of addiction, treatments for these chronic medical disorders heavily depend on behavioral change and medication compliance to achieve their potential effectiveness. In a review of over seventy outcome studies of treatments for these disorders (summarized in table 14.2) patient compliance with the recommended medical regimen was regarded as the most significant determinant of treatment outcome. Less than 50 percent of patients with insulin-dependent diabetes fully comply with their medication schedule,[24] and less than 30 percent of patients with hypertension or asthma comply with their medication regimens.[25,26]

Table 14.2
Compliance and relapse in selected medical disorders

	Compliance and relapse
Insulin-dependent diabetes mellitus	
Medication regimen	<50 percent
Diet and foot care	<30 percent
Relapse[a]	30–50 percent
Hypertension[b]	
Medication regimen	<30 percent
Diet	<30 percent
Relapse[a]	50–60 percent
Asthma	
Medication regimen	<30 percent
Relapse[a]	60–80 percent

[a]Retreatment within 12 months by physician at emergency room or hospital.
[b]Requiring medication.
Sources are references 33 and 34; for a complete list of references, please write to CPOB.

The difficulty is even worse for the behavioral and diet changes that are so important for the maintenance of short-term gains in these conditions. Less than 30 percent of patients in treatment for diabetes and hypertension comply with the recommended diet and/or behavioral changes that are designed to reduce risk factors for reoccurrence of these disorders.[27,28] It is interesting in this context that clinical researchers have identified low socioeconomic status, comorbid psychiatric conditions, and lack of family support as the major contributors to poor patient compliance in these disorders (see reference 27 for discussion of this work). As in addiction treatment, lack of patient compliance with the treatment regimen is a major contributor to reoccurrence and to the development of more serious and more expensive "disease-related" conditions.

For example, outcome studies show that 30 to 60 percent of insulin-dependent diabetic patients and about 50 to 80 percent of hypertensive and asthmatic patients have a reoccurrence of their symptoms each year and require at least restabilization of their medication and/or additional medical interventions to reestablish symptom remission.[24-28] Many of these reoccurrences also result in more serious additional health complications. For example, limb amputations and blindness are all too common consequences of treatment nonresponse among diabetic patients.[29,30] Stroke and cardiac disease are often associated with exacerbation of hypertension.[31,32]

There are, of course, differences in susceptibility, onset, course, and treatment response among all the disorders discussed here, but at the same time, there are clear parallels among them. All are multiply determined, and no single gene, personality variable, or environmental factor can fully account for the onset of any of these disorders. Behavioral choices seem to be implicated in the initiation of each of them, and behavioral control continues to be a factor in determining their course and severity. There are no "cures" for any of them, yet there have been major advances in the development of effective medications and behavioral change regimens to reduce or eliminate primary symptoms. Because these conditions are chronic, it is acknowledged (at least in the treatment of diabetes, hypertension, and asthma) that maintenance treatments will be needed to ensure that symptom remission continues. Unfortunately, other common features are their resistance to maintenance forms of treatment (both medication and behavior aspects) and their chronic, relapsing course. In this regard, it is striking that many of the patient characteristics associated with noncompliance are identical for these acknowledged "medical" disorders and addictive disorders, and the rates of reoccurrence are also similar.

Addiction Treatment Is a Worthwhile Medical Endeavor

A change in the attitudes of physicians is necessary. Addictive disorders should be considered in the category with other disorders that require long-term or life-long treatment. Treatment of addiction is about as successful as treatment of disorders such as hypertension, diabetes, and asthma, and it is clearly cost-effective. We believe that the prominence and severity of concerns about the public health and public safety associated with addiction have made the public, the press, and public policy officials understandably desperate for a lasting solution and disappointed that none has yet been developed. As with treatments for these other chronic medical conditions, there is no cure for addiction. At the same time, there is a range of pharmacological and behavioral treatments that are effective in reducing drug use, improving patient function, reducing crime and legal system costs, and preventing the development of other expensive medical disorders. Perhaps the major difference among these conditions lies in the public's and the physician's perception of diabetes, hypertension, and asthma as clearly medical conditions, whereas addiction is more likely to be perceived as a social problem or a character deficit. It is interesting that despite similar results, at least in terms of compliance or reoccurrence rates, there is no serious argument against support by contemporary health care systems for diabetes, hypertension, or asthma, whereas this is very much in question with regard to the treatments for addiction. Is it not time that we judged the "worth" of treatments for chronic addiction with the same standards that we use for treatments of other chronic diseases?

References

1. Mattick, R. P., & Hall, W. (1996). Are detoxification programmes effective? *Lancet, 347,* 97–100.

2. Schuckit, M. A. (1994). Low level of response to alcohol. *American Journal of Psychiatry, 151,* 184–189.

3. Gerstein, D., & Harwood, H. (1990). *Treating drug problems* (Vol. 1). Washington, DC: National Academy Press.

4. Gerstein, D., Judd, L. L., & Rovner, S. A. (1979). Career dynamics of female heroin addicts. *American Journal of Drug and Alcohol Abuse, 6,* 1–23.

5. Miller, W. R., & Hester, R. K. (1986). The effectiveness of alcoholism treatment methods: What research reveals. In W. R. Miller & N. Heather (Eds.), *Treating addictive behaviors: Process of change.* New York: Plenum Press.

6. Armor, D. J., Polich, J. M., & Stambul, H. B. (1976). *Alcoholism and treatment.* Santa Monica, CA: RAND Corporation Press.

7. McLellan, A. T., Luborsky, L., O'Brien, C. P., & Woody, G. E. (1980). An improved evaluation instrument for substance abuse patients: The Addiction Severity Index. *Journal of Nervous and Mental Disease, 168,* 26–33.

8. Institute of Medicine. (1989). *Prevention and treatment of alcohol problems: Research opportunities.* Washington, DC: National Academy Press.

9. Ball, J. C., & Ross, A. (1991). *The effectiveness of methadone maintenance treatment.* New York: Springer-Verlag.

10. Higgins, S. T., Budney, A. J., Bickel, W. K., Foerg, F., Donham, R., & Badger, G. J. (1994). Incentives improve outcome in outpatient behavioral treatment of cocaine dependence. *Archives of General Psychiatry, 51,* 568–576.

11. Fiore, M. C., Smith, S. S., Jorenby, D. E., & Baker, T. B. (1994). The effectiveness of the nicotine patch for smoking cessation. *Journal of the American Medical Association, 271,* 1940–1946.

12. Gerstein, D. R., Harwood, H., & Suter, N. (1994). *Evaluating recovery services: The California Drug and Alcohol Treatment Assessment (CALDATA)*. California Department of Alcohol and Drug Programs Executive Summary: Publication no. ADP94–628.

13. Moos, R. H., Finney, J. W., & Cronkite, R. C. (1990). *Alcoholism treatment: Context, process and outcome*. New York: Oxford University Press.

14. Simpson, D., & Savage, L. (1980). Drug abuse treatment readmissions and outcomes. *Archives of General Psychiatry, 37*, 896–901.

15. Hubbard, R. L., Marsden, M. E., Rachal, J. V., Harwood, H. J., Cavanaugh, E. R., & Ginzburg, H. M. (1989). *Drug abuse treatment: A national study of effectiveness*. Chapel Hill: University of North Carolina Press.

16. DeLeon, G. (1994). *The therapeutic community: study of effectiveness* (Treatment Research Monograph 84–1286). Rockville, MD: National Institute for Drug Abuse.

17. Havassy, B. E., Wasserman, D., & Hall, S. M. (1995). Social relationships and cocaine use in an American treatment sample. *Addiction (Abingdon, England), 90*, 699–710.

18. McLellan, A. T., Druley, K. A., O'Brien, C. P., & Kron, R. (1980). Matching substance abuse patients to appropriate treatments: A conceptual and methodological approach. *Drug and Alcohol Dependence, 5*, 189–193.

19. Alterman, A. I., & Cacciola, J. S. (1991). The antisocial personality disorder in substance abusers: Problems and issues. *Journal of Nervous and Mental Disease, 179*, 401–409.

20. Fuller, R. K., Branchey, L., Brightwell, D. R., et al. (1986). Disfulfiram treatment of alcoholism. *Journal of the American Medical Association, 256*, 1449–1455.

21. O'Brien, C. P., Woody, G. E., & McLellan, A. T. (1986). A new tool in the treatment of impaired physicians. *Philadelphia Medicine, 82*, 442–446.

22. Volpicelli, J. R., Alterman, A. I., Hayashida, M., & O'Brien, C. P. (1992). Naltrexone in the treatment of alcohol dependence. *Archives of General Psychiatry, 49*, 876–880.

23. O'Malley, S. S., Jaffe, A. J., Chang, G., Schottenfeld, R. S., Meyer, R. E., & Rounsaville, B. (1992). Naltrexone and coping skills therapy for alcohol dependence. *Archives of General Psychiatry, 49*, 881–887.

24. Graber, A. L., Davidson, P., Brown, A., McRae, J., & Woolridge, K. (1992). Dropout and relapse during diabetes care. *Diabetes Care, 15*, 1477–1483.

25. Horowitz, R. I. (1990). Treatment adherence and risk of death after a myocardial infarction. *Lancet, 336*, 542–545.

26. Dekker, F. W., Dieleman, F. E., Kaptein, A. A., & Mulder, J. D. (1993). Compliance with pulmonary medication in general practice. *European Respiratory Journal, 6*, 886–890.

27. Clark, L. T. (1991). Improving compliance and increasing control of hypertension: Needs of special hypertensive populations. *American Heart Journal, 121*, 664–669.

28. Kurtz, S. M. (1990). Adherence to diabetic regimes: Empirical status and clinical applications. *Diabetes Educator, 16,* 50–59.

29. Sinnock, P. (1985). *Hospitalization of diabetes. Diabetes data, national diabetes data group.* Bethesda, MD: National Institutes of Health.

30. Herman, W. H., & Teutsch, S. M. (1985). *Diabetic renal disorders. Diabetes data, national diabetes data group.* Bethesda, MD: National Institutes of Health.

31. Schaub, A. F., Steiner, A., & Vetter, W. (1993). Compliance to treatment. *J Clin Exp Hypertension, 15,* 1121–1130.

32. Gorlin, R. (1991). Hypertension and ischemic heart disease: The challenge of the 1990s. *American Heart Journal, 121,* 658–663.

33. National Center for Health Statistics. (1989). *Public use datatape documentation.* Hyattsville, MD: Author.

34. Harrison, W. H. (1993). *Internal medicine.* New York: Raven Press.

15

Ethical Considerations in Caring for People Living with Addictions

Laura Weiss Roberts and Kim Bullock

The care of people living with addiction is ethically complex work. Addiction is stigmatized in our society (1,2), and clinical services for addiction-related conditions are underdeveloped, raising many ethical issues related to respect, confidentiality, and justice. Addictions of all kinds are associated, by definition, with a lack of personal control over the addictive behavior and are often linked with intermittent or enduring cognitive deficits, creating concerns about affected individuals' capacities for autonomy and shared decision-making with caregivers (3–6). Some addictions are associated with risky and/or illegal activities, introducing very difficult considerations related to dangerousness, self-neglect, or self-injury and potential harm toward others (7). Moreover, the history of treatment for addiction has been riddled with approaches that emphasize punitive consequences, raising issues pertaining to beneficence, nonmaleficence, and medical professionalism (8). Finally, addiction often co-occurs with other health conditions, which may be difficult to recognize and burdensome to treat because of the addiction, raising ethical issues related to clinical competence. For these reasons, every aspect of clinical care for addictive disorders should be viewed as having important ethical meaning and implications.

Ethical dilemmas in clinical care occur usually because of a conflict between two "good" things or positive values. Such conflicts may involve balancing the need to confront a patient directly about an emerging substance use problem while he or she is going through a difficult divorce, that is, to act with honesty, with the wish to be empathic and supportive of the patient during a stressful life experience, that is, to act with compassion, beneficence, and nonmaleficence. Likewise, a clinician who is a provider in a court-mandated treatment intervention or a psychiatrist who performs pretransplant evaluations may be in the difficult position of influencing the decision of whether a patient returns to jail or is denied

Table 15.1
Bioethics principles especially relevant to the care of addiction disorders

Respect for persons	Treating another individual with genuine consideration and attentiveness to that person's life history, values, and goals
Autonomy	The ability to make deliberated or reasoned decisions for oneself and to act on the basis of such decisions
Beneficence	An obligation to benefit patients and to seek their good
Compassion	Literally, "suffering with" another person, with kindness and an active regard for his or her welfare
Confidentiality	The obligation of physicians not to disclose information obtained from patients or observed about them without their permission. Confidentiality is a privilege linked to the legal right of privacy and may at times be overridden by exceptions stipulated in law.
Dignity	The belief that every person, intrinsically, is valued and worthy of respect
Honesty	A virtue in which one conveys the truth fully, without misrepresentation through deceit, bias, or omission
Justice	The ethical principle of fairness. Distributive justice refers to the fair and equitable distribution of resources and burden through society
Nonmaleficence	The duty to avoid doing harm

a lifesaving liver transplant because of ongoing addiction issues and lack of treatment adherence. Situations such as these challenge the self-concept of conscientious physicians as professionals who "do good." Table 15.1 describes relevant ethical principles in addiction care.

Newer approaches to treatment have done much to advance the field of addiction care and, with it, the underlying ethics of this special clinical work. Motivational interviewing is particularly oriented toward supporting patient strengths (respect, autonomy) and the reduction of harm (nonmaleficence) associated with consequences of addiction. It is affirming (beneficence) and empathic (compassion) in its approach and has a strong evidence base of effectiveness (beneficence). It emphasizes transparency (honesty) while sidestepping the problem of punitive limit setting or enabling pathological behaviors (nonmaleficence).

People living with addictions often become "difficult" patients (9). Providers may have naturally negative reactions (countertransference) when treating patients who minimize or lie about their substance use patterns or who do not adhere to prescribed treatments. These issues may be of greatest concern when patients resemble their caregivers, for example, when the patient is a colleague or an accomplished professional. Patients who are perceived as drug seeking and who recruit a psychiatrist into "rescuing" them with medications that have addictive potential are particularly troubling. When patients are unkempt, disheveled, impulsive, threatening, agitated, or belligerent, providers can react quite strongly.

The key to ethically competent care of patients with complex problems is to remember that "difficult" attributes are a clinical sign—a manifestation of an illness process that should be recognized for its informational value in the care of the patient (figure 15.1). A psychiatrist who exhibits true professionalism will seek a therapeutic response to the situation, which may be as basic as ensuring the safety of the patient, keeping the patient engaged in care, and avoiding reactions that may be anchored in prejudicial attitudes rather than self-reflective clinical skills. Figure 15.2 describes steps for optimal clinical ethical decision making, and Table 15.2 provides special considerations in the care of people with addictions, including ethical responses.

Roughly 9 percent of the population fulfilled the diagnostic criteria for substance dependence or abuse in the past year according to results from the 2009 National Survey of Drug Use and Health. Lifetime estimates of addiction are now thought to be as high as 35 percent, which is higher than earlier estimates of closer to 15 percent (10,11). Experimenting with substances occurs early. Among eighth graders, 37 percent report having tried alcohol, 16 percent have tried marijuana, and 28 percent have tried some illicit drug other than marijuana (12). More than

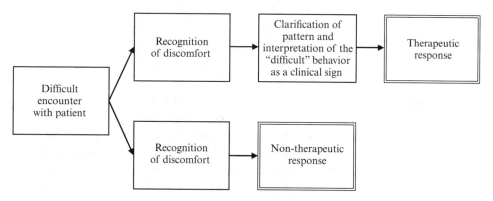

Figure 15.1
Responding therapeutically to the "difficult" patient. (Adapted from McCarty et al. [9])

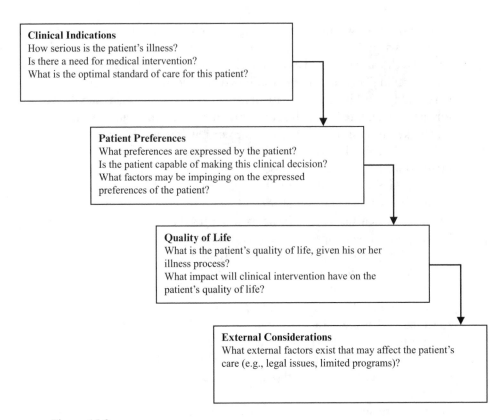

Clinical Indications
How serious is the patient's illness?
Is there a need for medical intervention?
What is the optimal standard of care for this patient?

Patient Preferences
What preferences are expressed by the patient?
Is the patient capable of making this clinical decision?
What factors may be impinging on the expressed preferences of the patient?

Quality of Life
What is the patient's quality of life, given his or her illness process?
What impact will clinical intervention have on the patient's quality of life?

External Considerations
What external factors exist that may affect the patient's care (e.g., legal issues, limited programs)?

Figure 15.2
Steps for clinical ethical decision making. (Reprinted from figure 17-2, from Concise Guide to Ethics in Mental Health Care, Roberts LW, Dyer AR. American Psychiatric Publishing, 2004, p. 307.)

1 million persons with addiction received treatment at outpatient mental health centers and 714,000 in a private doctor's office.

For these reasons, addictions represent a critical concern for public health and a clinical area of competence necessary for all practicing psychiatrists. People with addictions deserve appropriate care, characterized by the ideals of the profession including dignity, respect, and compassion. This aspiration represents a profound challenge, particularly given the underdeveloped system of care that exists in this country for people with addictions. For example, of the 23.5 million persons in need of treatment for an illicit drug or alcohol use problem, only 11.2 percent received treatment in 2009 (13). This fact alone suggests that psychiatrists will find themselves having to "stretch," that is, to serve in extended

Table 15.2
Example of special considerations with ethical implications in the care of people living with addictions

---

Social stigma—Addiction is associated with social isolation, diminished standing and rejection in personal relationships, and self-loathing.
Ethical responses: Greater efforts to introduce the topic of addictions in a respectful, nonjudgmental manner; to support treatment adherence; and to protect patient confidentiality are necessary.

Health disparities—Addiction is associated with economic disadvantage, inadequate development of clinical services in most communities, heightened barriers to care, loss of employment, and loss of insurance.
Ethical responses: Greater efforts to clarify the economic circumstances of the patient, to mobilize resources, to create facilitated pathways into confidential care, to support economic viability, and to access social programs are necessary in clinical and community leadership activities.

Legal issues—Addiction is associated with behaviors that may introduce legal "stakes" into the clinical situation, generating concerns that may range from interpersonal violence to truthfulness in clinical documentation.
Ethical responses: Greater efforts to balance duties to patients with legal imperatives (e.g., duty to report or comply with legal directives) and to explain these considerations to patients carefully and honestly are necessary, especially if monitoring and treatment are part of a legal intervention.

Clinical complexity—Addiction is associated with multiple and diverse health problems that may be masked, difficult to recognize, and increase burdens of care for patients and providers alike.
Ethical responses: Greater efforts to be extremely thorough in evaluating potential physical and mental health issues and to make few assumptions about the extent of the addiction and/or co-occurring conditions are necessary.

---

roles without adequate preparation or support to provide adequate clinical care for people living with addictions. Because addictions are increasingly prevalent, psychiatrists' strengths, including their deeply held professionalism, will be increasingly called upon to address the complex concerns of this underserved population in the years ahead.

References

1. Roberts, L. W., & Dunn, L. B. (2003). Ethical considerations in caring for women with substance use disorders. *Obstetrics and Gynecology Clinics of North America, 30,* 559–582.

2. Luoma, J. B., Twohig, M. P., Waltz, T., Hayes, S. C., Roget, N., Padilla, M., et al. (2007). An investigation of stigma in individuals receiving treatment for substance abuse. *Addictive Behaviors, 32,* 1331–1346.

3. Schlimme, J. E. (2010). Addiction and self-determination: A phenomenological approach. *Theoretical Medicine and Bioethics*, *31*, 49–62.

4. Hall, W., Carter, L., & Morley, K. I. (2004). Neuroscience research on the addictions: A prospectus for future ethical and policy analysis. *Addictive Behaviors*, *29*, 1481–1495.

5. Caplan, A. L. (2006). Ethical issues surrounding forced, mandated, or coerced treatment. *Journal of Substance Abuse Treatment*, *31*, 117–120.

6. Buchman, D. Z., Skinner, W., & Illes, J. (2010). Negotiating the relationship between addiction, ethics, and brain science. *AJOB Neuroscience*, *1*, 36–45.

7. Stone, D. B. (2000). *Alcohol and Other Drugs*. Rockville, MD: Substance Abuse and Mental Health Services Administration.

8. Saunders, J. L., Barros-Bailey, M., Rudman, R., Dew, D. W., & Garcia, J. (2007). Ethical complaints and violations in rehabilitation counseling: An analysis of commission on rehabilitation counselor certification data. *Rehabilitation Counseling Bulletin*, *51*, 7.

9. McCarty, T., & Roberts, L. W. (1996). The difficult patient. In R. H. Rubin, C. Voss, D. Derksen, A. Gateley, & R. W. Quenzer (Eds.), *Medicine: A Primary Care Approach* (p. 397). Philadelphia: Saunders.

10. Kessler, R. C., & Wang, P. S. (2008). The descriptive epidemiology of commonly occurring mental disorders in the United States. *Annual Review of Public Health*, *29*, 115–129.

11. Substance Abuse and Mental Health Services Administration. (2010). Results from the 2009 National Survey on Drug Use and Health (Vol. 1). *Summary of National Findings*. Rockville, MD: Department of Health and Human Services.

12. Johnston, L. D., O'Malley, P. M., Bachman, J. G., & Schulenberg, J. E. (2010). Monitoring the future: national survey results on drug use, 1975–2009. (Vol. 1). *Secondary school students* (NIH Publication No. 10–7584). Bethesda, MD: National Institute on Drug Abuse.

13. Geppert, C. M. A., & Roberts, L. W. (2008). *The Book of Ethics: Expert Guidance for Professionals Who Treat Addiction*. Center City, MN: Hazelden Foundation.

V

Mental Illness and the Courts

This part offers a sampling of articles that highlight ethical questions emerging at the intersection of law and mental health care. The first three articles coalesce around conflicts that mental health care practitioners face, and the fourth illustrates how legal systems may in fact reinforce bias against mentally ill persons. We turn to the paradigmatic case of *Tarasoff* v. *Regents of the University of California*, in which a young man murdered Tatiana Tarasoff, completing a plan he had described to his therapist.

The invocation of *Tarasoff* has become somewhat of an ethical clarion for the so-called duty to warn. Across all medical specialties, *Tarasoff* serves as the paradigm case against which questions of dangerousness versus confidentiality are judged. But thirty-five years on, there is a tendency among teachers and trainees to misremember and oversimplify *Tarasoff* as a case involving a psychologist who chose to limit disclosure and protect patient confidentiality rather than protect the public good. This was not so.

The 1975 essay by health law professor William Curran reminds us of the forgotten facts and complexities of *Tarasoff*. A basic question turns not on whether a clinician can or ought to breach confidentiality when a patient presents as clearly harmful to self or the community, but rather in ascertaining when such an ethical duty is appropriately and fully discharged. As Curran argues, the California Supreme Court in *Tarasoff I* (1974) inflated a basic allowance of disclosure of certain dangerousness—one that had existed well before *Tarasoff I and II*—into in impractical and supererogatory duty to protect a third party. Thus, Curran highlights a struggle that individual practitioners and behavioral health agencies must constantly grapple with: the trade-off between the therapeutic alliance and community safety. This article marks only the beginning of the continuing debate and discussion regarding the nature and limits of the so-called *Tarasoff* rules, which today vary considerably from state to state. Over the years, the complexities of those rules have been predictably revisited in the aftermath of tragedies, such as the 2012 mass shooting in an Aurora, Colorado, movie theater.

Next, Claire Pouncey and Jonathan Lukens argue in a conceptual analysis that legal attitudes about the autonomy of mentally ill persons often conflict with the core values of both psychiatry and the recovery movement. The authors first provide background on the recovery movement. They then argue that the enterprise of psychiatry—despite historical transgressions—is in fact aligned with the recovery movement's central tenet of respect for autonomy and patient self-determination. This is true, they claim, except in one important area: forensic psychiatry. Pouncey and Lukens expose a paradox of both forensic psychiatry and the recovery movement, asking, "How can we advocate treating persons with mental illness as full moral agents for the purpose of providing social goods, while simultaneously treating them as compromised moral agents when the same illness earns them social sanction?"

While Pouncey and Lukens describe conflicted professional roles at a macroscopic level, Robert Woody provides a concise analysis of the ethical problem of dual roles for the individual clinician *qua* forensic examiner. While not foreclosing on the possibility that clinicians may also serve as examiners, Woody highlights the difficulty in making the transition from healer to witness. He expresses concern that many clinicians enter the legal fray ill equipped to manage the myriad professional conflicts that inevitably ensue. He provides a schedule of five roles for the forensic mental health practitioners that are in general mutually exclusive.

We then shift from the theme of conflict to an examination of stigma within the legal context by Michelle Black and Jocelyn Downie. They present qualitative data on how mental illness and mentally ill persons are described by Canadian judges, whose descriptions are found to be fraught with inaccuracies at best and bias at worst.

One might expect the legal lexicon to be a scientifically enlightened one—a highly technical and precise language that draws not on anachronisms and aspersions but rather on sophisticated verbiage. Black and Downie point out dozens of examples of stigmatizing language that judges have used in their opinions and have been recorded in legislation. In so doing, the authors teach us a larger lesson: destigmatization and social change are slow processes, and even at the highest levels of educated society, beliefs about mentally ill persons stubbornly persist. Words reveal persistent beliefs: that mentally ill persons are their illnesses ("the schizophrenic"), that they should be ashamed of their maladies (by not "admitting" to being ill), or that they should be "arrested" or "incarcerated" in "lunatic" asylums.

We include this study for both its forensic content and because it reveals how deeply embedded stigmatizing beliefs and paradigms run. Whether we look at statehouses, courts, or clinics, stigmatizing beliefs abound—a revelation that is generalizable across all sectors of behavioral health care. In the context of the courtroom, these abstract beliefs become reality as they profoundly affect vulnerable parties.

16

Confidentiality and the Prediction of Dangerousness in Psychiatry

William J. Curran

The California Supreme Court continues to make financial awards to patients in suits against physicians with seemingly little regard for the effect of these awards and decisions upon the practice of medicine and the availability of insurance to cover this largesse of the judiciary, and without regard for the social consequences of this "money-for-everything" attitude.

The particular case, *Tarasoff* v. *Regents of the University of California* has already become infamous among mental health programs in California and among college and university student medical programs all over the country as it has taken its course through the various levels of trial and appeals courts in the Golden State.[1]

The facts of the situation are undisputed. A student at the University of California's Berkeley campus was in psychotherapy with the student health service on an outpatient basis. He told his therapist, a psychologist, that he wanted to kill an unmarried girl who lived in Berkeley but who was then on a summer trip to Brazil. The psychologist, with the concurrence of another therapist and the assistant director of the Department of Psychiatry, reported the matter orally to the campus police and on their suggestion sent them a letter requesting detention of the student and his commitment for observation to a mental hospital. The campus police picked up the student for questioning but, "satisfied" that he was "rational," released him on his "promise to stay away" from Miss Tarasoff. The police reported back to the director of psychiatry, Dr. Powelson. Dr. Powelson asked for the return of the psychologist's letter to the police and directed that all copies of the letter be destroyed. Nothing more was done at the health service about the matter. Two months later, shortly after Miss Tarasoff's return, the student went to her home and killed her.

The parents of Miss Tarasoff brought suit for damages against the university and against the therapists and the campus police, as employees of the university and individually. In suing Dr. Powelson, the plaintiffs sought not only general money damages for negligence in failing to warn the girl and her parents and to confine the student, but exemplary or punitive damages (which could be assessed in huge amounts as multiples of the general damages or in any amount at the determination of the jury) for malicious and oppressive abandonment of a dangerous patient.

The superior court dismissed all these grounds for legal action against the defendants. The supreme court, in a four-to-two decision, reversed the decision and found that on these facts, a cause of action was stated for general damages against all the therapists involved in the case and the assistant director and the director of psychiatry and against the university as their employer for breach of the duty to warn Miss Tarasoff. The court dismissed the claim for exemplary damages against the therapists. It also dismissed the action against the police as protected from a suit by statutory immunity, as well as the suit against the therapists for failure to confine the student under a commitment order, again because of a statutory immunity. The court implied that without the immunity, both of these actions might have been meritorious.

It seems to me most physicians would throw up their hands in dismay over this result and massive contradictions in the assessment of who was and who was not legally responsible for this death. If I were to describe in detail the reasoning of the court, the confusion of the medical mind would be compounded a thousand times.

The court asserted that the *Principles of Medical Ethics* of the American Medical Association, section 9, did not bar breaching the confidentiality of this patient "in order to protect the welfare of this individual [the patient] or the community." From this premise, the court jumped wholeheartedly to a positive duty to warn Miss Tarasoff. This is not what the Principles said. The traditional code of medical ethics allows a physician in his sound discretion to breach the confidentiality but does not require it. It is almost impossible to draft an ethical principle to force a duty on physicians to breach confidences. Must they always warn of death threats, but have discretion on less dangerous threats? Must they warn if the patient is psychotic, but not if he is less disturbed? Does this case mean that every time a patient makes a threat against an unnamed person, the therapist must take steps to find out who it is and warn him or her (of anything at all, from vague threats to murder) or suffer money damages in the thousands or tens of thousands if the threat, or an aspect of the threat, is carried out?

This case was greatly confused by the array of immunities from suits created under California law. It can be strongly argued that the thrust of these immunity statutes regarding the duty to warn should also have been applied to the therapists, since the statutes were intended to encourage police and mental health personnel to release patients and not confine them on the basis of unreliable diagnoses of dangerousness. In the past, it was thought that too many mental patients were confined for years and years because of their threats to other people, rarely carried out, and because of the conservatism of mental health personnel in exercising any doubt about dangerousness in favor of confinement as the safest way to prevent harm to third parties.

It seems clear that the therapists here thought that they had done all they could to protect their patient and the community by reporting the case to the police. They had exercised their discretion to warn the community and to breach the confidence of the patient, for his own sake, and that of the unknown girl. They could hardly warn her, since she was not even in the country at the time. Also, the threat to Miss Tarasoff might actually have been vaguely directed. The student could well have turned his anger and violence toward another person or toward himself. The only basic recourse was to recommend temporary observational commitment. The practice was to take this to the campus police. It was the police who acted, and they decided to release the student with a warning and a promise to stay away from the girl. How many thousands of such warnings—and releases—do police departments make every year? How many people then proceed to kill? The immunity statute was established to encourage release in these circumstances. But the statutory armor had a hole in it. The director of psychiatry was found by the court to have a "duty" to warn the girl, irrespective of the police action. The court utilized some precedents, none clearly applicable to this case, to justify its decision. It seems, however, that the real rationale was the aggravated nature of the case—a killing—in which the family was left without someone else to sue. The therapists, particularly Dr. Powelson, could have warned the girl if they had wanted to go against the police action and if they had thought the specific threat to Miss Tarasoff so serious as to warrant that action. The court did not apply any test to ascertain the custom of psychiatrists and mental-health programs actually in such situations. The Court declared the duty as a matter of law, regardless of the accepted practices of the profession. As in the *Helling* decision[2] discussed in an earlier column,[3] the court made the physician a guarantor against harm to this party, here not even a patient, on the basis of its own concept of monetary justice.

References

1. Tarasoff v. Regents of the University of California. (1974). 529 P.2d 553.
2. Helling v. Carey and Laughlin. (1974). 519 P.2d 981.
3. Curran, W. J. (1974). Glaucoma and streptococcal pharyngitis: Diagnostic practices and malpractice liability. *New England Journal of Medicine, 291,* 508–509.

17

Madness versus Badness: The Ethical Tension between the Recovery Movement and Forensic Psychiatry

Claire L. Pouncey and Jonathan M. Lukens

Introduction

With its consistent message that persons with severe mental illness can and should be responsible for their own life choices, the recovery movement in the United States has made progress in overcoming the stigma of mental illness, advancing the civil rights of persons with severe mental illness, and providing better and more accessible treatment for mental illness. However, in deliberately emphasizing the capabilities of persons with mental illness for self-determination, recovery advocates leave unaddressed important questions about how, when, and to what extent mental illness can limit a person's capacity to make sound choices, or even her moral accountability. Although both psychiatry and medical ethics share the ideals of the recovery movement, these disciplines recognize that severe mental illness can limit agency. In relation to forensic psychiatry in particular, this creates an uncomfortable tension because the recovery movement has not explored how its principles can extend from civil matters to criminal law. The recovery movement's silence on the limits of moral agency in persons with severe mental illness creates an ethical disconnect between forensic psychiatry, medical ethics, and recovery principles. This discussion will argue for the importance of combined efforts from these three disciplines to address problems of agency in severe mental illness. We will show that the three approaches to understanding moral agency in persons with severe mental illness are not inherently antithetical but do need to better inform one another.

The Recovery Movement

Beginning in the 1950s, mental health policy in the United States changed dramatically as new psychiatric medications became available, the civil rights and rehabilitation movements gained momentum, and the government made funding available for community-based treatment of persons with mental illness. In this time of political, social, medical, and economic flux, there was a strong trend toward deinstitutionalizing persons with severe mental illness and providing adequate community-based treatment for them. Throughout the 1960s and into the 1970s, new federal funding led to the establishment and expansion of community mental health centers throughout the United States [1–3]. However, policy reformers paid insufficient attention to the challenges many formerly institutionalized persons faced in the community, especially in terms of finding appropriate housing, work opportunities, outpatient treatment, and community acceptance [4], and many persons who had spent years in institutions failed to thrive in the community setting. In addition, mental illness carried a great deal of social stigma, creating overwhelming barriers to full social integration.

The psychiatric rehabilitation movement emerged in this setting as an effort to expand the limited scope of mental health treatment by arguing that effective, comprehensive treatment of mental illness must address psychosocial as well as psychiatric needs. In order to meet the full range of psychosocial needs of persons with severe mental illness, psychiatric rehabilitation emphasized illness management and community reintegration, along with psychiatric treatment. It focused on developing mechanisms for social intervention, such as interpersonal skills, access to social services and resources, and improved practical and legal mechanisms for maximizing patient self-determination. This movement empowered persons with severe mental illness to collaborate with community care providers to plan their own treatment, and the focus changed from the passive treatment of medical deficits to the development of personal strengths [5].

Whereas the psychiatric rehabilitation movement arose as an effort among care providers and policymakers to improve community services, the mental health consumers' movement began as a self-help initiative among persons who were being transitioned from institutional to community-based care by creating self-help groups and peer-managed programming for persons with mental illness [6]. The consumers' movement advocated not just effective treatment and resources but also basic human rights. It strived to empower persons with mental illness with lexical changes, making them active "consumers" of mental health services rather than passive psychiatric "patients." It fought against social discrimination and stigma by emphasizing the capabilities of mental health service consumers rather than their disabilities. In doing so, the consumers' lobby became a strong voice for mental health advocacy, conveying to both consumers and the public that how we provide care is as important as what care we provide.

The psychiatric rehabilitation movement and the mental health consumers' movement thus laid the foundation for the modern recovery movement, which merges the multifaceted psychosocial treatment approach of the psychiatric rehabilitation program with the consumer-focused civil rights agenda of the consumers' movement. However, the concept of "recovery" has been defined in myriad ways, and those definitions have shifted over time, which has led to an inherent ambiguity in the movement and resistance from organizations that do not fully understand the movement's mission.

Note that the recovery movement is *not* an updated version of the antipsychiatry movements of the 1960s and 1970s. Although psychiatry still has critics who question whether mental illness exists or whether psychiatry has any real treatments to offer, the recovery movement does not conceptually preclude or practically exclude psychiatry. Recovery advocates share the belief that mental illness exists, and that it can impair rational processes. It departs from the psychiatric tradition in that the recovery movement circumscribes psychiatry's role to one of many possible means to improve the quality of life for persons with severe mental illness. It advocates that persons with mental illness are persons, full moral and political agents, and the movement discourages both consumers and health care professionals from seeing persons with mental illness as mere embodiments of a diagnosis or a collection of symptoms. In other words, the recovery movement does not disparage psychiatry as merely assigning empty diagnostic labels, but it views persons as more than their diagnoses, and it sees psychiatry as one of many methods to instill in consumers a full sense of agency and social participation.

Although mental health policy in the United States has rallied around the recovery movement, the "recovery" concept is difficult to characterize consistently or define clearly. The *National Consensus Statement on Mental Health Recovery* lists ten "fundamental components" that would make a mental health program recovery based: self-determination, person-centered care, empowerment (including the protection of civil rights), holism, nonlinearity, respect, focus on strengths rather than weaknesses, peer support, responsibility, and hope [7]. Davidson et al. note the imprecision and inconsistency with which both the term "recovery" and these specific goals can be interpreted [8,9]. They endorse an understanding of recovery with respect to mental health as "recovery in" rather than "recovery from" serious mental illness, thus distinguishing mental health recovery from curing mental illness. Rather than attempting to eliminate psychiatric symptoms or illness, recovery "calls for the provision of accommodations and supports that enable people with psychiatric disabilities to lead safe, dignified, and full lives in the community" [8].

Jacobson and Greenley distinguish between "internal and external conditions [that] produce the process called recovery" [10]. Internal conditions are those within the individual, many of which were advocated by the consumer movement: hope, healing, empowerment, and connection. *Hope* is the belief that recovery from severe mental illness is possible, *healing* is the process of controlling symptoms and refusing to see them as defining features of oneself, *empowerment* entails assuming a greater role in one's treatment, and *connection* entails finding "roles to play in the world."

External conditions are the components of a supportive sociopolitical environment that includes respect for human rights, a "positive culture of healing," and recovery-oriented services, echoing the agendas of both the psychosocial rehabilitation and the consumer movements. *Human rights* entail an equitable distribution of power between consumers and providers, as well as the satisfaction of basic needs from goods that range from food and shelter to health care parity. A *positive culture of healing* is one that allows social inclusion and the amelioration of stigma for persons with severe mental illness. *Recovery-oriented services* are those that integrate treatments provided by both health care professionals and consumer peers.

Others view recovery as "an ongoing, dynamic, interactional process that occurs between a person's strengths, vulnerabilities, resources, and the environment" [11]. It is client centered, in that the consumer decides how her recovery goals, as well as her success in reaching them, ought to be defined. It consists in an approach to treatment in which service consumers and service providers collaborate. Anthony defines recovery as the "development of new meaning and purpose in one's life as one grows beyond the catastrophic effects of psychiatric disability"; he communicates the importance of reconceptualizing one's life to accept the presence of persistent mental illness, while also expecting a rich, rewarding, and meaningful life [12].

We find that recovery is best understood not as an intervention or end point, but rather as a set of values and aims that constitute a treatment ideology. As such, we believe that the term *recovery* delivers an important, influential, but often rhetorical message that advocates will need to refine in order for the ideals to be implemented.

Community Psychiatry, and Civil Commitment

Psychiatry generally shares the recovery movement's ideals, but comes to them from a different direction. In particular, community psychiatry—the psychiatric subspecialty that works most closely with the population of severely mentally ill persons—has in large part embraced the concept of recovery. However, psychiatry was not part of the original psychiatric rehabilitation or consumer self-help movements from which the recovery movement grew, and so psychiatrists tend to be less familiar with the term *recovery* or the concepts used to describe the basic principles (e.g., "consumer oriented") [13]. Psychiatry is not antithetical to recovery, but there is a great deal of misunderstanding on both sides that impedes communication and collaboration.

Both recovery advocates and psychiatrists believe that mental illness exists and that it can interfere with a person's rational capacities and abilities to make sound decisions that promote his own best interests. Although psychiatry has been accused of defending an inappropriate "medical model" of mental illness that posits a reductionist and over-simplified view of mental illness, most of psychiatry instead embraces a biopsychosocial model, which acknowledges bidirectional causal influence among persons, their environments, and their psychological and biological constitutions [14]. Furthermore, psychiatry distinguishes different kinds and degrees of mental illness, thus recognizing that even patients with similar diagnoses, symptoms, and life events cannot be treated identically. Finally, psychiatry recognizes that most mental illnesses have symptoms that wax and wane over a person's lifetime, so that previously debilitating symptoms may remit, or a person who is functioning well overall may relapse through no fault of his own. Psychiatry thus shares the view of recovery advocates that people do develop mental illnesses (i.e., as opposed to mere "problems in living" [15]), but that carrying a certain diagnosis does not permit assumptions or predictions about a person's ability to function in the world.

Psychiatry is the only medical profession represented among the behavioral health professions and is the perpetrator of some of the institutional abuses against which the community mental health, psychosocial rehabilitation, consumer self-help, and recovery movements have reacted so strongly. So some critics of psychiatry might be surprised to learn that psychiatry shares some of the fundamental values of the recovery movement, as reflected in the *Principles of Medical Ethics with Annotations Especially Applicable to Psychiatry*, published by the American Psychiatric Association [16]. These principles are shared in full with other medical disciplines, and there are areas of significant overlap with the ethics codes of other behavioral health professions, as well as with the recovery movement. As does all of medicine in the United States, psychiatry respects patients' abilities and rights to be involved in making their own medical and life decisions—this is the widely embraced ethical principle of patient self-determination. In addition to self-determination, the *Principles of Medical Ethics* require that physicians both lobby for political change and protect patients' civil rights, which also align strongly with recovery values. Psychiatrists endorse these principles as an integral part of professional training, rather than as a response to consumer demand or a particular social reform movement.

However, physicians also are aware that symptomatic patients are not always capable of fully autonomous decision making, often because the problems that bring them to treatment impair cognitive and reasoning processes. Physicians always ought to maximize patient self-determination, but also must balance it against the simultaneously held values of beneficence and nonmaleficence. That is, doctors must help their patients, or at least refrain from harming them.

However, the subjects of physicians' beneficence can always interpret those actions as paternalistic, coercive, or otherwise harmful. Many of the reforms addressed in the recovery movement can be recast in terms of the rival values of self-determination and beneficence. Before the 1960s, few biological treatments were available for severe mental illness, especially for treating acute psychotic episodes. The days of indefinite hospitalizations in large state institutions were based on the limited psychiatric knowledge of the times, together with a societal belief that providing institutional care was beneficent. This is not to excuse some of the known abuses that took place in psychiatric institutions during the first half of the twentieth century; in retrospect, we now know that institutionalized patients suffered many harms, including violation of fundamental liberty rights. Some critics of psychiatry will likely consider this too charitable an interpretation of an unfortunate part of U.S. history. Our aim here is not to excuse offenses, but to illustrate how psychiatrists may have erred on the side of beneficence when they believed severely ill patients had limited capacities for self-determination.

Another principle of medical ethics helps explain some of the tension between psychiatry's persistent use of the term *patient*, and the preference of those persons to be called *clients, consumers,* or *stakeholders.* Recall that both the "consumer/survivor" and psychiatric rehabilitation programs struggled for persons with psychiatric illness to be thought of as full agents rather than as the sum of their symptoms. Recall, too, the recovery movement's promulgation of person-centered care. These efforts are meant to reconceptualize for care providers, as well as for consumers and their families, persons with mental illness as not merely passive recipients of diagnoses and treatments but as full participants in the process of deciding how to live with certain vulnerabilities. Furthermore, referring to oneself as a consumer provides a mechanism for asserting the independence and autonomy that the recovery movement urges others to recognize. Despite these efforts, psychiatrists are the holdouts among behavioral health professionals in using the word *patient* to describe the persons they treat; psychologists and social workers, among others, have adopted the terms *client* or *consumer* to describe those who utilize their services.

Medical professionalism instills in all physicians an obligation to serve the needs of the patient who cannot be abandoned once a doctor-patient relationship has been established. As stated in section 8 of the *Principles of Medical Ethics,* "A physician shall, while caring for a patient, regard responsibility to the patient as paramount" [16]. Doctors have resisted conceiving of their professional relationships as contracts with clients or as commercial services for sale to consumers, because doing so interferes with the sense of professional responsibility that has been ingrained since early in medical training. Furthermore, it is part of psychiatry's professional identity to maintain its status as a medical discipline: just as other medical specialties continue to treat "patients," so does psychiatry. For psychiatrists to treat "clients" or "consumers" rather than "patients" dilutes their sense of responsibility to persons with mental illness. However, it is easy to see how psychiatry's critics could interpret this resistance as an attempt by psychiatry to remain politically dominant among the behavioral health professions, especially since the growth of multidisciplinary teams is diffusing the power of the psychiatrist [13].

The responsibility for patients that psychiatry assumes for itself is simultaneously endorsed by the public's reliance on psychiatry to settle certain civil legal issues, most notably, civil commitment. Many of the public battles fought by recovery advocates over the past sixty years concern the extent to which autonomy can be attributed to persons with

244 *Claire L. Pouncey and Jonathan M. Lukens*

severe mental illness, the extent to which medication or hospitalization can be imposed against a person's wishes, and the extent to which the powers of the state and the psychiatric profession can be curtailed in order to empower the persons who suffer with mental disabilities. The Supreme Court of the United States has weakened states' abilities to confine people involuntarily and without the provision of treatment. However, psychiatrists still have a legal obligation to involuntarily commit persons who are dangerous as well as suffering from symptoms of a mental illness. Psychiatrists and other behavioral health professionals bear legal responsibility for protecting the public from patients whose mental illnesses make them dangerous by hospitalizing them involuntarily [17,18]. And psychiatrists must ascribe a diagnosis in order to do so. Psychiatric diagnoses are thus used to justify coercion, and psychiatry is forced into the role of the paternalistic enforcer. This social expectation creates a dual agency for the individual psychiatrist and an uncomfortable tension for the profession, both of which may be misinterpreted as a play for power and a violation of recovery values.

Ironically, patients who are involuntarily committed to hospitals are often those who stand to benefit most from the application of recovery principles. There has been some progress toward implementing systems that maximize patient self-determination even while they experience symptoms, such as instituting outpatient commitment laws and advance directives for mental health care. Such measures are of limited value, since in order to be effective, the patient must still desire treatment during her symptomatic episodes, an assumption that may not hold true. When a person experiences active symptoms that lead her to decline treatment, psychiatrists are less likely to respect patient preferences than they would be in a less critical situation [19]. Although the values that guide the recovery movement and psychiatry align in several central ways, there is reason for consumer criticism about psychiatrists' willingness to act paternalistically, if not coercively. However, it is important to note that such situations arise only when a patient is symptomatic and dangerous and is refusing the treatment that the psychiatrist *and the state* believe is necessary. Community psychiatry's dual allegiance to the public as well as to the patient occurs by mandate, not by choice.

Apart from civil commitment requirements and psychiatry's insistence on calling the persons who seek their care "patients," the professional values of psychiatry and those of the recovery movement align in several crucial respects. The significant divergences arise from psychiatry's concomitant commitments to other professional values. However, the alignment is further strained in forensic psychiatry in ways that present a real challenge to the recovery movement.

Forensic Psychiatry, Recovery, and Culpability

Forensic psychiatry, another psychiatric subspecialty, shares psychiatry's basic commitments but differs from community psychiatry in ways that are relevant to the recovery movement. Although public concerns sometimes temper the community psychiatrist's moral obligations to a patient, there is still a physician-patient relationship between them. In contrast, forensic psychiatrists sometimes work outside of any such relationship. Rather, forensic psychiatrists often work for the state, providing treatment within prisons or other forensic facilities, or they may be hired by an attorney to provide expert testimony either for or against a person with mental illness at trial. This creates a new set of ethical tensions for the forensic psychiatrist. Since forensic psychiatrists are involved in criminal as well as civil matters, psychiatrists who assess or treat prisoners or detainees do so in an inherently coercive setting in which self-determination is already strongly curtailed. Furthermore, when a psychiatrist testifies for the prosecution in a criminal trial, successful testimony may actually harm the patient, thus apparently violating the medical ethical principles of beneficence and nonmaleficence. In either case, the psychiatrist is not working directly for the patient, and at times may work against the mentally ill person, thus precluding a formal doctor-patient relationship.

Forensic psychiatry also contrasts with community psychiatry in that it often uses diagnosis in ways that counteract recovery principles. We saw that civil commitment uses psychiatric diagnosis in part to authorize involuntary commitment; forensic psychiatrists similarly use diagnosis to support recommendations regarding workers' compensation, child custody, or criminal culpability. In such cases, forensic psychiatry provides (1) a person's diagnosis and (2) psychiatric theory about how the symptoms associated with that diagnosis are likely to influence behavior. The state uses the forensic psychiatrist's report to decide whether to restrict the personal freedoms or entitlements in question. Although forensic psychiatrists strive to maintain neutrality and objectivity in making these assessments [20], such practices appear to legitimize the recovery movement's concern that persons with mental illnesses are not recognized as full agents but simply as the sum of their symptoms.

One important role of the forensic psychiatrist is to elucidate any causal role played by mental illness when persons with mental illness commit criminal acts. Sometimes psychiatrists serve as expert witnesses in criminal proceedings to testify whether the offender's mental illness makes her incompetent to stand trial, that is, to determine whether psychiatric symptoms render that person incapable of understanding the legal proceedings against her or of assisting in her own defense [17]. At other times, forensic psychiatrists are called upon to testify whether mental illness may have caused the criminal behavior in question. In such "insanity defense" cases, courts and juries use psychiatric testimony to decide whether the mental illness mitigates or exonerates the offender's responsibility for the act in question [21]. While the forensic psychiatrist does not ultimately decide the guilt or innocence of the offender, the role of the forensic expert is relevant to the recovery movement because it revives questions about whether and to what extent we can attribute social deviance to mental illness. Despite decades of sociological critique that psychiatry cannot infer the existence or presence of mental illness from deviant behavior alone [22], the forensic psychiatrist presupposes that severe mental illness can cause not just deviant but criminal behavior. Note that this is not the same as claiming that all social deviances are attributable to mental illness or that mental illness *always* causes deviant behavior. The lingering question is on what grounds and in what situations a psychiatrist can legitimately infer that mental illness caused criminally deviant behavior.

The corollary question is at what point society in general and psychiatry in particular are justified in questioning the moral and legal agency of a person whose mental illness severely influences his behavior. This question about agency is an old one in ethics, and it cuts to the heart of the recovery movement's position. As we have seen, the recovery movement's core value is to presume that all persons with mental illness are fully self-determining agents. However, recovery advocates do recognize that even in treatment, people with severe mental illness can expect a recurrence of symptoms at various times throughout their lives, and they are not to be blamed for those recurrences. But the recovery movement remains agnostic about how to reconcile patient autonomy and accountability, leaving policymakers to wonder how we should understand the transient changes to moral and legal agency that severe psychiatric symptoms can cause.

The situation can be characterized in Kantian terms. We can cast the recovery movement's central values as a commitment to both the moral worth of persons with mental illness and to their full participation in a community of moral agents who jointly decide how to conduct themselves in society. How does that community respond when a member violates the moral law? One response is that the person knowingly acted immorally, and should therefore suffer the consequences of doing so. But one also might consider whether the rational capacity a person requires in order to function as a full moral agent was compromised, giving that person's actions a different moral valence. That is, we ascribe culpability to rational moral agents who knowingly violate the moral law, but the misdeed itself can lead us to question whether the person who committed it was rational at the time. When rationality is called into question, a moral transgression might be less blameworthy in the eyes of the community, but the person must relinquish status as a full moral agent. Yet it is just this sense of agency that the recovery movement wants to protect for persons with severe mental illness.

Although the recovery literature encourages mental health care providers to treat persons with mental illness as fully rational agents, it is silent on the question of how to understand immoral and illegal acts committed by those persons when their agency seems to be transiently compromised by mental illness. The *National Consensus Statement on Mental Health Recovery*'s "fundamental components" include both self-direction and responsibility [7], suggesting that both our civil and our criminal social systems should treat persons with severe mental illness as they treat anyone else. However, with respect to criminal behavior, the mutual emphasis on responsibility and self-determination creates a paradox: whereas mental illness can be used to mitigate culpability when it causes illegal behaviors, the recovery movement could be expected to advocate against the position that mental illness exculpates illegal or immoral acts. With respect to socially aberrant or abhorrent behavior, these fundamental components suggest that the influence of mental illness on behavior should not excuse illicit acts.

Such a conclusion seems to contradict the basic message of the recovery movement, that even with psychiatric vulnerabilities, persons with mental illness have equal moral worth and deserve assistance to function fully in society. Besides access to services, jobs, education, housing, and treatment, this assistance includes a long history of special consideration under the law and efforts to divert mentally ill persons from prisons. The recovery movement now faces a dilemma: How can we advocate treating persons with mental illness as full moral agents for the purpose of providing social goods, while simultaneously treating them as compromised moral agents when the same illness earns them social sanction? Worded differently, if recovery entails reducing the stigma of socially deviant behavior and discouraging professional and governmental programmatic efforts to coerce conformity, can it consistently reconcile the use of psychiatric symptoms to excuse immoral or illegal acts?

However we phrase it, the question is not rhetorical. In 2003, the ongoing efforts of the recovery movement were rewarded in the United States when the President's New Freedom Commission on Mental Health submitted a report [23] that endorsed recovery values. It does not, however, provide substantive recommendations for how such ideals might be realized. While the New Freedom Commission's report promulgates the assignation of full agency to persons with mental illness, it does not explicitly address the question of *moral* or *legal* agency. Davidson interprets the report as an argument for recovery principles to guide all mental health services, *except* for forensic services for offenders with mental illness, which might strive instead for "containment or community safety" [8, p. 643]. Indeed, the report presupposes that some mental health care will be provided to prisoners, and it calls for providing appropriate diagnosis and treatment for offenders who are in jail. This suggests that having a serious mental illness does not automatically excuse criminal behavior. The report also advises that persons with symptomatic mental illness who have not committed crimes be diverted out of the legal system and provided with treatment in a safer and more appropriate setting. This reinforces the recovery principle that unpredictable behavior caused by severe mental illness is not in itself cause for confinement. However, the report also calls for providing "supervised community care" for "nonviolent offenders" [8, p. 43]. This possibility suggests that nonviolent criminal offenses committed by persons with severe mental illness may be at least partially excused by the illness or that the illness may mitigate the punishment. The report does not specify *which* symptoms exculpate *which* otherwise unjustified behaviors, nor does it justify modified punishment for offenders with mental illness.

The insanity defense thus raises an important challenge for recovery, even as it seems to legitimize the movement's concerns about the appropriate role of psychiatry in mental health care. Forensic psychiatry provides an opportunity for some offenders to receive treatment rather than punishment, which is consistent with the recovery movement's call to minimize the social mistreatment of persons with mental illness. But it seems to violate the recovery movement's insistence that mentally ill persons are full agents who can "lead, control, exercise choice over, and determine their own path of recovery" [7] when it uses compromised agency as the basis for mitigating responsibility for social wrongs.

Can Bioethics Be a Resource for the Recovery Movement?

Describing the tension between the recovery movement and the practices of forensic psychiatry in terms of Kantian agency elucidates both epistemological and ethical aspects of the problem. The epistemological questions concern how we can know about mental illnesses apart from their observable behavioral manifestations and what counts as evidence for or against that knowledge. These questions have been addressed extensively in the philosophy of psychiatry, and we will not review them here [24–26]. Additionally, some provocative empirical research is being done to identify what personal capacities and abilities are affected in persons with severe mental illnesses [27, 28], as well as how recovery principles might be enacted in forensic psychiatry [29, 30].

The question of agency in severe mental illness is fundamental, but neither the recovery movement nor bioethics has devoted much attention to it, either severally or jointly. We find this inattention surprising. Like the psychiatric rehabilitation and consumer self-help movements, academic bioethics also grew from the civil rights concerns of the 1950s and 1960s. It has been the source of influential discussions of practical questions about patients' rights, self-determination, quality of life, advance directives, substituted judgment, and truth telling to patients, which are all topics that have been addressed with respect to the recovery movement. Also, like the recovery movement, bioethics has contributed both directly and indirectly to social reforms, some of which have been applied to behavioral health, such as the initiation of advance directives for mental health care. The bioethics literature also includes a charged debate about how to define "mental disorder," and how to understand mental disorders as similar to or different from medical diseases [25,26,31,32]. Most pertinent, central questions about capacity and agency have been addressed in bioethics [33–37]. However, despite the parallel histories and mutual interests, the field of bioethics has not specifically engaged with the recovery movement to address concerns about patients' rights and moral agency, nor has it significantly clarified conceptual issues about self-determination, accountability, and culpability with respect to forensics.

We believe that academic bioethics, law, forensic psychiatry, and recovery-oriented social reformers would do well to collaborate. If social programs for the mentally ill are to be "transformed," as the New Freedom

Commission's report suggests they should be, part of that transformation should include opportunities and mechanisms for multidisciplinary collaboration. These could include joint workshops, conferences, and research projects to address both conceptual and practical obstacles to implementing recovery ideals. It is important that scholars, recovery advocates, and public policymakers explore together how our society will address moral agency and legal responsibility among persons with severe mental illness. Although activists may not welcome views from the ivory tower, the recovery movement is likely to benefit from historical perspectives, theoretical arguments, and conceptual analyses. Forensic psychiatry might be called upon to contribute insights about the heterogeneity among disorders, symptoms, and the persons who exhibit them in order to avoid overgeneralizations that hinder progress in adopting other recovery values. Ethical and legal scholarship might help to compare legal, moral, and political conceptions of agency. Finally, recovery advocates will keep the interests of stakeholders at the forefront of the exploration while benefiting from expertise about how to execute the particulars of the vision. We believe it will take input from multiple voices to implement recovery ideals without confusion or contradiction.

This joint effort could go on to address further questions that affect the implementation of recovery-based policies, such as, Are all volitional behaviors morally equivalent? Who has responsibility for deciding a person's capacity to do good or to abide by a basic social contract? or What mechanisms exist for transforming systems and educating the public about recovery implementation? Interdisciplinary programs could be developed to educate police, forensic facility staff, courts, and juries. A joint effort may also elucidate how prisoners with mental illness could benefit from recovery principles. Other questions are sure to follow.

Our goal here is not to set an agenda, but to call attention to how values and rhetoric can shape policy only up to a point. We have provided one example of how the current practices of one mental health subspecialty elucidates a contradiction in the basic recovery message. This single paradox posed by the mutually endorsed values of agency and responsibility should alert activists and policymakers that some fundamental problems need to be addressed before the recovery vision can be enacted.

References

1. Lerman, P. (1985). Deinstitutionalization and welfare policies. *American Association of Political and Social Science*, 479, 132–155.

2. Grob, G. N. (1992). Mental health policy in America: Myths and realities. *Health Affairs*, *11*, 7–21.

3. Frank, R., & Glied, S. (2006). *Better but not well: Mental health policy in the United States since 1950*. Baltimore, MD: Johns Hopkins University Press.

4. U.S. Department of Health and Human Services. (1999). *Mental health: A report of the surgeon general*. Rockville, MD: U.S. Department of Health and Human Services.

5. Corrigan, P. W., Mueser, K. T., Bond, G. R., Drake, R. E., & Solomon, P. (2008). *Principles and practices of psychiatric rehabilitation: An empirical approach*. New York: Guilford Press.

6. Solomon, P. (2004). Peer support/peer provided services underlying processes, benefits, and critical ingredients. *Psychiatric Rehabilitation Journal*, *27*, 392–403.

7. U.S. Department of Health and Human Services. (2009). *National consensus statement on mental health recovery*. U.S. Department of Health and Human Services. http://store.samhsa.gov/home. Accessed 12 August 2009.

8. Davidson, L., O'Connell, M., Tondora, J., Styron, T., & Kangas, K. (2006). The top ten concerns about recovery encountered in mental health system transformation. *Psychiatric Services (Washington, D.C.)*, *57*, 640–645.

9. Davidson, L., O'Connell, M. J., Tondora, J., Lawless, M., & Evans, A. C. (2005). Recovery in serious mental illness: A new wine or just a new bottle? *Professional Psychology, Research and Practice*, *36*, 480–487.

10. Jacobson, N., & Greenley, D. (2001). What is recovery? A conceptual model and explication. *Psychiatric Services (Washington, D.C.)*, *52*, 482–485.

11. Mulligan, K. (2003). Recovery movement gains influence in mental health programs. *Psychiatric News*, (January): 10.

12. Anthony, W. (1993). Recovery from mental illness: The guiding vision of the mental health service system in the 1990s. *Psychiatric Rehabilitation*, *16*, 12–23.

13. Rogers, J. A., Vergare, M. J., Baron, R. C., & Salzer, M. S. (2007). Barriers to recovery and recommendations for change: The Pennsylvania consensus conference on psychiatry's role. *Psychiatric Services (Washington, D.C.)*, *58*, 1119–1123.

14. Engel, G. L. (1980). The clinical application of the biopsychosocial model. *American Journal of Psychiatry*, *137*, 535–544.

15. Szasz, T. (1964). *The myth of mental illness: Foundations of a theory of personal conduct*. New York: Harper & Row.

16. American Psychiatric Association. (2009). *The principles of medical ethics with annotations especially applicable to psychiatry* (Rev. ed.). Washington, DC: Author. http://www.psych.org/MainMenu/PsychiatricPractice/Ethics/ResourcesStandards/PrinciplesofMedicalEthics.aspx. Accessed September 17, 2009.

17. Perlin, M. L. (Ed.). (1999). *Mental disability law: Cases and materials*. Durham, NC: Carolina Academic Press.

18. Appelbaum, P. S. (1994). *Almost a revolution: Mental health law and the limits of change.* New York: Oxford University Press.

19. Hamann, J., Mendel, R., Cohen, R., Heres, S., Ziegler, M., Bühner, M., et al. (2009). Psychiatrists' use of shared decision making in the treatment of schizophrenia: Patient characteristics and decision topics. *Psychiatric Services (Washington, D.C.), 60,* 1107–1112.

20. American Association of Psychiatry and the Law. (2005). *Ethics guidelines for the practice of forensic psychiatry.* Washington, DC: Author. http://www.aapl.org/ethics.htm. Accessed 23 September 2009.

21. Appelbaum, P. S., & Gutheil, T. G. (2007). *Clinical handbook of psychiatry and the law* (4th ed.). Philadelphia: Lippincott, Williams & Wilkins.

22. Aneshensel, C. S., & Phelan, J. C. (1999). *Handbook of the sociology of mental health.* New York: Kluwer Academic/Plenum.

23. U.S. Department of Health and Human Services. (2003). *President's New Freedom Commission on Mental Health: Achieving the promise: Transforming mental health care in America. Final report.* Rockville, MD: U.S. Department of Health and Human Services.

24. Sadler, J. Z. (2005). *Values and psychiatric diagnosis: International perspectives in philosophy and psychiatry.* New York: Oxford University Press.

25. Fulford, K. W. M. (1989). *Moral theory and medical practice.* Cambridge: Cambridge University Press.

26. Murphy, D. (2006). *Psychiatry in the scientific image.* Cambridge, MA: MIT Press.

27. Lieberman, J. A., Drake, R. E., Sederer, L. I., Belger, A., Keefe, R., Perkins, D., et al. (2008). Science and recovery in schizophrenia. *Psychiatric Services (Washington, D.C.), 59,* 487–496.

28. Ware, N. C., Hopper, K., Tugenberg, T., Dickey, B., & Fisher, D. (2008). A theory of social integration as quality of life. *Psychiatric Services (Washington, D.C.), 59,* 27–33.

29. Hillbrand, M., & Young, J. L. (2008). Instilling hope into forensic treatment: The antidote to despair and desperation. *Journal of the American Academy of Psychiatry and the Law, 36,* 90–94.

30. Wexler, D. (2008). *Rehabilitating lawyers: Principles of therapeutic jurisprudence for criminal law practice.* Durham, NC: Carolina Academic Press.

31. Boorse, C. [1976] (1982). What a theory of mental health should be. In R. B. Edwards (Ed.), *Psychiatry and ethics,* 29–48. Buffalo, NY: Prometheus Books.

32. Sedgwick, P. (1973). Illness—Mental and otherwise. *Hastings Center Studies, 1,* 19–40.

33. Appelbaum, P. S. (2007). Clinical practice: Assessment of patients' competence to consent to treatment. *New England Journal of Medicine, 357,* 1834–1840.

34. Appelbaum, P. S., Lidz, C. W., & Klitzman, R. (2009). Voluntariness of consent to research: A conceptual model. *Hastings Center Report, 39,* 30–39.

35. Drane, J. F. (1985). The many faces of competency. *Hastings Center Report,* *15,* 17–21.

36. Jefferson, A. L., Lambe, S., Moser, D. J., Byerly, L. K., Ozonoff, A., & Karlawish, J. H. (2008). Decisional capacity for research participation in individuals with mild cognitive impairment. *Journal of the American Geriatrics Society, 56,* 1236–1243.

37. Raad, R., Karlawish, J., & Appelbaum, P. S. (2009). The capacity to vote of persons with serious mental illness. *Psychiatric Services (Washington, D.C.), 60,* 624–628.

18

Ethical Considerations of Multiple Roles in Forensic Services

Robert Henley Woody

Over the past few decades, the practice of forensic psychology has advanced rapidly along an ambiguous pathway (Otto & Heilbrun, 2002): "The purview of forensic psychology continues to expand, demonstrating the breadth and differentiating scope of practice in this specialty field" (Craig, 2005, p. 3). Being in a "professional" specialty necessitates that a code of ethics provide a framework for provision of services to consumers (Brint, 1994). Alignment with behavioral science opens the door for mental health practitioners of every ilk to enter into the courtroom to provide forensic services (*Daubert v. Merrell Dow Pharmaceuticals, Inc.*, 1993).

The recent vicissitudes of the marketplace (e.g., the negative impact on the incomes of clinical practitioners) have introduced new temptations for some mental health practitioners to venture into new areas of practice. Since managed care is not involved, the fees for forensic services are often higher than pay for clinical services. This enticement leads some practitioners to enter forensic work with minimal or inadequate professional preparation. Consequently, forensic services may pose problems: "courtrooms are foreign territory for psychologists, psychiatrists, and social workers" (Melton, Petrila, Poythress, & Slobogin, 1997, p. 4), and "although therapists' concerns for their patients and for their own employment is understandable, this practice constitutes engaging in dual-role relationships and often leads to bad results for patients, courts, and clinicians" (Greenberg & Shuman, 1997, p. 50).

Barring Clinicians from the Courtroom

The objectives for clinical and forensic services are substantially different. Greenberg and Shuman (1997) believe that therapists are likely to encounter irreconcilable role conflicts when they become forensic experts, such as offering psycholegal opinions in court proceedings; their solution is for the psychologist to not try to be both a clinician and a forensic expert (Greenberg & Shuman, 2007). Strasberger, Gutheil, and Brodsky (1997) voiced this same restrictive view.

Granted, a problem may be created by a mental health practitioner's not having competence for all the roles that are requested or seemingly justified: "Just because a psychologist whose primary professional identity is that of 'therapist' is also competent at providing forensic examinations, and, conversely, just because a psychologist whose primary professional identity is that of 'forensic examiner' is also competent at providing therapy, does not lead to the conclusion that he or she should provide both services to the same individual" (Greenberg & Shuman, 2007, p. 129). Whether therapy or another form of clinical service, the mental health practitioner should be cautious about the potential dissonance created by multiple roles.

Solid clinical training and a high level of practice competency do not assure that there will be the expertise needed to adequately participate in legal proceedings. Thus, an ethical and best practice risk may arise because "with increasing frequency, psychologists, psychiatrists, and other mental health professionals are participating as forensic experts in litigation on behalf of their patients" (Greenberg & Shuman, 1997, p. 50).

The combined roles of clinician and forensic expert also raise the specter of objectivity being compromised. As Greenberg and Shuman (2007) state: "When a therapist also serves as a forensic expert, the therapist is part of the fabric of the case" (p. 130). This supports that forensic testimony by any clinician may be vulnerable to a conflict of interest, which points to the ethical standard:

Psychologists refrain from taking on a professional role when personal, scientific, professional, legal, financial, or other interests of relationships could reasonably be expected to (1) impair their objectivity, competence, or effectiveness in performing their functions as psychologists or (2) expose the person or organization with whom the professional relationship exists to harm or exploitation. (APA, 2002, p. 1065)

Similarly, the specialty guidelines for forensic psychology say: "Forensic practitioners refrain from taking on a professional role when personal, scientific, professional, legal, financial, or other interests or relationships could reasonably be expected to impair their objectivity, competence, or effectiveness in providing forensic services," and "When offering expert opinion to be relied upon by a decision maker, or when teaching or conducting research, forensic practitioners demonstrate commitment to the goals of accuracy, *objectivity*, fairness, and independence" [italics added] (Committee on the Revision of the Specialty Guidelines for Forensic Psychology, 2006, p. 5).

The notion underlying the "fabric of the case" caveat is that connecting clinical testimony to the outcome of the legal case may lead to a quasi-contingency effect. That is, the mental health practitioner will be susceptible to skewing the information toward a legal outcome that will be self-beneficial. Any semblance of a contingency that has a financial implication seems counter to ethics, as well as the specialty guidelines for forensic psychology:

Forensic practitioners avoid undue influence upon their methods, procedures and products that might result from financial compensation or other gains. Because of the threat to objectivity presented by the acceptance of contingent fees, forensic psychologists avoid providing professional services on the bias of contingent fees when those services involve the offering of evidence to a court or administrative body, or when called upon to make sworn statements or other affirmations to be relied upon directly by a court or tribunal. (Committee on the Revision of the Specialty Guidelines for Forensic Psychology, 2006, p. 12)

Although some mental health practitioners may be able to sidestep or negate any adverse effects from linking clinical and forensic objectives, it is an issue that merits consideration. After all, the specialty guidelines say: "Forensic practitioners recognize that providing both forensic and therapeutic services with regard to the same individual, or with closely related individuals, is *likely to create a role conflict and an apparent conflict of interest*" [italics added] (p. 11), and "Forensic practitioners treat all participants and weigh all data, opinions, and rival hypotheses impartially" (p. 5).

Mental health practitioners should not, of course, be kept totally from forensic services; for example, it may be that the practitioner's involvement was initiated for a clinical reason, and when a legal case develops, information from the clinical services will be of great importance to the legal matters. Barring a clinician from entering into a forensic role, as could potentially be accomplished by a statute or administrative code rule pertaining to a state license, has widespread impact. Heltzel (2007) recognizes that practitioners need to be aware of the ethical challenges that arise in forensic testimony but believes that any hard and fast restriction on a clinician's participation in legal proceedings would be detrimental to public interest. Speaking against regulation by a state licensing agency, Heltzel states:

Furthermore, for state boards of psychology to define a therapist's expert opinions as inherently unethical would be to usurp a prerogative and responsibility of a court to weight the credibility of any expert testimony. Such an approach would deny clients the use of the opinion of the therapist, which might be regarded as a free speech or civil rights issues. Certainly, the patient and court would lose access to an important source of vital information if a patient's therapist is prevented from expressing wellfounded expert opinions. . . . To deny treatment providers the ability to testify would impose significant costs on patients and the judicial system because of the necessity of requiring additional assessments from high-priced specialists. (p. 128)

Being "professional" services, the rationale for multiple roles is strengthened by the benefits that would potentially accrue to society in general and clients in particular (Brint, 1994).

In view of the arguments presented above, it seems shortsighted to simply proscribe more than one role for a mental health practitioner in a legal case. The ethics code from the APA (2002) states: "Multiple relationships that would not reasonably be expected to cause impairment or risk exploitation or harm are not unethical" (p. 1065). Relevant to forensic services, the ethics code acknowledges that a psychologist may encounter "extraordinary circumstances to serve in more than one role in judicial or administrative proceedings" (p. 1065). If nothing else, unless the practitioner is unfettered in knowledgeable and professional involvement, society and the clients may be unable to obtain certain benefits (e.g., consider the rural area that has precious few mental health practitioners available or the elevated fees that will be incurred by bringing in additional experts, when a therapist's testimony might suffice).

Reconciling Differences between Clinical and Forensic Roles

To be effective in forensic services, the mental health practitioner must be able to reconcile differences between the clinical and forensic roles. The prerequisite is the practitioner having knowledge of the legal system and being professionally comfortable working within it. The forensically naive expert "can get overly caught up in thinking that their testimony is about winning" (Brodsky, 2004, p. 11).

The role of the expert witness is not to promote winning for one of the parties, it is to assist the trier of fact (the judge or the jury):

If scientific, technical, or other specialized knowledge will assist the trier of fact in understanding the evidence or in determining a fact in issue, a witness qualified as an expert by knowledge, skill, experience, training, or education, may testify about it in the form of an opinion; however, the opinion is admissible only if it can be applied to evidence at the trial. (Florida Statutes 90.702)

Some therapists may find it difficult to shift from communications that reflect primary concern for a client's clinical needs to giving priority to assisting the court (especially when the objectives of the judicial system are contrary to the clinical needs of the client).

A lack of familiarity with the legal system and a willingness and ability to embrace it, even if contrary to the client's clinical needs, can result in disciplinary problems for the mental health practitioner. A high number of complaints to ethics committees, licensing boards, or courts of law are lodged against the allegedly ill-informed or improperly functioning psychologist in courtroom. Clearly specialized training in forensic issues is essential (e.g., knowing the rules and procedures relevant to a particular legal case).

In the forensic context, it is fundamental that a mental health practitioner adhere to relevant ethics, be adequately versed in behavioral science, and understand the unique characteristics of the legal system. As discussed, the clinician's involvement in forensic services points to multiple roles that can create conflict of interest, of which some may be irreconcilable (Greenberg & Shuman, 1997, 2007; Woody, 2002a, 2002b).

From the point of view of ethics, it is preferable that the clinician maintain a clear and singular role testifying in a forensic case. For example, in child custody cases, "multiple roles, even if requested by the court [or legal counsel] or the parents, should be opposed, and if insisted upon, a motion to withdraw from the case should be submitted to the court" (Woody, 2000, p. 50). However, in accord with the earlier rationale, it seems logical to accept that, although it might be potentially risky, the clinician may appropriately enter into a forensic role as well.

The Pitfalls for Multiple Roles

In a legal case, the crux of the problem for the mental health practitioner is that the attorney's primary objective is to champion the legal interests of the litigant (the petitioner/plaintiff/complainant versus the respondent/defendant). On the other hand, "the forensic psychologist's main goal is to help the court" (Craig, 2005, p. 12). Because of these differing purposes, "it is apparent that mental health professionals are frequently misused, overused, and, on occasion, underused by the legal system, depending upon the specific issues" (Melton et al., 1997, p. viii).

Interprofessional Relationships

Beyond differing purposes, the various professionals working repeatedly in legal cases (e.g., judges, attorneys, mental health practitioners) eventually become acquainted, commonly at a personal level. Personal-social relationships may develop, especially if the context is a small community. Gould (2006) expresses concern about these "extralegal relationships" giving "the *perception* of impropriety" (p. 371) and says: "Once a shadow has been cast upon either your credibility or the objectivity of your data, it is difficult to rehabilitate the external perception of your neutrality" (pp. 371–372). The values, public policies, and laws of modern society and the standards and ethics of the contemporary mental health professions oppose even the appearance of impropriety being attached to public and professional services (Morgan & Reynolds, 1997). It is known that attorneys and judges often face this same sort of "perception of impropriety" and must struggle with how to ameliorate any negative effects.

Professional Bias

Accepting multiple roles introduces the possibility of professional bias. Berliner and Conte (1993) state: "Professional bias, whether it results from the psychological needs of the professional, *the commercial sale of professional opinion as in some expert testimony* or other factors appears to be a significant problem in this field" [italics added] (p. 112).

Conflict of Interest

As discussed earlier, a threshold issue for the practitioner involved in multiple clinical-forensic roles is the possibility of a conflict of interest: "a situation in which individuals or groups are drawn to the pursuit of goals or outcomes that are incompatible with the goals they are supposed to be pursuing" (VandenBos, 2007, p. 215). In psychology, this is also referred to as "double agentry": "the situation in which the therapist's allegiance to the patient is in conflict with the demands from the institution or from other professionals" (p. 298).

In discussing ethical lapses, Benjamin and Gollan (2005) recognize that "it has been common for psychologists or other mental health providers to provide psychotherapeutic and evaluative functions within the same case, despite the resulting conflicts of interest or the appearance of conflict generated by combining therapeutic and forensic roles" (p. 30); however, they assert that such multiple relationships should be avoided. Babitsky and Mangraviti (1997) include conflicts of interest among the common ethical violations by expert witnesses.

Thus, if someone in the legal system (e.g., a particular attorney) presses the practitioner into a forensic role that includes legal advocacy, it is feasible that the clinical or other mental health role will become secondary and/or in conflict with the preferences of the legal source. As an example of this potential dilemma, Benjamin and Gollan (2005) advise against the forensic psychologist's having ex parte communications with any legal source since "contact with only one of the professional legal people involved in the case . . . may lead to the appearance of unfairness or prejudice" (p. 44).

Ethical Implications

For psychologists entering into forensic services, there are two documents that, when combined, create what might be considered an ethical framework for the issue of multiple roles in forensic psychology: Ethical Principles of Psychologists and Code of Conduct (APA, 2002) and Specialty Guidelines for forensic Psychologists (Committee on Ethical Guidelines for Forensic Psychologists, 1991, 2008). Practitioners from the other mental health disciplines should consider the relevant code ethics. Further, every practitioner should be mindful of statutory law and administrative code rules that define propriety for practice in the given jurisdiction.

Essentially all ethical documents deem it necessary to recognize potential conflicts of interests that may occur in multiple relationships. For example, the APA ethical code has a general principle that states: "When conflicts occur among psychologists' obligations or concerns, they attempt to resolve these conflicts in a responsible fashion that avoids or minimizes harm"; and psychologists should "seek to manage conflicts of interest that could lead to exploitation or harm" (p. 1062). As mentioned earlier, the APA ethics code also contains a standard about refraining from taking on a professional role that might impair objectivity, competence, or effectiveness or bring about harm or exploitation (see APA, 2002, p. 1065). Similarly, the specialty guidelines make it clear that when a legal proceeding requires multiple roles, "forensic psychologists take reasonable steps to minimize the potential negative effects of these circumstances" (Committee on Ethical Guidelines for Forensic Psychologists, 1991, p. 659). Although not ethically wrong per se, accepting multiple roles can be expected to elevate the risk of a conflict of interest and open the door to a possible question about the practitioner's professional ethics and standards.

Possible Forensic Roles

To develop protective knowledge, the mental health practitioner should understand the various roles that occur in the forensic context. By defining each role clearly, the professional can identify the factors that could complicate ethical decision making. As Knapp, Gottlieb, Berman, and Handelsman (2007) point out: "Often apparent conflicts between the law and ethics can be avoided if psychologists anticipate problems ahead of time or engage in integrative problem solving" (p. 58).

Due to the needs of the legal system and a mental health practitioner's wealth of knowledge and practical skills, there is a myriad of possible forensic roles. The American Board of Forensic Psychology (ABFP, 2007) indicates that the practice of forensic psychology includes psychological evaluation and expert testimony regarding criminal and civil forensic issues; assessment, treatment, and consultation regarding individuals who pose high risk for aggressive behavior; research, testimony, and consultation on psychological issues impacting on the legal process; specialized treatment service to individuals involved with the legal system; consultation to lawmakers about public policy issues with psychological implications; consultation and training to law enforcement, criminal justice, and correctional systems; consultation and training to mental health systems and practitioners on forensic issues; analysis of issues related to human performance, product liability, and safety; court-appointed monitoring of compliance with settlements in class-action suits affecting mental health or criminal justice settings; mediation and conflict resolution; policy and program development in the psychology-law arena; teaching, training and supervision of graduate students, psychology, and psychiatry interns/residents, and law students (note that the items are paraphrased or partially quoted from the referenced source). In accord with the ABFP definition, Bartol and Bartol (2004) provide a detailed list of functions or services appropriate for forensic psychologists.

From the foregoing services, Wrightsman and Fulero (2005) deduce three roles: being a trial consultant for jury selection, case preparation, and pretrial publicity; conducting forensic evaluations; and offering expert testimony. This trichotomy of forensic services appears overly simple.

It seems that there are, in fact, five roles for mental health practitioners in forensic cases. The five roles are (1) academic/behavioral science expert, (2) fact witness as a treating therapist, (3) expert witness based on a clinically oriented assessment, (4) pretrial and/or trial consultant, and (5) professional critic of other experts. Any combination of the roles might contribute to a possible conflict of interest.

Being an academic/behavioral science expert should, in some ways, be inherent to all of the other roles. After all, the mental health practitioner is invited into a legal case to bring academic and scientific knowledge that will assist the trier of fact. As a treating therapist for a client who becomes embroiled in litigation, assuming that the client's mental factors are relevant and material to a legal issue before the court, factual information from the clinical context has broad acceptance and possible benefit for the court.

Giving factual testimony as a scholar or treating therapist is relatively low in risk because the role of the witness predated involvement in the particular legal case. The problem or potential for significant (elevated) risk arises when the mental health practitioner also attempts to do a forensic assessment of a person who had previously been solely a therapy recipient (i.e., the assessment would not be for therapeutic purposes), serve as a pretrial and/or trial consultant, and/or testify (critique) other experts who testify. Any of the roles could, however, be enhanced by offering relevant academic or scientific information.

For the mental health practitioner who offers expert opinion testimony, the possibility of advocacy of a particular legal outcome may develop. When a mental health practitioner assists one of the attorneys as a pretrial and/or trial consultant, there seems no doubt that a partisan stance has been adopted; if this consulting role moves to one of the other roles (e.g., being expert witness about treatment or assessment), the possibility of an ethical violation is profound. If one of the attorneys asks (or gets the court to order) a mental health practitioner who has, say, testified for whatever reason (e.g., academic or consultant) or in whatever manner (fact or expert) to also serve as a professional critic of another expert, the dual role has been bathed in legal advocacy, and the appearance of impropriety comes into focus.

Establishing Competency for Forensic Services

As discussed, all mental health practitioners are not prepared to engage in forensic services. Although the particular legal matter or forensic role will determine the competency that is needed, suffice it to say that the mental health practitioner's effectiveness in forensic services requires formal and extensive training and supervision relevant to both law and mental health services. The old adage "a little knowledge is a dangerous thing" is too often evident in forensic services. Further, society is currently plagued by a number of quasi-professional sources that issue (some would say "sell") a diploma or certification that will allow a mental health practitioner to move into forensic service but provide little or no true assurance of competency (Woody, 1997, 2007). It is counter to professionalism to engage in forensic services without well-established competency.

Conclusion

Attorneys and judges alike tend to want to maximize usage of a mental health practitioner's knowledge, skills, and expertise. In other words, the legal system wants the "biggest bang for the buck." Taken alone, this is an inappropriate and inadequate reason for the practitioner to risk violating professional ethics and standards.

When mental health practitioners are pressed into multiple roles that "could reasonably be expected to (1) impair their objectivity, competence, or effectiveness in performing their functions as psychologists or (2) expose the person or organization with whom the professional relationship exists to harm or exploitation" (APA, 2002, p. 1065), the action of choice would be to immediately attempt to resolve and manage the risk of a conflict in a responsible fashion to avoid or minimize harm. In many instances, the most honorable alternative would be to withdraw from (1) all but one role or (2) fully from the case. Further, the practitioner should recall the ethical standard: "If psychologists' ethical responsibilities conflict with law, regulations, or other governing legal authority, psychologists make known their commitment to the Ethics Code and take steps to resolve the conflict" (p. 1063).

There is no disgrace in owning uncertainty about conflict resolution: "Even the most seasoned and knowledgeable clinicians may be unsure of how to proceed in some situations" (Barnett, 2007, p. 7). The responsible approach is to seek to be proactive (e.g., analyze the forensic situation to identify possible pitfalls or risks), that is, the "process should try to foresee multiple relationship problems in an effort to prevent them . . . [which] is far preferable to coping with them afterwards" (Gottlieb, Robinson, & Younggren, 2007, p. 247).

References

American Board of Forensic Psychology. (2007). [Brochure]. Savannah, GA: Author.

American Psychological Association. (2002). Ethical principles of psychologists and code of conduct. *American Psychologist, 57*(12), 1060–1073.

Babitsky, S., & Mangraviti, J. J., Jr. (1997). *How to excel during cross-examination: Techniques for expert that work*. Falmouth, MA: SEAK.

Barnett, J. E. (2007). The ethical decision-making process in everyday practice. *Professional Psychology, 38*(1), 7–9.

Bartol, C. R., & Bartol, A. M. (2004). *Introduction to forensic psychology.* Thousand Oaks, CA: Sage.

Benjamin, G. A., & Gollan, J. K. (2005). *Family evaluation in custody litigation: Reducing risks of ethical infractions and malpractice.* Washington, DC: American Psychological Association.

Berliner, L., & Conte, J. R. (1993). Sexual abuse evaluations: Conceptual and empirical obstacles. *Child Abuse and Neglect, 17,* 111–125.

Brint, S. (1994). *In an age of experts: The changing role of professionals in politics and public life.* Princeton, NJ: Princeton University Press.

Brodsky, S. L. (2004). *Coping with cross-examinations and other pathways to effective testimony.* Washington, DC: American Psychological Association.

Committee on Ethical Guidelines for Forensic Psychologists. (1991). Specialty guidelines for forensic psychologists. *Law and Human Behavior, 15*(6), 655–665.

Committee on the Revision of the Specialty Guidelines for Forensic Psychology. (2006). *Special guidelines for forensic psychology.* Unpublished manuscript.

Craig, R. J. (2005). *Personality-guided forensic psychology.* Washington, DC: American Psychological Association.

Daubert v. Merrell Dow Pharmaceuticals, Inc. (1993). 113 S. Ct. 786.

Gottlieb, M. C., Robinson, K., & Younggren, J. N. (2007). Multiple relations in supervision: Guidance for administrators, supervisors, and students. *Professional Psychology, 38*(3), 241–247.

Gould, J. W. (2006). *Conducting scientifically crafted child custody evaluations* (2nd ed.). Sarasota, FL: Professional Resource Press.

Greenberg, S. A., & Shuman, D. W. (1997). Irreconcilable conflict between therapeutic and forensic roles. *Professional Psychology, 28,* 50–57.

Greenberg, S. A., & Shuman, D. W. (2007). When worlds collide: Therapeutic and forensic roles. *Professional Psychology, 38*(2), 129–132.

Heltzel, T. (2007). Compatibility of therapeutic and forensic roles. *Professional Psychology, 38*(2), 122–128.

Knapp, S., Gottlieb, M., Berman, J., & Handelsman, M. M. (2007). When laws and ethics collide: What should psychologists do? *Professional Psychology, 38*(1), 54–59.

Melton, G. B., Petrila, J., Poythress, N. G., & Slobogin, C. (1997). *Psychological evaluations for the courts: A handbook for mental health professionals and lawyers* (2nd ed.). New York: Guilford.

Morgan, P. W., & Reynolds, G. H. (1997). *The appearance of impropriety.* New York: Free Press.

Otto, R. K., & Heilbrun, K. (2002). The practice of forensic psychology. *American Psychologist, 57*(1), 5–18.

Strasberger, L., Gutheil, T., & Brodsky, A. (1997). On wearing two hats: Role conflict in serving as both psychotherapist and expert witness. *American Journal of Psychiatry, 154*, 448–456.

VandenBos, G. R. (Ed.). (2007). *American Psychological Association dictionary of psychology*. Washington, DC: American Psychological Association.

Woody, R. H. (1997). Dubious and bogus credentials in mental health practice. *Ethics and Behavior, 7*(4), 337–345.

Woody, R. H. (2000). *Child custody: Practice standards, ethical issues, and legal safeguards for mental health professionals*. Sarasota, FL: Professional Resource Press.

Woody, R. H. (2002a). Clinical psychology in the courtroom: Part I. Proper and multiple roles in forensic services. *Clinical Psychologist, 55*(3), 11–15.

Woody, R. H. (2002b). Clinical psychology in the courtroom: Part II. Being a professional critic. *Clinical Psychologist, 55*(4), 13–18.

Woody, R. H. (2007). Bogus and dubious credential revisited: Professionalism requires action. *In Practice, 27*(3), 140–141.

Wrightsman, L. S., & Fulero, S. M. (2005). *Forensic psychology* (2nd ed.). Belmont, CA: Wadsworth.

19

Watch Your Language: A Review of the Use of Stigmatizing Language by Canadian Judges

Michelle Black and Jocelyn Downie

"The difference between the almost right word and the right word is really a large matter—it's the difference between the lightning bug and the lightning."[1] —Mark Twain

Introduction

It might be expected that with more knowledge about the causes and consequences of psychological disorders, we would see a reduction in stigmatizing behaviors toward those who have mental illness. However, according to a U.S. Surgeon General's Report and other, more recent research, there is actually even more stigma now than there was forty years ago.[2] The history of mental illness can be captured by Kale's description of the history of epilepsy: "4000 years of ignorance, superstition, and stigma followed by 100 years of knowledge, superstition, and stigma."[3] This is troubling because stigmatization may lead to a person being stereotyped and/or discriminated against, for example, through loss of job or housing opportunities, denial of societal rights (e.g., to hold elective office in the United States[4]), and being made more reluctant to seek psychiatric care.[5]

A commonly identified culprit in the stigmatization of mental illness is the media.[6] Television shows, movies, and news outlets regularly convey images of people with (often unnamed) mental illnesses as dangerous individuals to be feared. They also play regularly to any number of the other prevalent stereotypes of individuals with mental illness.[7] Less well recognized is the role of the courts in the stigmatization of mental illness. However, it has been reported that U.S. judges have a history of using and/or allowing stigmatizing language in their courtrooms.[8] We therefore decided to investigate the use of such language in Canadian cases.

Canadian courts are highly respected institutions and, given the powerful position of judges in our society, we wondered whether stigmatizing language was being used in and by them. To determine whether the language used by Canadian judges in their decisions was stigmatizing with respect to mental illness, we conducted a computer-based qualitative research review. We found that although judges are generally respectful in their decisions, there were a number of instances in which judges used stigmatizing language.[9] To explain how we came to this conclusion, we first define our terms and describe our methodology. We then describe and discuss our results. We then offer some reflections on possible reasons for these results and, finally, call upon all Canadian judges to stop the use of stigmatizing language with respect to persons with mental illness.

Terminology

It is important to first carefully define our terms—specifically, *stigma* and *stigmatizing language*. Stigma as a concept has evolved over time, with researchers taking the dictionary definition ("a mark of shame or discredit"[10]) and transforming it into a much more complex concept. The early work of Goffman is seen as a critical foundation from which much of the expansion of the concept of stigma has been built.[11] Goffman defined *stigma* as an attribute with particular results; stigma is "an attribute that is deeply discrediting" within a particular social interaction that results in the stigmatized person being reduced from "a whole and usual person to a tainted, discounted one."[12] Since Goffman's early work, a substantial literature on stigma has been produced; Link and Phelan attribute the ever-growing supply of definitions and information arising in this context to the variety of circumstances in which stigma research has been conducted and to the multidisciplinary nature of such research.[13]

A survey of the increasingly complex definitions of *stigma* can be somewhat bewildering. Sartorius, for example, describes stigma as "the negative attitude (based on prejudice and misinformation) that is triggered by a marker of illness—e.g., odd behaviour or mention of psychiatric treatment."[14] Corrigan carries the concept a step further to assert that "stigma is the cue that signals a specific attitude-behavior link."[15] On this view, the attitude is the driving force behind the behaviors. According to Link and colleagues, "stigma exists when elements of labeling, stereotyping, separation, status loss, discrimination, and emotional reactions occur together in a power situation that allows them."[16] Thus, stigma is seen as a mark, an attitude, a behavior, an attitude-behavior link, or a result. It is seen to rest in the subject or the object of the stigmatization. We are not in a position to resolve the definitional debates of this specialized field. We therefore acknowledge the complexity but take as our working definitions the following:

- *Stigma* means "a mark of shame or discredit."
- *Stigmatizing* means "causing or bestowing stigma."
- *Stigmatizing language* is language that marks mental illness as something for which one should feel shame, conveys negative judgments about persons by virtue of their mental illness, and relies upon or reinforces negative stereotypes of persons with mental illness.

Methods

Following the Supreme Court of Canada's decision in *R v. Swain*,[17] Parliament amended sections of the Criminal Code of Canada (Criminal Code) dealing with mental disorders.[18] For example, and of particular relevance for this article, in section 16 of the Criminal Code, the word *insanity* was replaced with the term *mental disorder*.[19] Thus, an accused could be found "not criminally responsible on account of mental disorder" instead of "not guilty by reason of insanity." The substance of section 16 remained essentially the same; the wording was the biggest change. The changes to the wording of section 16 were made after conducting consultations with, among others, "health officials" and non-governmental organizations, including the Canadian Mental Health Association, which felt that a change in the wording would "bring it in line with current psychiatric views."[20]

We hypothesized that despite deliberate changes in the wording of the legislation and despite increased knowledge about the etiology of mental illness and the importance of choosing words carefully, stigmatizing language would continue to be found in the text of judges' decisions. To test our hypothesis, we first established a list of words and phrases that can be stigmatizing in the context of talking about persons with mental illness. We then searched for these terms in the decisions of judges in Canadian courts available through LexisNexis Quicklaw. We searched all Canadian cases reported after the enactment of Bill C-30 on February 4, 1992.

The specific terms for which we searched were *admit, confess, arrest, imprison* (with *mental health, mental illness,* or *mental issue* in the same paragraph); a selection of archaic terms, including *insane* (truncated so deviations such as *insanity* would also be picked up), *lunatic, imbecile, idiot, nutter, shrink, headshrinker,* and *moron* (with *mental health, mental illness,* or *mental issue* in the same sentence); and *schizophrenic.*[21] Generally, these terms were chosen because, in the context of decisions involving persons with mental illness, they can be (whether indirectly or directly, whether intentionally or not) stigmatizing toward those with mental illness. More detailed explanations of the problems with the use of such language can be found in the Results/Discussion section.

Results/Discussion

We should first note and indeed emphasize that the judges' decisions dealing with persons with mental illness are generally crafted to show a high level of respect for those with mental illness. Many cases do not use any stigmatizing language and some of the terms for which we searched were not found.[22] However, there remain disturbing uses of stigmatizing language in judicial decisions. The following results and discussion include examples of the use of stigmatizing language and explain more fully why we and others consider such use to be stigmatizing and, therefore, to be avoided.[23]

Inaccurate Terminology
Admit
Admit is a term that is sometimes used by judges when speaking of people acknowledging their mental illness:

> I would add that a decision to consent to treatment on P.C.'s[24] behalf would not violate P.C.'s determined refusal to admit that he suffers from mental illness, since such a decision would not be made by P.C.[25]

> K.J.D.'s refusal to admit that she is "sick" or suffering from a mental illness may arguably support the conclusion that she does not have insight into her illness.[26]

> Mrs. S. tried very hard to avoid the issue of her mental condition at the time. At one point she said that it would only be raised if it was necessary. The irresistible conclusion is that at the time she was suffering from a serious mental illness which she did not care to admit.[27]

> I do not believe that counselling while on a conditional sentence order would cause Mr. S. to accept that he has a mental problem of some sort. I am forced to conclude that a jail sentence is more likely to achieve that necessary end. I think this is an aspect of specific deterrence, a perhaps somewhat unusual aspect, but it is necessary before rehabilitation can take place for Mr. S. to admit a problem and be willing to actively attempt to deal with it.[28]

Dr. W. pointed to a further inconsistency in Mr. M.'s behaviour. Most paranoid schizophrenics are reluctant to admit they are ill once they are in treatment, and will resist taking medication and try to hide their illness. However, Mr. M. tended to call out to anybody who would listen that he was ill.[29]

In Dr. D.'s opinion, Mr. W.'s behaviour presents certain risks to himself and to others, and requires treatment, which should be administered by force if he refuses it. Dr. D. assesses these risks on the basis of Mr. W.'s past behaviour, his refusal to admit that he has any mental illness, his inability to understand how medical treatment can improve his mental state, and his innate mistrust of the Institute's staff.[30]

Since the stigma surrounding mental illness is still so strong, people who have received a diagnosis of mental illness might feel that it is something to which they might have to "admit." However, judicial use of this term perpetuates the notion that mental illness is something of which to be ashamed, or to keep as a secret. This cannot be due to a lack of acceptable alternatives—there are many words or phrases, such as *acknowledge*, *show appreciation (for)*, and *recognize*, that convey the appropriate meaning without the connotation of shameworthiness.

Arrest

Arrest is a term that is sometimes used by judges when describing the apprehension of persons with mental illness not on suspicion of having committed criminal offenses but, rather, for the purpose of having them taken into the mental health system for purposes of psychological assessment.

Subsequently, police attended at the accused's location and arrested him under the authority of the Mental Health Act and transported him to hospital.[31]

There were indications from D.K. that her husband was upset and depressed. As a result, the respondent was arrested under the Mental Health Act, R.S.N. 1990 c. M-9 and brought to the police lockup in St. John's for assessment by a doctor.[32]

It was at this point, some 30 minutes after awakening the Accused, that Constable K. stated that he had "reasonable and probable grounds to believe" that she was a danger to herself, and he therefore arrested her under the Mental Health Act.[33]

However, the term *arrest* is inappropriate when describing the process of detaining a person under mental health legislation for psychological assessment.[34] The word *arrest* is, of course, an appropriate term to use when describing police actions in relation to, for example, a theft. However, none of the provincial/territorial mental health acts actually contain the word *arrest*.[35] Despite this, as illustrated above, the word *arrest* continues to be used by judges when describing the apprehension of someone for the purposes of having them submit to a psychiatric evaluation under mental health legislation.

Surprisingly, judges persist in using the word *arrest* even when they are aware that it is not present in the statute. For example, one judge used the subheading, "Arrest under the Mental Health Act," and then proceeded to outline the provisions of that part of the act: "The Mental Health Act . . . provides that a person suffering from a mental disorder, defined in s. 1(g) of the Act, may be apprehended under s. 10 or s. 12 of the Act."[36] Despite having just given a word-for-word recitation of the relevant part of the statute, and despite the fact that the word *arrest* does not appear in the section, the judge still referred to the process as an "arrest."

Similarly, another judge discussed at some length the purpose behind the Mental Health Act, but still referred to the action taken as being an "arrest" rather than detention or apprehension:

> I presume that on each occasion the complainant was arrested pursuant to s. 17 of the Mental Health Act. A purposive analysis of the arrest power under s. 17 of the Mental Health Act reveals that it is meant to be employed as the initial stage in a course of treatment for an individual in certain circumstance[s] including whether the police officer is of the opinion that "the person is apparently suffering from mental disorder of a nature or quality" that will likely result in serious bodily harm or serious physical impairment to that person or another person.[37]

Another judge acknowledged that there is some value to distinguishing between arresting a person and taking a person into custody, but maintained that being "arrested" per the Criminal Code and being taken into custody per the Mental Health Act are essentially the same thing:

> I recognize the social value of distinguishing between people who have been taken into custody for health reasons and those who have been arrested because they allegedly committed a criminal offence. However, the reality remains that generally police officers are authorized to act in the same manner under the Act as they would under the Criminal Code, R.S.C. 1985, c. C-46, when performing an arrest. There is really no substantive distinction between the act of forcibly taking someone into custody, and the act of arresting someone. Both generate risks to the individual, the police and the public. Specifically, as compared to a criminal offence, taking a person into custody who has mental health problems potentially generates similar or sometimes greater risks to officer and public safety. Such a risk is clearly present when the officers are responding to a threat by a person to cause bodily harm to himself or to another person.[38]

The judge here failed to appreciate the seriously stigmatizing impact on individuals with mental illness of suggesting that there is no meaningful substantive difference between being suspected of having committed a crime and being thought to be mentally ill. With the focus on the effects on police officers and the public, the judge lost sight of the effect on the persons with mental illness.

Certainly, there are times when a person who happens to have a mental illness will be arrested because he or she is alleged to have committed a crime. But when the judge explicitly indicates that the person was "arrested" per mental health legislation, it is an inaccurate and stigmatizing statement.

Imprison

Just as it is stigmatizing and inaccurate to say that a person has been arrested under mental health legislation, so too is it objectionable to indicate that a person is being "imprisoned" at a psychiatric institution, even when he or she is there involuntarily. Nonetheless, such language can be found in the case law:

Considering that the defendant Hospital is not empowered to imprison its patients or force treatment upon them, absent Certification under the Mental Health Act which is the province of physicians, I query the seriousness of this argument.[39]

If a person is being detained at a hospital for a psychiatric evaluation or treatment, he or she is not being imprisoned. It is important to distinguish between the two concepts, as speaking of imprisonment and arresting people under mental health legislation perpetuates the notion that people with mental health problems are, or are like, criminals and have done something blameworthy.

Archaic Language
Insane

Just as it is no longer acceptable to refer to someone as "crazy," it is also unacceptable to use such terms as *lunatic, imbecile, idiot,* and *insane.*[40] While it might be argued that some of these words do continue to appear in legislation, it is unnecessary to use these words unless quoting directly from the statute. As mentioned in the Introduction, deliberate steps have been taken to remove the word *insanity* from the mental disorder provisions of the Criminal Code, so one would (and reasonably could) expect a concurrent shift in the language of the courts. However, it is still possible to find objectionable archaic language in the case law:

It is obvious that it is fundamental to Mr. C.'s case in the present action that he is not insane and was not insane when he was judicially found to be insane.[41]

Either she [the accused] is insane or she is evil, one or the other, which one is it?[42]

In this case, the Crown argues that while the foregoing comments were specific to an insanity defence, they apply equally to this case where the defence lies in a lack of intent.[43]

First of all, we must point out that, after rejecting the defence of insanity, the jury could still have considered the appellant's mental condition in deciding whether the Crown had proven beyond a reasonable doubt that she had the specific intent to commit murder when she killed her son.[44]

The Alberta Court of Appeal set aside the conviction and ordered a new trial on the ground that the trial judge had erred in his interpretation of the insanity provision of s. 16(1) of the Criminal Code, R.S.C., 1985, c. C-46. The Crown appeals to this Court against that order, seeking reinstatement of the conviction for murder.[45]

Before dealing with those two submissions I want to say that, in my opinion, the Judge was correct in not putting either insanity or self-defence to the jury. There was no evidence that Mr. H. met the test of insanity set out in s. 16 of the Criminal Code of Canada or that he was acting in self-defence.[46]

(Nor is it likely that someone can really intend to get so intoxicated that they would reach a state of insanity or automatism.)[47]

In what might appear to be a step in the right direction, a judge in one case put the word "insane" in quotes, thus appearing to recognize its problematic nature. However, the footnote accompanying the word belies even a moderately positive interpretation of the step: "I use the word 'insane' when speaking at a general level to refer to anyone who is exempt from criminal liability under s. 16 of the Criminal Code."[48] As of the decision date, *insane* was no longer a term used in section 16.

One response to our criticism of the continued use of the term *insane* might be that the new terminology (i.e., *mental disorder*) is ungainly. This is in fact a criticism that some have levied against "people-first language" (discussed below under the subheading "Non–People First Language")—that people-first language "is unwieldy and repetitive, and any ear tuned to appreciate vigorous, precise prose must be offended by its impact on a good sentence."[49] Similar criticisms, under the guise of economy of language, have been implied in terms of the section 16 provisions:

However, in order to more accurately reflect the provisions of section 16 of the Criminal Code [Justice Bastarache] stated that the terms "mental disorder" automatism and "non–mental disorder" automatism should be used instead of insane and non-insane automatism. Professor Paciocco refers to non-mental disorder automatism more economically as "sane automatism" which is a term that I prefer."[50]

But we are not just talking about the quality of prose or the elegance of a sentence. More important, we are also talking about the dignity of people who should not be identified by words that are insulting and harmful. Despite what the judge said in the previous example, there is no necessity to be economical in the judgment. Respectful, yes. Accurate, yes. Economical, no.

Unlike the judges quoted above, other judges acknowledge the change in the Criminal Code ("The current wording of s. 16 which references 'mental disorder' recently replaced earlier language defining insanity"[51]), and they make use of the new terminology ("it is the defence's primary position that Mr. S.A.T.C. is not criminally responsible for his actions in the sense that the defence of mental disorder which is set forth in section 16 of the Criminal Code of Canada applies.")[52]. Clearly, it is possible to phase out the use of this antiquated term.

Lunatic

Archaic words such as *idiot* and *lunatic* were once acceptable terms.[53] Now, they are rarely to be found, although some (particularly *lunatic*) are still lurking in various statutes[54] and some judges seem comfortable with continuing to use the term *lunatic*:

As long ago as 1955, our Court of Appeal observed in Hardman v. Falk, [1955] 3 D.L.R. 129 at p. 133:

The contract of a lunatic is voidable not void: see York Glass Co. v. Jubb (1925), 134 L.T. 36. Courts of equity will not interfere if a contract with a lunatic is made in good faith without any knowledge of the incapacity of the lunatic and no advantage is taken. If the contract is fair and the respondent had no knowledge that the appellant was a lunatic, the appellant is without a remedy: see Wilson v. The King, [1938] 3 D.L.R. 433 at p. 436, S.C.R. 317 at p. 322. [Robertson J.A.]

So, too, I suggest would the party contracting with the lunatic in circumstances such as those here be without a remedy."[55]

Even though the word *lunatic* is still found in some current federal and provincial legislation, judges have the opportunity to substitute more acceptable words or to use quotation marks (and cite the statute) as an acknowledgment that the use of such words as acceptable labels has expired. In the above example, the judge was not even citing a statute and therefore should have chosen a different word.

Non–People First Language
Schizophrenic

Unfortunately, judges often describe people in terms of their illness:

Mr. P. is a disadvantaged individual. He has been diagnosed as a paranoid schizophrenic.[56]

Mr. C. also suffers from a major mental illness. He is a paranoid schizophrenic.[57]

M.M. (who is now deceased) was a developmentally delayed, schizophrenic woman who spent time at the Kingston Centre mall. [58]

He, Mr. S., certainly understands the importance of him being labeled a schizophrenic as opposed to one being labeled as suffering from antisocial personality disorder.[59]

S.M. is 38 years old. She is single and is a chronic schizophrenic.[60]

A patient in a mental hospital asked to make a will. . . . The testator, a paranoid schizophrenic, exhibited bizarre behaviour on the evening of his psychiatric examination and before and after executing the will.[61]

He is a schizophrenic and has been schizophrenic since his young–late teen years, early twenties.[62]

He also accepted that schizophrenics have an impairment of the executive functions of the brain which can manifest itself in difficulty spontaneously processing information as they encounter it, resulting in a slowed down thought process. He stressed, however, that it is highly variable as to how impaired a schizophrenic might be. Some are highly functional and others show significant deficits manifested by episodic memory deficits and a compromise of executive control processes.[63]

It is very common for schizophrenics to resist taking anti-psychotic medications because the illness compromises insight into the illness, its presence and the need for treatment.[64]

The problem with identifying people with mental illnesses by the diagnosis which they happen to have (as, e.g., "a schizophrenic") is that it is the first (and sometimes only) way in which they are identified, which can lead to the dehumanizing of those persons. The dehumanization of people with mental illness is common and makes it too easy for anyone outside of the illness to think of the person as "a schizophrenic" rather than a person who has schizophrenia; the person is the disease, rather than the person has the disease. Yet, as Otto Wahl points out, we don't do this with so-called physical illnesses—we don't call people "cancerous" or "heart diseased."[65] To avoid labeling people as their illness, many sources suggest using "people-first language," which recognizes that anyone, regardless of their physical or mental condition, is a person first and foremost. Rather than calling a person "a schizophrenic," he or she should be referred to as "a person with schizophrenia." This could, of course, be generalized to other psychiatric disorders (e.g., refraining from calling someone "a psychotic").

Reflections on Reasons for Results

While we start from the assumption that judges are not *trying* to stigmatize, a search through the case law suggests that inappropriate words and phrases are still being used. Certainly judges have been known, at times, to fail to recognize the extent of other kinds of social development happening around them. Take, for example, Justice McClung's deplorable words in the *Ewanchuk* case. There, McClung said (among other things) that the sexual assault committed by the offender was "less criminal than hormonal." He also said that the woman "did not present herself to Ewanchuk . . . in a bonnet or crinolines."[66] Madame Justice L'Heureux-Dube criticized McClung's language for perpetuating the myths and stereotypes about sexual assault against women:

> The *Code* was amended in 1983 and in 1992 to eradicate reliance on those assumptions; they should not be permitted to resurface through the stereotypes reflected in the reasons of the majority of the Court of Appeal. It is part of the role of this Court to denounce this kind of language, unfortunately still used today, which . . . perpetuates archaic myths and stereotypes about the nature of sexual assaults.[67]

Similarly, we would argue that the language some judges use today continues to perpetuate the myths and stereotypes about mental illness, despite the change in language that was deliberately made in the *Criminal Code* following the 1991 *Swain* decision.

So why are some judges still using such language? It may be a combination of factors. There is some evidence to suggest that judges can be influenced by the media as well as by certain internal biases.[68] Further, judges hear such language coming from the expert witnesses—the psychologists and psychiatrists who treat the accused. Consider each of these possible influences in turn.

A great number of studies have examined the extent to which the media stereotypes people with mental illness, with the predominant stereotype being that of the dangerous "mental" patient.[69] In books, television, news programs, movies, newspaper articles, and even children's programming, the media inundate society with misrepresentations of mental illness. The media have played a powerful and negative role in perpetuating the myths and stereotypes of mental illness and judges, like the rest of us, are not immune to the influences of biasing information.[70] Thus, since our society (if the media can be taken as a measure of what our society will pay for and condone) still appears to feel quite comfortable with negative images of people with mental illness, it is possible that judges too are susceptible to such images.

Judges have also been shown to be just as prone to certain biases as other decision makers. Guthrie and colleagues conducted a series of experiments through which they found that judges show comparable amounts of hindsight bias (tending to think that someone should have "known better") and egocentric bias (believing that they are less capable than others of making mistakes) than did decision makers in other studies.[71] While Guthrie et al. caution that their experiment does not necessarily translate directly into the courtroom, they suggest that there are indeed existing examples of occasions when a judge's biases influenced certain decisions made in court. These biases to which the judge may be susceptible could result in the judge having a particular, predetermined view of the people in his or her court, and this may lead to the incorporation (or the lack of filtering) of stigmatizing language.

Finally, it is conceivable that judges hear stigmatizing language within the courtroom coming from the people who certainly ought to know better—those who work in the mental health field itself. Research studies have demonstrated that caregivers and those in the mental health field can be extremely stigmatizing.[72] Indeed, the Mental Health Commission of Canada is launching a ten-year antistigma campaign, and its first two focus groups are children and those employed in the mental health field.[73] But just as it is of course not acceptable for judges to blindly accept testimony, they need not also unthinkingly repeat testimony. A judge could use alternate words or terms or at least put quotes around language that is stigmatizing and distance the court from it. Similarly, a judge should feel entitled and responsible for challenging the language of the witness when it is derogatory toward those with mental illness.

Conclusion

In closing, it is important to stress that we do not believe that judges are actively trying to be stigmatizing. On the whole, in fact, judges appear to use appropriate and respectful language. Still, we trust judges to use respectful language since, as leaders of our community, they are unquestionably in a position to influence the way society thinks about mental illness.[74] That is why we look to them to set the linguistic tone, and why we suggest that some of them must be more careful with the words they choose. In his book *Telling Is Risky Business,* Otto Wahl offers a list of things that we all can do to help reduce stigma and one of the items on his list is to "watch our language."[75] This is precisely what we would ask of all Canadian judges.

Notes

1. Letter to George Bainton, 10/15/1888; online from http://www.twainquotescom/index.html.

2. US Surgeon General's Report, US Department of Health and Human Services (1999: 8); Rüsch, N., Angermeyer, M. C., & Corrigan, P. W. (2005). Mental illness stigma: Concepts, consequences, and initiatives to reduce stigma. *European Psychiatry, 20,* 529–539 [Rüsch].

3. Kale, R. (1997). Bringing epilepsy out of the shadows: Wide treatment gap needs to be reduced. *British Medical Journal, 315,* 2–3.

4. Hemmens, C., Miller, M., Burton, V. S. Jr., & Milner, S. (2002). The consequences of official labels: An examination of the rights lost by the mentally ill and mentally incompetent ten years later. *Community Mental Health Journal, 38,* 129–140; Corrigan P. W., Watson, A. C., Heyrman, M. L., Warpinski, A., Gracia, G., Slopen N., & Hall, L. L. (2005). Structural stigma in state legislation. *Psychiatric Services, 56,* 557–563 [Corrigan].

5. *Rusch, supra,* note 2; Overton, S.L., & Medina, S. L. (2008). The stigma of mental illness. *Journal of Counseling and Development, 86,*143–151 [Overton]; Corrigan, P. (2004). How stigma interferes with mental health care. *American Psychologist, 59,* 614–625.

6. For an interesting discussion of the media's portrayal of mental illness, see Wahl, O. F. (1995). *Media madness: Public images of mental illness.* New Brunswick, NJ: Rutgers University Press. [Wahl].

7. For example, *lazy, incurable, malingering, lacking intelligence, unpredictable, weak,* etc. See Kate McLaughlin online at http://www.katemclaughlin.net/dispel-the-myths-overcome-the-stigma/.

8. Perlin, M. (1999). Half-wracked prejudice leaped forth: sanism, pretextuality, and why and how mental disability law developed as it did. *Journal of Contemporary Legal Studies, 10,* 3–35.

9. We also looked broadly at decisions referencing "mental illness" as a background context for the study and based this conclusion on that review.

10. *Merriam-Webster's collegiate dictionary* (10th ed.). (1993). Springfield, MA: Merriam-Webster.

11. Goffman, E. (1963). *Stigma: Notes on the management of spoiled identity.* Englewood Cliffs, NJ: Prentice Hall.

12. Ibid., p. 3.

13. Link, B. G., & Phelan, J. C. (2001). Conceptualizing stigma. *Annual Review of Sociology, 27*, 363–385 [Link].

14. Sartorius, N. (2007). Stigma and mental health. *Lancet, 370*, 810–811.

15. Corrigan, P. W. *Beat the stigma and discrimination! Four lessons for mental health advocates.* Online at http://www.dmh.ca.gov/PEIStatewideProjects/docs/CorriganBeattheStigmaandDiscrimination.pdf.

16. Link, B. G., Yang, L. H., Phelan, J. C., & Collins P.Y. (2004). Measuring mental illness stigma. *Schizophrenia Bulletin, 30*, 511–541.

17. R. v. Swain, 1 S.C.R. 933 (1991), S.C.C.

18. Bill C-30, An Act to Amend the Criminal Code; enacted February 4, 1992.

19. Other changes included, for example, the elimination of the lieutenant governor's warrants. Ibid.

20. *House of Commons Debates*, Volume III (14 October 1991) at 3296 (Hon. Kim Campbell).

21. This last term was used as an example of non–people-first language. See below for a discussion on this issue.

22. For example, *confess* (as in "confessing" to having a mental illness), *imbecile, idiot, nutter, shrink, headshrinker,* and *moron.*

23. It must be emphasized here that we conducted a qualitative not a quantitative study. Our research question was whether this kind of language was still being used rather than to what extent it was still being used. We restricted our approach in this way to make the project feasible (there would simply be an unmanageable number of cases to review if one wanted to draw conclusions about prevalence) and because we felt that the ongoing existence of use was a problem worth discussing independent of the prevalence of use.

24. In an effort to avoid further exposure of the individuals involved, we use only their initials.

25. C. v J., 59 O.R. (3d) 737 (2002), ON.C.A.

26. K.J.D. v. C., O.J. 2462 (2006), ON.Sup.Ct.Jus.

27. S. v. L., O.J. 3957 (2001), ON.Sup.Ct.Jus.

28. R. v. S., B.C.J. 2988 (2004), B.C.Prov.Ct.

29. R. v M., A.J. 1640 (2002), AB.Q.B.

30. Institut Philippe Pinel de Montréal v. W., Q.J. 1041 (1997), QC.C.S.

31. R. v. A., O.J.1591 (2006), ON.Ct.Jus.

32. R. v. K., 355 (1993), NL.S.C.

33. R. v. M., B.C.J. 2400 (2008), B.C.Prov.Ct.

34. See, e.g., the Psychiatric Patient Advocate Office, online at: http://www.ppao.gov.on.ca/sys-arr.html.

35. Although, in the French version of the Yukon Mental Health Act, the word *arrêtée* is used; in English the word used is *apprehend Mental Health Act*, R.S.Y. 2002, c. 150 s. 41(1).

36. R. v. C., A.J. 292 (2005), AB.Prov.C.

37. R. v. R.L., O.J. 4095 (2007), ON.Sup.Ct.

38. R. v. T., M.J. 252 (2007), MB.Q.B.

39. W.V.W. v. Misericordia Hospital, A.J. 875 (1999), AB.Q.B.

40. National Alliance on Mental Illness, online at http://www.nami.org/.

41. C. v. D., O.J. 1942 (1995), ON.Ct.

42. R v. B. (2009), unreported, ON.Ct.Jus.

43. R. v. A., B.C.J. 570 (2008), B.C.S.C.

44. R. v. D., N.B.J. 55 (2002), N.B.C.A.

45. R. v. O., 2 S.C.R. 507 (1994), S.C.C.

46. R. v. H., N.B.J. 37 (1996), N.B.C.A.

47. R. v. D., 3 S.C.R. 63 (1994), S.C.C.

48. R. v. L. O.J. 4016 (1997), ON.C.A.

49. Vaughan, C. E. (2009). People-first language: An unholy crusade. *Braille Monitor*, online at http://www.nfb.org/images/nfb/Publications/bm/bm09/bm0903/bm0903tc.htm.

50. R v. B., M.J. 172 (2004), MB.Prov.Ct.

51. R. v. S.A.T.C., S.J. 492 (1996), SK.Q.B.

52. Ibid.

53. Matloff, J. (2008). Idiocy, lunacy, and matrimony: Exploring constitutional challenges to state restrictions on marriages of persons with mental disabilities. *American University Journal of Gender, Social Policy and Law, 17,* 497–520.

54. e.g., Provincial Subsidies Act, R.S.C. 1985, c.P-26, Devolution of Estates Act, R.S.N.B. 1973, c.D-9, Watershed Associations Act, R.S.S. 1978, c.W-11, Registry Act, R.S.N.B. 1973, c. R-6.

55. R. v. R., B.C.J. 9 (1998), BC.S.C.

56. R. v. P., Nu.J. 17 (2007), NuCt.Jus.

57. R. v. C., O.J. 5857 (1998) ON.Ct.Jus.

58. R. v. C., O.J. 3609 (2007), ON.Sup.Ct.Jus.

59. R. v. S., O.J. 2765 (2009), ON.Ct.Jus.

60. Nova Scotia (Minister of Community Services) v. M.N.S.J. 367 (1995), NS.Fam.Ct.

61. P. v. S., N.J. 217 (1999), NL.S.C.T.D.

62. R. v. B., A.J. 245 (2006), AB.Prov.Ct.

63. R. v. I., O.J. 312 (2008), ON.Sup.Ct.Jus.

64. R v. W., O.J. 744 (2007), ON.Sup.Ct.Jus.

65. Wahl, O.F. (1999). *Telling Is Risky Business.* New Brunswick, NJ: Rutgers University Press, p 220.

66. R. v. Ewanchuk, A.J. 150 (1998), AB.C.A.

67. R. v. Ewanchuk, 1 S.C.R. 330 (1999), S.C.C.

68. Guthrie, C., Rachlinski, J. J., & Wistrich, A. J. (2001). Inside the judicial mind. *Cornell Law Review*, 86, 777–830 [Guthrie]; Robbennolt, J. K., & Studebaker, C. A. (2003). News media reporting on civil litigation and its influence on civil justice decision making. *Law and Human Behavior*, 27, 5–27 [the authors note that this phenomenon in judges particularly requires more study].

69. Corrigan, P. W., Watson, A. C., Gracia, G., Slopen, N., Rasinski, K., Hall, & L. L. (2005). Newspaper stories as measures of structural stigma. *Psychiatric Services*, 56, 551–555; Clement, S., & Foster, N. (2008). Newspaper reporting on schizophrenia: A content analysis of five national newspapers at two time points. *Schizophrenia Research*, 98, 178–183; Day, D. M., & Page, S. (1986). Portrayal of mental illness in Canadian newspapers. *Canadian Journal of Psychiatry*, 31, 813–817; Klin, A., & Lemish, D. (2008). Mental disorders stigma in the media: Review of studies on production, content, and influences. *Journal of Health Communication* 13, 434–449; *Wahl, supra* note 6.

70. Landsman, S., & Rakos, R. F. (1994). A preliminary inquiry into the effect of potentially biasing information on judges and jurors in civil litigation. *Behavioral Sciences and the Law*, 12, 113–126; Wistrich, A. J., Guthrie, C., & Rachlinski, J. J. (2005). Can judges ignore inadmissible information? The difficulty of deliberately disregarding. *University of Pennsylvania Law Review*, 153, 1251–1345.

71. *Guthrie, supra* note 68.

72. The Standing Senate Committee on Social Affairs, Science and Technology. (2006). *Out of the shadows at last: Transforming mental health, mental illness and addiction services in Canada*. Online at http://www.parl.gc.ca/39/1/parlbus/commbus/senate/Com-e/SOCI-E/rep-e/rep02may06-e.htm; *Overton, supra* note 4; Barney, L. J., Griffiths, K. M., Christensen, H., & Jorm, A. F. (2009). Exploring the nature of stigmatising beliefs about depression and help-seeking: Implications for reducing stigma. *BMC Public Health*, 9, 61; Thornicroft, G., Rose, D., & Kassam, A. (2007). Discrimination in health care against people with mental illness. *International Review of Psychiatry*, 19, 113–122.

73. See Mental Health Commission of Canada online at: http://www.mentalhealthcommission.ca/.

74. The case in note 39 received much attention from local press, with newspapers running such subheadlines as: "'Either she's insane or she's evil,' judge says in handing commuter 12 months [sic] probation plus fines for burning victim in morning rush." *Globe and Mail* online at: http://v1.theglobeandmail.com/servlet/story/RTGAM.20090601.escenic_1163315/BNStory/. National Coverage from other sources inevitably included the line cited in note 39.

75. *Wahl, supra* note 65, p. 178.

VI
Therapeutic Boundaries

The proper bounds of the therapeutic relationship have long been the subject of ethical inquiry. In *The Oath*, Hippocrates identifies and proscribes certain boundary breaches:

> Into whatever houses I enter, I will go into them for the benefit of the sick, and will abstain from every voluntary act of mischief and corruption; and, further from the seduction of females or males, of freemen and slaves.

From graft to sex, Hippocrates recognizes the range of potential boundary issues. Indeed, volumes have been produced pertaining to the ethics of sexual boundary violations in both medicine generally and mental health care specifically. In this final part, we present a sampling of material related to ethically fraught nonsexual boundaries, not to minimize the gravity of sexual violations but to attend to other kinds of novel and questionable boundary crossings. For example, new questions about the permissibility of interacting with patients and clients outside the conventional therapeutic space have emerged. Social media are pushing historical limits on therapist-patient interactions and testing the consensus about the impermeability of once seemingly settled boundaries.

To begin, we turn to a conceptual piece by philosopher Jennifer Radden in which she challenges the basic idea of what constitutes a "boundary violation" through a critical examination of boundary-violation discourse. Radden argues that conceptual clarification of what it means to violate a boundary is needed before we can ascertain whether a boundary violation has in fact happened and, if so, what should be done about it. She notes that the literature and research examining the ethics of boundaries in mental health care have been steeped in equivocation around the basic meanings of the concept of boundaries. Often, failure to adequately judge a boundary violation happens because careful examination of the behavior in question is undercut by a lack of attention to context. Radden argues that any analysis of potential boundary violations should be done within the social and moral context of the clinician's particular role. Such "role morality" is the fulcrum on which ethical judgments may be leveraged and is foundational to Radden's other influential writings about virtue ethics in psychiatry.

The next several articles present case vignettes and discussions to illustrate the complexity in negotiating the ethical limits of boundaries. The essays dovetail by way of encouraging pragmatic, context-dependent decision-making strategies to avoid and resolve boundary questions. David Brendel and his colleagues, writing as members of the ethics committee of McLean Hospital, discuss a common problem that mental health care providers face: clients who wish to give them gifts. Through a series of reality-based vignettes, the authors reveal the complexity of the gifting relationship and provide a method for "negotiating the poles of rule-bound rigor and individually tailored flexibility [that] is a significant practical challenge when a patient or patient's family offers the psychiatrist a gift."

Arnold Lazarus seeks to negotiate these same poles by arguing that in some cases, rules and well-intentioned ethical guidelines that map out particular boundaries may in fact be detrimental to the patient's therapeutic success. Lazarus describes several episodes throughout his career in which he breached the standard nonsexual boundaries of psychotherapy by playing tennis and socializing with those in his care or by accepting small gifts from them. These interactions, Lazarus contends, were simply part of a healthy human relationship that is built on trust, benevolence, and care. Lazarus expresses deep suspicion of what he perceives to be an overreliance of so-called risk-management principles that take "precedence over humane interventions."

Frederic Reamer, former chair of the National Association of Social Workers ethics task force, offers us what Lazarus so vehemently objects to: a code-based, risk management protocol for clinical social workers to help them negotiate dual relationships and boundary issues. It is arguable that psychotherapy and clinical social work are categorically different professions, and, moreover, clinical social work is doubly fraught with boundary issues given the nature of the clinician-client relationship. If so, then a clear ethics protocol is both helpful and necessary. It would seem that codified guidance—when not mistaken for an oracle—should serve as a valuable touchstone in helping clinicians begin to examine boundary concerns in their own practice. We include this article to offer both interdisciplinary dialogue about boundary concerns and juxtapose different ethical approaches.

The last two articles in this book introduce and begin to address novel questions that have emerged in an age of social media: How do we understand and respect professional and personal space in an age when the traditional boundaries between private and public life are evaporating before our very eyes?

Brian Clinton, Benjamin Silverman, and David Brendel examine the question of how and if it is appropriate for clinicians to search the Internet for information about their patients—a practice they call patient-targeted Googling (PTG). Using a pragmatic framework, they offer several questions to help clinicians think through their true intentions and the clinical and ethical consequences of PTG. More broadly, the authors suggest that the profession of psychiatry—and all allied mental health care professions—must come to terms with emerging risks to patient privacy, which serves as the bedrock of all therapeutic relationships.

Such emerging risks are described by Glen Gabbard, Kristin Kassaw, and Gonzalo Perez-Garcia who survey the state of the Internet and social media and propose a set of guidelines to help clinicians better manage increasingly hazy boundaries. As technology makes it easier and easier to openly gaze into the once-private lives of family members, friends, colleagues, patients, and complete strangers, how ought clinicians behave to maintain a safe, bounded space within which to practice, and what should they reasonably expect from their patients in return?

20

Boundary Violation Ethics: Some Conceptual Clarifications

Jennifer Radden

Boundary-violation discourse may be said to be the *lingua franca* of psychiatric and other psychotherapeutic ethics today. Informal discussions about unacceptable behavior are rarely characterized in any but these terms. Although this language is perhaps overused, psychotherapeutic practice places more stringent restrictions on boundary transgressions than are found in other areas of medical practice.

Boundary-violation discourse is integral to forensic psychiatry, in which boundary-violating behavior is evaluated as impermissible or in other ways legally actionable. Here, behavior judged to be boundary-violating leads to professional censure. It also gives rise to malpractice charges because of its damaging effects, such as suicide and regression to severe psychiatric illness. Because the courts and the examination rooms of professional boards and the setting where boundary-violation judgments are decided in specific cases, forensic psychiatrists are at the forefront in interpreting and shaping boundary-violation discourse. Moreover, the role conflict encountered by the therapist asked to serve as an expert witness is a kind of boundary transgression peculiar to the forensic setting.[1]

Reference to boundary violations permits ethical evaluation of an important dimension of professional practice. But boundary-violation discourse often seems confused, ambiguous, and even contradictory. And boundary-violation judgments are marked by inconsistency, subjectivity, and disagreement. In an attempt to offer conceptual clarification of boundary-violation discourse, I begin with some basic methodological considerations: (1) difficulties defining or formulating criteria for boundary-violating behavior, (2) conceptual ambiguities in the fundamental metaphor of boundaries crossed and violated, and (3) misunderstandings of the explanatory status of the claim that certain actions constitute boundary violations. Two additional features of boundary-violation discourse require clarification. One is the status of the disputes and disagreements about boundary-violation judgments, analyzed here by appeal to theories of professional role morality (i.e., ethical constraints on conduct dictated by professional role). The last, the larger social meaning of much boundary-violating behavior, which allows us to see boundary-violation discourse as a form of social critique, is introduced through a brief discussion of boundary-violating behavior in relation to gender. The interwoven confusions addressed derive from two sources: the variety of factors involved in boundary-violation judgments and ambiguities and insufficiencies in the language in which those judgments are expressed.

Although my discussion in this article focuses on preliminaries, its implications for forensic psychiatry should be apparent. Because boundary-violation discourse is so integral to forensic psychiatry, it is especially important that forensic psychiatrists and expert witnesses appreciate the complexity and assumptions that go into evaluating particular questionable actions as wrongful in this way.

Types of Boundary-Violating Behavior

One source of the confusion that attaches to boundary-violation discourse is the variety of behaviors denoted as boundary violating. These include physical contact between treater and patient (nonsexual touching, such as pats and hugs, as well as sexual intimacy); forms of self-disclosure on the part of the treater about personal matters, such as the insertion of aspects of the treater's personal life into the therapeutic discussion; breaches of confidentiality by the treater; what would otherwise be known as conflicts of interest (e.g., when the treater initiates or permits a social or business relationship to exist at the same time as the therapeutic one, or when role reversal allows the patient to provide support or other gratification for the therapist); and finally, an assortment of improprieties associated with the therapeutic engagement (fee setting, gift giving, and appointment times and places, for example). In its broadest interpretation (one I consider misleadingly broad), the notion of boundary violation seems to encompass almost any form of exploitation and/or any behavior likely to diminish the therapeutic effectiveness of the engagement.

Added to the confusing breadth of attributions about boundary violations is another factor. Reference to boundaries occurs in two closely related contexts. "Internal," or psychic, boundaries, including so-called self-boundaries or ego boundaries, enter into much psychodynamic discourse about patients in therapy.[2] Those whose "external" boundaries are said to be violated by inappropriate actions on the part of their treaters also possess internal boundaries, evaluated as loose, rigid, weak, and strong. Opportunities for confusion and ambiguity thus are multiplied.

The Definition Problem

To the unwieldy breadth of this usage, which makes conceptualization difficult, is added another problem: Judgments of boundary violation seem to be extremely context sensitive. Gutheil and Gabbard have argued that contextual framing is always required to tell us when, as they put it, a possibly innocuous boundary crossing becomes an unethical boundary violation.[3] Context includes "the treater's professional ideology, the presence or nature of informed consent by the patient, the point in therapy in which behavior occurs, the respective cultures of the dyad, and such environmental factors as whether therapy occurs in a small town or in an urban center, and whether public transportation is available." The authors illustrate: "A therapist who gives a patient a ride home in a blizzard might be judged differently, depending on whether the therapy occurs in a prairie town or a major city with a subway, whether the patient feels coerced by the therapist to accept the ride, and whether the therapist also gives the patient rides when the weather is mild."[3] Context also explains how repeated boundary crossings can be transformed into boundary violations by their progressive impact or by their incremental increase.[4]

This context sensitivity precludes the possibility of codifying those boundary crossings that should be classified as boundary violations, according to these authors, thus making it impossible for us to provide a covering definition to demarcate the class of boundary-violating behavior.

Writing several years earlier, Brown[5] offered a similar critique of boundary-violation discourse to that offered by Gutheil and Gabbard,[3] noting the context-sensitive nature of these judgments, and arguing for the "futility of trying to identify (and then avoid) all behaviors which are potentially boundary-violating." Rather than a concrete model of boundary violations, Brown proposed conceptual criteria. Boundary violations occur in those instances in which (1) the client is "objectified," violating the Kantian prohibition on treating others as objects rather than as persons, (2) the therapist's impulses are gratified through the behavior, (3) the needs of the therapist are made paramount over those of the client, or (4) the client feels violated.

Brown's model goes some way toward avoiding the definitional problem raised in Gutheil's and Gabbard's[3] discussion. Not one of Brown's criteria is unproblematic, however. Although capturing something important about the kinds of behavior usually judged to be boundary violating, the objectification of the client is itself an obscure criterion, the satisfaction of which would appear to be met by one or several of criteria 1 through 3. But criterion 2, the therapist's impulses are gratified through the behavior, also raises difficulties of interpretation. It may be true that boundary violations occur when behavior is engaged in solely to gratify the therapist's impulses. Yet it seems implausible to designate as boundary violating all behavior that gratifies the therapist's impulses. Behavior engaged in for some other therapeutic purpose may happen to gratify those impulses as well. (Indeed, without some satisfactions remaining to treaters, it seems doubtful any would stay in the field.) Brown's criterion (3), the needs of the therapist are made paramount over those of the client, does seem to capture some subset of the behavior widely judged to be boundary violating, but not all boundary-violating behavior fits this criterion. Boundaries may be violated in a misplaced effort to help, or through inappropriate sympathy, for example, and it would appear overly cynical to judge all such behavior as placing the needs of the therapist over those of the client. Brown's criterion 4, the patient feels violated, is also unsatisfactory. Paranoid or oversensitive clients are likely to feel violated in the absence of any actual violation. The treater may have an ethical imperative to uncover and discuss those feelings of violation, but she would be unlikely to be judged culpably responsible for them.

Other discussions of boundary violations rely heavily on two additional conceptual features not named by Brown: that the behavior in question is (or is potentially) exploitative and/or that it is detrimental or at least not conducive to therapeutic success.[6] A lack of understanding or empathy on the part of the treater may jeopardize therapeutic success without violating any conceivable boundaries, and an analysis into exploitative and potentially exploitative behavior also yields less than a satisfactory definition of boundary-violating behavior. On any assessment, the range of exploitative behavior seems to exceed the range of boundary-violating behavior. (Although wrong and exploitative, a treater's overcharging the patient or providing unnecessary or inadequate care, for example, would not generally be regarded as violating boundaries, although this is certainly unethical behavior of some kind.)

Confirming Gutheil's and Gabbard's[3] claims, then, a clear conceptual definition of boundary violations appears elusive. Nonetheless, this effort at definition is premature. Preliminary clarifications of the primary conceptual features of this discourse are called for, especially the metaphor—if metaphor it is—sustaining this discourse of boundaries and boundary violations.

What Is Bounded?

Touching, sexual and otherwise, crosses bodily boundaries. Sometimes, therefore, the subject of these claims—that which is bounded—appears to be the body. Breaching a patient's confidence, on the other hand, crosses nonconcrete boundaries. The subject here appears to be the psyche, person, or self of the patient—or her secrets. In other behavior labeled boundary violating such as inappropriate self-disclosure by the treater, or the example noted earlier of giving the patient a ride, it seems clearest to say that the dyad, the relationship between treater and patient, is the subject. (This echoes Gabbard's remark that boundary violations concern the "edge or limit of appropriate behavior by the psychiatrist in the clinical setting.") In the literature on boundary violations, as well as in less formal discussions, each kind of subject (body, self, or psyche relationship) is implied, often in the same discussion, and no consistent or defined usage reveals itself.

In relation to boundaries, the subjects of self and psyche are better avoided. They are the subjects in that parallel internal boundary discourse that, because it at least seeks to be descriptive rather than evaluative and about the patient rather than the dyad, is not to be confused with the discourse of boundary violations under analysis here. For clarity and economy, it can be stipulated that the therapeutic relationship is that which is bounded. This allows us to honor the extension of boundary talk to include cases such as treater self-disclosure and giving the patient a ride and yet also captures more concrete violations, such as sexual and nonsexual bodily contact.

The claim that the therapeutic relationship, or what is sometimes identified as the therapeutic "frame," is the possessor of boundaries is found in some of the literature on boundary violations.[8,9] But what does such a claim mean? At risk of atomizing what is better seen in relational terms, I suggest it means that the relationship requires roles for each participant. A role can be defined as a circumscribed (bounded) and rule-dictated way of behaving in a circumscribed context, when presupposed are (1) that persons adopt different roles with different social contexts and (2) that there may be role incompatibilities that prevent a person's adopting more than one role at a time. Incompatibility between roles depends on how precisely the behavior prescribed for each is defined and how strongly each is differentiated. The precisely defined and differentiated roles of theater, where one may play Miranda or Prospero but not play Miranda and Prospero at the same time, illustrate obvious cases of role incompatibility. Once the differentiation of the two roles has been made clear, the "two hats" required of a therapist called to testify can also be seen to represent role incompatibility, as can other instances of dual-role activity, such as the therapist's engaging in a sexual or independent business relationship with the client while therapy is ongoing.

Professional Role Morality

Boundary violations, in this analysis, are role violations. An account of boundary-violating action in terms of role violation offers little substantive progress alone. But it has positioned us to explore an important link—that between boundary violations and what moral philosophers have called professional role morality. (Professional role morality refers to the set of moral and ethical imperatives derived from professional conduct, status, or role.) This link enables us to sort and stack the several moral principles and theories informing boundary-violation restrictions and to better understand the special importance of boundaries for psychiatric practice. It is also useful as we approach the question of disagreement over boundary violations.

The role morality sometimes attributed to doctors, lawyers, and government servants in the practice of their professional duties introduces a kind of moral double standard, in that it prescribes different conduct for professionals than for other people. One version of this system is known as strong role morality.[11] Strong role morality asserts that what is morally permissible or even morally required by a professional role is not necessarily required and is sometimes not even permitted according to that common or broad-based morality[12] applicable to the rest of the community. Even when some action conflicts with the values and ends of broad-based morality, such as the patient's usefulness to society, (role) morality for the doctor or healer is dictated by the goal of maintaining the patient's health.[11-13]

Not all role morality is so strong, however. A profession's role morality may also require more, not less, stringent obligations than those dictated by broad-based morality. Weak role morality, which is widely accepted as characteristic of the professions, is often used as a marker of professional status.[11-14] Weak role morality never overrides the dictates of broad-based morality, however; it just adds to them. Strong role morality has often been challenged. Some refuse to accept that any professional roles could contravene the dictates of broad-based morality, and certainly the dangers surrounding the "just doing my (professional) duty" defense have been amply exposed.[15] But weak role morality is not vulnerable to the same criticisms.

Some of the expectations and limitations of roles denoting so-called boundary violations apply across all professional relationships. But there are also role expectations and limitations that are developed within and specific to the particular professional practice involved. The relationship between lawyer and client imposes constraints different from those in the relationship between doctor and patient, for example. While keeping in mind the constraints imposed by any professional relationship, we must identify and acknowledge those attaching only to relationships in medicine. Psychiatric relationships bring additional constraints, with more precise and narrowly drawn role expectations than govern relationships in the other fields of medicine. What is morally permissible in the relationship between internist and patient may be a boundary violation in the relationship between psychiatrist and patient, for example.

Recognizing this nesting of moral obligations, we can see that the relationship between psychiatrist and patient is constrained in three different ways. First, it must comply with general standards of professional ethics (by avoiding noncontractual exploitation of the patient and conflicts of interest, for example). Second, it must uphold the particular set of values guiding all medical practice, in which the patient's health is paramount and such principles of biomedical ethics as autonomy, benevolence, and nonmaleficence are adhered to.[16] Finally, there must be role constraints distinctive to psychiatric practice.

At least some of the psychiatrist's special constraints pertain to the means of achieving or maintaining not merely physical but also mental health. In psychiatry as traditionally construed, the therapeutic relationship or "alliance" means that the healing relationship is regarded either as the primary medium through which healing takes place, or at least as a *sine qua non*, without which healing could not take place.

It is because so much emphasis is placed on the use of the relationship within psychiatry that the role constraints particular to psychiatrists focus on the niceties of maintaining the boundaries of the therapeutic relationship. This point has been noted by Gabbard[7] in an illuminating discussion of the therapeutic rationale for limiting boundaries. Boundaries, he explains, are:

[the] structural characteristics of the relationship that allow the therapist to interact with warmth, empathy, and spontaneity within certain conditions that create a climate of safety . . . the external boundaries of the treatment are established so that the psychological boundaries between patient and therapist can be crossed through a number of means that are common to psychotherapeutic experience . . . [including] identification, empathy, projection, introjection, and projective identification.

Summing up, then, the psychiatrist's ethical concerns are several: those imposed by his or her role as a professional, those by his or her role as a doctor, and those by his or her role in a practice in which the professional goal and good is mental health and the particular professional instrument is (often) the therapeutic relationship. Rather than imposing conflicting ethical duties, the three levels of weak role morality constraints impose a nested set of demands, all incumbent on the psychiatrist.

Explanatory Status

The judgment that "X is a boundary violation" is frequently introduced as an explanation of professionally and ethically unacceptable conduct. But taken alone, this phrase promises more than it can deliver. Further grounding is required. The force of the judgment depends on implicit assumptions—observational, theoretical, and ethical assumptions—that are often the source of bias, disagreement, and conflicting opinion. Rather than "action X is wrong because it is a boundary violation," we should recognize that it is because it is wrong that X is (regarded as) a boundary violation and should be able to sort out why it is regarded as wrong.

Boundary-violation language requires allegiance to additional assumptions of several kinds, and these can be identified and sorted. Observational assumptions underlying these judgments are often causal hypotheses predicting the consequences of certain conduct, as we have seen (the belief that some particular action would likely diminish or enhance therapeutic effectiveness, for example). Such assumptions, in turn, rest on further, often theoretical, assumptions.

The theoretical assumptions implicit in boundary-violation discourse are of at least two kinds: psychological and moral. The respective cases of (1) post-termination sex between client and treater, familiar from the forensic setting, and (2) the treater's self-disclosure, familiar from the clinical setting, illustrate each of these kinds of assumption. Adherence to psychodynamic theoretical tenets may preclude any post-termination sex on the grounds that such activity forever represents a proto-incestuous union. Without adherence to such theoretical tenets, in contrast, no such theoretically grounded objection to post-termination sex would be maintained (although nontheoretical objections may remain, such as concern that the sex would jeopardize any later resumption of therapy).

Therapist self-disclosure is often regarded as boundary violating.[17] Within feminist therapy, in contrast, in which the relationship is construed as importantly and self-consciously egalitarian, reducing what have been called "artificial and unnecessary barriers to equality"[5] through therapist self-disclosure is an essential part of the engagement, not a boundary violation. The feminist therapist's emphasis on equality reflects underlying values. Whether therapist self-disclosure is judged to be boundary violating depends, at least in part, on what moral theoretical tenets are presupposed.

More generally, then, theoretical presuppositions, psychological in the first case and moral in the second, ground and justify the claim that post-termination sex and self-disclosure, respectively, are or are not boundary violations.

Informal discussion with clinicians readily elicits the range of moral theoretical frameworks, models, and assumptions that underlie boundary-violation discourse. Six of the most common of these will be described. These alternative frameworks will perhaps only rarely yield substantively different judgments about whether a given action is to be regarded as a boundary violation. Nonetheless, they represent significantly differing moral theoretical standpoints and differing forms of moral reasoning. *Kantianism:* Brown's[5] attempt to define boundary violations appeals to the Kantian ideal of respecting personhood, which precludes treating others as objects. *Principles of biomedical ethics:* Judgments that a particular action constitutes a boundary violation are sometimes grounded by appeal to one or several of the other traditional principles of biomedical ethics, such as beneficence or autonomy. Thus, for example, boundary violations are regarded as wrong because they detract from the patient's autonomy. *Utilitarianism:* These judgments are grounded in the framework we associate with utilitarian ethics, in which boundary crossings that increase suffering or disutility count as boundary violations. *Contractualist model:* Some judgments of boundary violation reflect allegiance to the contractualist model of doctor-patient relationships. In such a model, boundary transgressions are wrong because they break the compact, formal or implicit, between therapist and patient. *Hippocratic oath:* The principle of nonmaleficence *primum non nocere,* often associated with the oath, sometimes underlies boundary-violation judgments. Harm to the patient must be avoided, and boundary-violating actions are judged wrong because they are likely to cause harm. The principle also underlies the oath's explicit injunction concerning confidentiality. Disclosing confidences is regarded as a boundary violation because of that injunction. *Fiduciary relationship:* Another underlying moral framework found in some of the literature on boundary violations introduces the value of trust and designates the therapeutic relationship as a fiduciary one involving a special trust.[10,18] Boundary-violations reflect perceived breaches of this special trust.

To sum up, the contextual features influencing boundary-violation judgments include a range of usually tacit assumptions—some observational, others theoretical—that can make good the force of any given boundary-violation prohibition or judgment. That prohibition or judgment is only as strong as, and is determined by, the force of these assumptions. "X is a boundary violation" is an empty assertion, requiring for its completion some context, including further presuppositions, tenets, or assumptions.

Disagreements about What Violates Boundaries

Few, if any, doubt that dual relationships,[9] such as engaging in sexual relations or forming a business partnership with a patient while therapy is ongoing, constitute wrongful professional conduct.[19] But away from these obviously egregious cases, opinion is not settled, as variations in the codes of professional ethics in the case of post-therapy sex have made abundantly clear.

Many within psychiatry are skeptical about the possibility of making progress or resolving ethical disagreements in these strongly contested cases. Such impasses are attributed to stubbornly subjective moral oppositions about which nothing further and nothing useful can be said. (Philosophers speak of irresolvable, unreasoned, "gut-level" subjective responses and attitudes such as these as "moral intuitions.")

But two aspects of the preceding discussion should serve to stem this skepticism about reaching agreement in these matters. The additional assumptions undergirding boundary-violation judgments is one; the distinction between different kinds of nested role obligation is the other.

Underlying Assumptions

That some intuitive moral differences may be present when there is disagreement about boundary violations is undeniable. But because judgments of boundary violations seem to rest on additional, implicit assumptions, it is more likely disagreement about these underlying assumptions than intuitive and immediate moral disagreement that explains differences of judgment regarding particular alleged boundary violations. Using surveys, Kardener et al.,[20] in a well-known study, established that 86 percent of psychodynamically oriented therapists and only 61 percent of behavioral therapists believe that erotic contact is never of benefit to the patient—a finding that illustrates the way that aspect of context, which includes theoretical orientation, influences such judgments. We saw earlier what is probably reflected in these differences. More psychodynamically oriented therapists would preclude erotic contact because of their theoretical beliefs about the nature of the transference. Behavior therapists could find fewer theoretical grounds for such an objection.

As Kardener et al.[20] illustrate, assumptions from psychological theory account for much disagreement about boundary violations. Such assumptions are themselves elaborate, multilayered observational and theoretical presuppositions not easily open to experimental verification. Although they also may constitute irresolvable sources of difference, they are not to be confused with intuitive moral disagreements.

Different Role Obligations

Some apparently irreducible disagreements may reflect a failure to acknowledge the complexity of the psychiatrist's several different kinds of role obligation, as the following (hypothetical) case illustrates. A new patient grants permission to the treater to contact her spouse. Months later, when the therapeutic relationship is ongoing and without again raising her intention with the patient, the treater telephones the spouse. The patient feels violated. Note that because the patient feels violated, this is deemed a boundary violation under Brown's[5] criteria. Under a contractual informed-consent model, however, no rule appears to have been breached, in that the explicit terms of engagement permitted this action on the part of the treater.

This may be less an irresolvable disagreement or a case of competing moral frameworks than a misunderstanding of role, nonetheless. The contractual model applies in this transaction just as it would in any— whether psychiatric, medical, or nonmedical—between professional expert and fee-paying client. General professional role requirements would have allowed the treater to contact the spouse as long as that explicit agreement had been established.

Granted, this case is complicated by the element of time, and a more enlightened and ethically sensitive approach understands informed consent to be an ongoing process subject to revision as therapy proceeds. Nonetheless, the basic legal notion of contract is time insensitive, or time spanning, and when issues of legal liability are concerned, the informed consent extends for the duration of the treatment.

But strictures specific to medicine and/or psychiatry may well prohibit contacting the spouse later. If the action were deemed one likely to diminish trust in the therapist, when such trust was regarded as essential to the effectiveness of the therapeutic relationship, for example, then the moral role obligations of the treater render this boundary crossing a boundary violation.

The Gender Context

An additional aspect of boundary-violating behavior and boundary-violation discourse not raised thus far concerns the gender bias within the broader system where these boundary violations take place and the larger social meaning of much boundary-violating behavior. Other forms of bias are also found in therapeutic relationships, of course. But because of the frequency of sexual boundary issues in a professional setting where females are often treated by males, the gender context deserves special attention. Feminist bioethics has stressed the extent to which medicine, with its patriarchal practices, is a system that has harmful effects on women.[21] Because women's experiences within medicine echo their experiences in society, these two sets of experiences are mutually reinforcing.

Karasu[22] has pointed to several features of our broader societal structures that form an interlocking, reinforcing systemic harm within psychiatry: androcentric theory, training practices, and—most pernicious—the replication within the therapeutic relationship between male therapist and female patient of a position in which women typically find themselves in their lives in general. Even allowing for the greater numbers of women in therapy and of men as therapists, a significantly higher number of women than men are the victims of those boundary violations concerning sexual contact.[23-25] This personal harm and exploitation inflicted on women represents an extremely troubling aspect of psychiatric practice. But as Karasu[22] illustrates, this is harm that is systemic as well as personal. Since it sustains a broader, systemic social wrong, boundary-violating sexual behavior constitutes wrongful conduct greater than the sum of its particular, personally harmful occurrences. In drawing attention to that systemic social wrong, boundary-violation discourse plays an important part in social critique.

Conclusions

To the extent that psychiatry employs traditional psychotherapeutic methods, its particular focus on relationship means that boundary-violation ethics are more elaborate and more critical in psychiatry than in other medical fields. This discussion has explored several features of boundary-violation discourse: conceptual ambiguities and unclarities in its fundamental metaphor, difficulties defining or formulating criteria for boundary-violating behavior, and the explanatory status of the judgment that some action constitutes a boundary violation. In addition, its link to professional role morality and its part in social critique were examined. Four points were particularly emphasized. First, claims about boundary violations do not stand alone; they depend on context. Thus, a boundary-violation ethic would be incomplete without the explicit acknowledgment of aspects of context, including the observational and theoretical assumptions on which, as a set of prohibitions, it rests. Second, by recognizing boundary-violation ethics as a form of weak role morality, it is possible to sort the moral theoretical tenets underlying the role constraints involved, some deriving from professional ethics that are most generally understood, some from biomedical ethics, and some particular to psychiatry. Third, boundary-violating behavior that is sexually exploitative often constitutes part of a systemic social wrong, as well as a personal violation. Finally, some disagreements over boundary violations stem from irreducible, intuitive differences of moral conviction. But many stem from other sources, including two in particular: a failure to recognize the different role constraints involved and differences in the theoretical beliefs underwriting boundary-violation judgments.

A special language is needed to acknowledge and codify the heightened attention to the ethical constraints on interpersonal exchange characteristic of clinical and forensic practice. But the confusions in boundary-violation judgments must be clarified, and the terms of boundary-violation discourse refined, before fully professional determinations about these very complicated interactions can be achieved.

References

1. Strasburger, L., Gutheil, T., & Brodsky, A. (1997). On wearing two hats: Role conflict in serving as both psychotherapist and expert witness. *American Journal of Psychiatry, 154,* 448–456.

2. Radden, J. (1996). Relational individualism and feminist therapy. *Hypatia, 11,* 72–96.

3. Gutheil, T., & Gabbard, G. (1998). Misuses and misunderstandings of boundary theory in clinical and regulatory settings. *American Journal of Psychiatry*, 155, 409–414.

4. Simon, R. I. (1999). Therapist-patient sex: From boundary violations to sexual misconduct. *Psychiatric Clinics of North America*, 22, 31–47.

5. Brown, L. (1994). Boundaries in feminist therapy: a conceptual formulation. In N. Gartrell (Ed.), *Bringing Ethics Alive: Feminist Ethics in Psychotherapy Practice* (pp. 29–38). New York: Harrington Park Press.

6. Garfinkel, P., Dorian, B., Sadavoy, J., & Bagby, R. M. (1997). Boundary violations and departments of psychiatry. *Canadian Journal of Psychiatry*, 51, 357–375.

7. Gabbard, G. (1999). Boundary violations. In S. Bloch, P. Chodoff, & S. Green (Eds.), *Psychiatric Ethics* (pp. 141–160). Oxford: Oxford University Press.

8. Gold, S., & Cherry, E. (1997). The therapeutic frame: On the need for flexibility. *Journal of Contemporary Psychotherapy*, 27, 147–155.

9. Plaut, S. M. (1997). Boundary violations in professional-client relationships: Overview and guidelines of prevention. *Sexual and Marital Therapy*, 12, 77–94.

10. Welfel, E. R. (1998). *Ethics in Counseling, and Psychotherapy: Standards, Research, and Emerging Issues*. London: Brooks/Cole Publishing Co.

11. Luban, D. (1988). *Lawyers and Justice: An Ethical Study*. Princeton, NJ: Princeton University Press.

12. Oakley, J., & Cocking, D. (In press.) *Virtue Ethics, and Professional Roles*. Cambridge, UK: Cambridge University Press.

13. Pellegrino, E., & Thomasma, D. (1993). *The Virtues of Medical Practice*. New York: Oxford University Press.

14. Churchill, L. (1989). Reviving a distinctive medical ethics. *Hastings Center Report*, 19, 815–817.

15. McIntyre, A. (1999). Social structures and their threats to moral agency. *Philosophy (London, England)*, 74, 311–329.

16. Beauchamp, T., & Childress, J. *Principles of Biomedical Ethics* (4th ed.). New York: Oxford University Press, 1994.

17. Barnett, J. (1998). Should psychotherapists self disclose? Clinical and ethical considerations. In L. VandeCreek, S. Knapp, & T. Jackson (Eds.), *Innovations in Clinical Practice: A Source Book* (Vol. 16, pp. 419–428). Sarasota, FL: Professional Resource Press.

18. Jorgenson, L., Hirsch, A., & Wahl, K. (1997). Fiduciary duty and boundaries: Acting in the client's best interests. *Behavioral Sciences and the Law*, 15, 49–62.

19. Appelbaum, P., & Jorgenson, L. (1991). Psychiatrist-patient sexual contact after termination of treatment: an analysis and a proposal. *American Journal of Psychiatry*, 148, 1466–1473.

20. Kardener, S., Fuller, M., & Mensh, I. N. (1973). A survey of physicians' attitudes and practices regarding erotic and non-erotic contact with patients. *Am J Psychiatry 130*, 1077–1081.

21. Sherwin, S. (1992). *Patient No Longer*. Philadelphia: Temple University Press.

22. Karasu, T. (1991). Ethical aspects of psychotherapy. In S. Bloch & P. Chodoff (Eds.), *Psychiatric Ethics*. Oxford: Oxford University Press.

23. Gabbard, G. (1989). *Sexual Exploitation in Professional Relationships*. Washington, DC: American Psychiatric Press.

24. Gartrell, N. (1994). *Bringing Ethics Alive: Feminist Ethics in Psychotherapy Practice*. New York: Harrington Park Press.

25. Barnes, F. (1998). *Complaints, and Grievances in Psychotherapy: A Handbook of Ethical Practice. New York*. Routledge.

21

The Price of a Gift: An Approach to Receiving Gifts from Patients in Psychiatric Practice

David H. Brendel, James Chu, Jennifer Radden, Howard Leeper, Harrison G. Pope, Jacqueline Samson, Gail Tsimprea, and J. Alexander Bodkin

No professional relationship is more complex than the one between a patient and a psychiatrist (*psychiatrist* here is used as a proxy for *mental health clinician*). This relationship is defined in large measure by the respective roles that they both play in their multifaceted interactions. Patients come for help with the hope and expectation that they will be treated with respect, compassion, and competence. Psychiatrists, meanwhile, expect that patients will strive to tell the truth about their conditions, adhere to treatment recommendations, and pay their bills. Treatment relationships in psychiatry conform, for the most part, to the typical conventions of any other professional practice. By staying within the confines of their respective roles, patients and psychiatrists establish interpersonal boundaries that lay the groundwork for a relationship in which, under ordinary circumstances, the patient obtains some relief from mental suffering while the clinician earns a living and derives gratification from a job well done.

Ethical dilemmas arise when the professional relationship is disrupted by the words or actions of the patient or the psychiatrist. Much has been written in the psychiatric literature in recent years about the ethical challenges that arise when clinicians engage in boundary crossings (departures from the usual professional relationship that do not harm, and might even help, the patient) and boundary violations (deviations that exploit or otherwise harm the patient).[1–4] There is broad acceptance in the field that certain actions on the part of psychiatrists, such as sexually or financially exploiting patients, are clearly unethical (and may also be illegal). Other actions that psychiatrists may take—for example, offering a patient a much needed ride home in the context of a calamity—represent boundary crossings that may be ethically justified or even obligatory.[5] Some boundary crossings fall into ethical gray areas and therefore merit careful reflection and deliberation.[6] Is it appropriate to hug a patient who is distraught and stricken by acute grief following the loss of a loved one? Or to hug a deeply grateful patient who is leaving treatment after many years of productive work together?

Such questions arise frequently in the course of everyday psychiatric practice and have no simple, routine answers. In order to grapple with these challenges in a thoughtful and ethical way, psychiatrists need to address them in the context of the actual treatment relationship and always with an eye toward identifying and acting in the patient's best interest. Doing so, however, is no easy task. The clinician must take a multiplicity of factors into account in these deliberations, and often must do so with little time to ponder all the dimensions and nuances of the situation at hand. When a patient asks unexpectedly for a hug, the clinician is forced to decide on the spot whether to grant or refuse the request and to articulate some words that might be clarifying or therapeutic for the patient. Under other circumstances, the clinician has time to consider the possible deviation from the usual conventions of practice; for example, if a patient asks the clinician to attend an event that is extremely meaningful to the patient (such as a graduation or wedding), the clinician may have time to reflect on the meaning of the request and the likely consequences of accepting or declining it, and be able to promote a dialogue about its significance.

The common scenario in which the patient offers his or her psychiatrist a gift raises all these questions about how to maintain appropriate professional boundaries. Ethical issues that arise when patients present clinicians with gifts of various kinds have been explored in both the general medical literature[7–11] and the psychiatric literature.[12–16] Gift giving in psychiatry is especially interesting and clinically potent in view of the powerful emotional aspects of the patient-psychiatrist relationship. As in the case of general medical practice, a psychiatrist has to consider the intention of the gift, its relative monetary (or other) value to the patient, and the anticipated effect of accepting or refusing it on the patient and the treatment itself. Medical practitioners and psychiatric practitioners alike are ethically obligated to consider patients' best interests when deciding about how to handle the offer of a gift.

In addition, the clinician may need to pay special attention to considerations that are unique to psychiatric practice. Is the treatment primarily pharmacotherapy and based on the traditional "medical model," or is it primarily a psychodynamic psychotherapy in which analysis of the transference is a key element? If the former, can the psychiatrist approach the situation as any other physician would? If the latter, does the psychiatrist

have a greater burden to explore the underlying intentions and unconscious meanings of the gift? Because of the potency of transference
dynamics in psychodynamic psychiatry, ethical analysis of how to respond
to a gift is especially complicated. On the one hand, if a main concern
in a patient's psychotherapy is rejection sensitivity or fear of abandonment, then the psychiatrist's refusal of a gift may touch the patient's core
emotional problems and have a deleterious impact on the therapy itself.
On the other, if a narcissistic patient often uses expensive gifts to bribe
or manipulate people in his or her personal life, then the presentation of
a gift to the psychiatrist would raise clinically important questions.
Appropriate treatment in such a case would entail a careful exploration
of the intention and meaning of the gift, regardless of whether the psychiatrist ultimately accepts or refuses it.

For each psychiatrist, the ethical deliberations about such scenarios
occur on a case-by-case basis, requiring careful analysis of how to
promote the patient's best interest while adhering to the spirit of the
professional relationship. Abstract moral principles provide insufficient
guidance in the specific gift-giving scenarios in which clinicians find
themselves. For example, while the general moral tenet that clinicians
should never exploit patients is indisputable, it does not constitute a
generalized approach to dealing with all gifts in psychiatric practice.
Clinicians certainly can avoid the risk of exploiting their patients by
never accepting a gift, and some clinicians may choose to adopt this
approach. But by adopting a uniform, standardized rule of this kind, they
may run the risk of violating other important principles of clinical ethics,
such as flexibility in the service of the particular patient's best interest at
a particular moment. For example, if a patient's offer of a modest gift to
a psychiatrist represents a significant therapeutic step toward a healthy
form of gratitude, does the psychiatrist want to preclude accepting that
gift based on the general principle that accepting gifts in clinical contexts
may exploit and harm some patients?

Psychiatrists must be rigorous in their ethical commitment to avoid
the exploitation of patients by accepting certain gifts, but also must be
flexible enough to step outside the boundaries of their narrowly defined
role when it is in the patient's best interest. Negotiating the poles of rule-
bound rigor and individually tailored flexibility is a significant practical
challenge when a patient or patient's family offers the psychiatrist a gift.
The psychiatrist, we propose, can resolve this dilemma by working in
the framework of "clinical pragmatism," an approach to clinical ethics
that specifies several core values that ought to be balanced in patient

care.[17-20] Regarding presentation of gifts to psychiatrists, a major core value of clinical pragmatism is that the psychiatrist should focus ethical deliberations as to whether to accept a gift on the specific results of that decision for the particular patient in question, not merely on abstract moral principles. How does one define a good result for a patient under these circumstances? The ethics of clinical pragmatism suggest that the psychiatrist must assess whether accepting or declining the gift advances the treatment relationship and helps the patient reach his or her treatment goals. But clinical pragmatism makes clear that the psychiatrist alone is not empowered to assess the outcome: the patient can and should participate in discussions about whether accepting or declining the gift would be helpful. In addition, there are others outside the treatment dyad who might have something to say about the psychiatrist's decision to accept or not accept a gift, including the patient's family members, the clinician's community of colleagues and peers, and professional review boards (which might get involved if the patient or family later files a complaint regarding exploitation or boundary concerns). When a patient presents a gift, the psychiatrist may become embroiled in a complex interpersonal, social, legal, and ethical web, with little guidance about how to achieve clarity of purpose and action.

The pragmatic framework does not specify whether a psychiatrist should accept or decline any particular gift, but it urges the clinician, at the very least, to address the following six questions whenever a patient or patient's family member offers a gift of any kind:

1. Would accepting the gift be exploitative insofar as it would benefit the clinician and possibly harm the patient financially, emotionally, or otherwise? If so, the clinician must decline the gift and strive to find a therapeutic way to discuss the refusal of the gift with the patient.

2. Is the gift of great monetary or other value to the patient, the clinician, or others in the community? If so, the clinician should not simply accept the gift without engaging in a robust dialogue about its meaning and implications with the patient (and possibly the patient's family) and also, perhaps, with professional colleagues or an ethics committee.

3. Is the gift extremely valuable or desirable to the clinician? If so, the clinician must reflect carefully on whether his or her clinical judgment or performance would be compromised by accepting it (e.g., might he or she become overly acquiescent and unable to confront the patient about difficult issues?). Also, clinicians ought to reflect on whether accepting the gift might erode their sense of themselves as professionals with a strong code of ethics.

4. Would accepting the gift run counter to professional norms in one's practice community? If so, the psychiatrist ought to consult with colleagues or an ethics committee, preferably before the gift is accepted.

5. Would declining the gift be hurtful, traumatic, or otherwise counter-therapeutic to the patient? Conversely, would accepting the gift possibly advance the treatment? If so, and if the gift is not of excessive value and does not raise the specter of exploitation or other harms, then the clinician can (and perhaps should) accept the gift.

6. Is the clinician's deliberation about accepting or declining the gift guided primarily by consideration of the patient's best interest? If not, then the clinician needs to reflect more (and possibly consult with colleagues) about why other motives might be informing his or her reaction to the gift. The prime consideration always must be the practical outcome for the patient of accepting or declining the gift.

In the following sections we present five cases that raise ethical dilemmas about patient gift giving in psychiatry and analyze each case from the standpoint of the pragmatic model. The cases describe a wide diversity of clinical scenarios in which the gift is offered; all five are composites of many different patients with whom we have worked clinically. Each case is followed by comments on relevant ethical principles and on the pragmatic approach to handling gifts from patients.

Case 1

Ms. Simon was a thirty-two-year-old married woman with depression, anxiety, and agoraphobia who had been receiving treatment from a psychiatrist for more than three years. Due to her symptoms, she had been unable to work for many years. The treatment consisted of psychodynamically oriented psychotherapy, along with some cognitive-behavioral techniques for managing the agoraphobia and acute episodes of anxiety.

In the therapy, Ms. Simon explored long-standing, conflicted feelings about her family of origin. She recalled that while growing up, her father had routinely ridiculed her mother; Ms. Simon had regularly sided with her father in order to win his approval. Her mother had died prior to Ms. Simon's beginning therapy. She felt quite guilty about her behavior toward her mother and reported that she missed her greatly.

Ms. Simon went through a period of crisis around the anniversary date of her mother's death. Longstanding conflicts between her and her husband flared when he was unresponsive to her distress. In therapy sessions, she reported increasing hopelessness and strong suicidal ideation but refused hospitalization. She felt no relief of symptoms from medication. During this period, her psychiatrist tried to be more available to Ms. Simon—including frequent telephone conversations. With ongoing therapy and support over the next few months, her depression and anger appeared to resolve considerably.

In December following the period of crisis, the psychiatrist received a package from Ms. Simon at her office. It contained a holiday card expressing gratitude for all the help that she had received during the past year. The card also explained that her mother had always sent gifts to those who had treated her well throughout the year and that the gift was similar to something that her mother had cherished. Opening the box, the psychiatrist found an exquisite vase by a well-known designer. Aside from the discussion that would need to take place about the thought behind the gift, the question of what to do with it remained.

This vignette describes the case of a three-year psychotherapy with powerful transference dynamics that culminate in the patient's presentation of an expensive gift to the therapist. When Ms. Simon experienced some marital conflict around the anniversary of her mother's death (which had occurred several years earlier), the therapist went beyond the call of duty in order to help the patient through an emotional crisis that was marked by hopelessness and suicidal ideation. Ms. Simon felt genuine gratitude for what the therapist had done for her during that difficult time. Under these circumstances, the gift may have been an appropriate and straightforward way for Ms. Simon to express her heartfelt thanks. Looked at in this uncomplicated fashion, the therapist might have simply accepted the gift, expressing thanks for it and reiterating that it had been a pleasure to help Ms. Simon in her time of need.

When examined from a technical clinical perspective, however, this case is more complicated because the proffering of the gift appears to have represented an important maternal transference reaction that called for in-depth analysis. Considering that Ms. Simon had felt guilty about her unkind treatment of her deceased mother, it is conceivable that the gift was intended to make amends for her past behavior toward her mother. If so, the giving of the gift might have embodied Ms. Simon's intense guilt and self-punishment, which would require recognition and working through if Ms. Simon was to heal herself emotionally and overcome her depression. It is conceivable, however, that the gift represented a major step forward in Ms. Simon's effort to resolve her guilt and grief regarding her mother. By acting in a way that her mother also would have acted (i.e., by giving a thoughtful gift), Ms. Simon may have been forming a healthy and growth-promoting identification with her deceased mother, whose memory she internalized as a good object. At the same time, the gift may have represented a significant paternal transference. By presenting such a lovely gift, Ms. Simon could have been trying to win the therapist's approval in the same way that she had attempted to win her father's approval by siding with him against her mother. One way or another, Ms. Simon's gift to her therapist had significant transference meaning that ought to have been thoroughly explored in the sessions.

The question whether to accept or decline the gift requires careful consideration in this case. We do not know the actual monetary value of the gift, but can presume that its cost would be substantial for many or most patients. Although she herself did not work outside the home, Ms. Simon was married to a successful attorney, and the vase may be similar in value to gifts that the two of them often gave on special occasions. If the therapist did not yet know Ms. Simon's financial circumstances, the occasion of the gift would probably constitute an appropriate moment to ascertain that information discreetly. Unless the monetary value was truly excessive by any common measure, the therapist's rejecting the gift could have proven to be hurtful and detrimental to the therapy, partly because the process of giving the gift may have represented a major psychological advance for Ms. Simon as she strove to introject her mother's good qualities and thereby overcome her long-standing guilt and depression. If so, then the therapist ought to have acknowledged and promoted Ms. Simon's progress by either (1) accepting the gift while also exploring its momentous intrapsychic significance, or (2) declining the gift (if its value was too great) but doing so graciously and with expressions of gratitude, admiration for her emotional growth, and encouragement to deepen an already rich psychotherapy process.

Case 2

Ms. Bradley was a twenty-four-year-old single woman who began treatment with a psychiatry resident for generalized anxiety and panic attacks. It soon became evident that medication was only somewhat helpful and that there were significant psychological issues that were relevant to her distress. In weekly psychodynamically oriented therapy, Ms. Bradley initially reported a happy childhood, but it was quickly apparent that she had very ambivalent feelings about her father. Although he could be loving, he was often harshly critical and at times somewhat abusive. She remembered his explosive anger when she would not behave herself as he thought she should. On one occasion when she was quite young, she recalled that he responded to her wetting the bed by pushing her face into the urine-soaked sheets and shouting, "This'll teach you to be dirty!" Ms. Bradley also began to understand that her father would subtly encourage her to be with him to the exclusion of others and would punish her when she paid attention to friends. He discouraged her from dating in her teenage years, implying that boys would not really care about her and that they wanted only sex.

The insights from her therapy seemed to help Ms. Bradley. Over the course of the next two years, she gradually improved. Although she continued to have some periodic anxiety and panic attacks, she began to feel more comfortable with herself. She received a promotion at work and began dating (and eventually married) a man whom she met through friends. Finally, fulfilling a long-standing dream, she became pregnant with her first child.

During the holiday season that began the third year of her treatment, Ms. Bradley handed her therapist a card. Along with a message expressing thanks, the card contained two crisp $100 bills. The resident, after expressing initial surprise, gratefully accepted the gift, thinking to himself that it would help to defray his own holiday expenses. When he subsequently discussed the gift with his supervisor, however, he was told that he could not accept the gift and should return it. He then returned the money with an explanation about professional roles and boundaries, and attempted to discuss the meaning of the gift. Ms. Bradley was devastated by his approach, saying that she felt "just like when my father pushed my face in the dirty sheets." Shortly thereafter, she terminated treatment.

At first glance, this case describes a conflict between ethical behavior (refusal to exploit a vulnerable patient who has offered a gift) and clinically sound behavior (sensitivity to a patient's personal needs and fragilities). One could argue that as the direct result of the clinician's following conventional rules of ethics, clinical care foundered and the therapy ended prematurely. It is plausible to argue that the clinician's behavior was not ethically sound, precisely because it failed to meet the professional obligation to serve the best interests of the patient. It is difficult to fairly assess the resident's initial impulse to accept his patient's gift.

Was his decision to accept the gift motivated by his desire to act in her best interest, which he felt would be well served by accepting the gift at this stage in their treatment relationship? Or was his initial acceptance of the gift driven by financial self-interest or a belief that he was entitled to the gift as a year-end bonus for work well done?

Some mixture of both motives, of course, is possible and even likely. But perhaps the focus of the ethical analysis in this case should be more on the supervisor than on the resident. One could imagine that powerful interpersonal dynamics in the relationship between the resident and supervisor led the resident, against his better judgment, to obediently acquiesce to his supervisor's instruction to return the gift. If so, then it would be reasonable to argue that the supervisor failed both clinically and ethically, as the instruction to return the gift appears rigid and antithetical to ethical precepts concerning the best interests of the patient and the psychotherapy supervisor's duty to provide thoughtful and flexible clinical guidance. The supervisor in this case appeared to be focused on relevant concerns about selfish exploitation of the patient by the resident. But the supervisor, unfortunately, did not help the resident to reason and act pragmatically, which would have also involved considering the result of declining the gift and attempting to interpret its meaning. It appears that the patient's best interest may have been compromised in this case by the supervisor's inflexible view on how to negotiate the presentation of a gift from a patient.

Case 3

Mr. Brown was a seventy-eight-year-old man who was initially admitted to an inpatient psychiatric hospital in the early 1950s for the evaluation and treatment of severe social withdrawal. He was chronically impaired throughout his life, receiving treatment for his psychiatric illness at various hospitals all across the country. He was unable to work and was supported by an inherited trust fund. During his later years, he was treated and housed in a residence at a psychiatric hospital. Mr. Brown remained at that facility for many years, during which time he was seen in supportive psychotherapy by a psychiatrist, who provided a consistent presence and helped him cope with, and adjust to, stresses in his life.

Mr. Brown was eventually transferred to a hospice, for care of terminal cancer. While preparing a transition plan for Mr. Brown's care in the hospice, the nursing home staff and his psychiatric treatment team requested that his psychiatrist continue to see him there for psychotherapy. During the first therapy session at the hospice, Mr. Brown asked the psychiatrist if she could be identified as his next of kin to make medical and financial decisions should he become incapacitated; he was estranged from his family and had no friends. She responded that she was uncomfortable being named his next of kin, because she was his therapist. When she suggested that perhaps he could consider asking his lawyer, Mr. Brown looked pained. He stated that he understood her reasoning, although he commented that she was like family to him, as his family disowned him years ago. He also made a vague reference to his will. A few weeks later, Mr. Brown died, and the psychiatrist was notified that he had bequeathed a considerable portion of his estate to her, with the remainder going to a variety of charities. The psychiatrist's discomfort with this turn of events was heightened by a conversation with a family member, who insinuated that she had unduly influenced Mr. Brown to feel negatively about his family.

Many of the factors that preclude accepting gifts from patients on ethical grounds presuppose that the patient is alive and, even if not currently being treated, may return for care at some later date. The case of Mr. Brown is unusual since the gift was only vaguely referred to while he was alive and since it was actually given (as a bequest) after his death. Although the practical effect of a gift on the patient and on the treatment relationship are, under the pragmatic model, key considerations influencing the ethics of accepting or rejecting gifts, that model does not apply in a straightforward way in this particular case.

Another factor that often influences the appropriateness of accepting a gift is the stage of the treatment: what is proffered after a treatment relationship lasting many years may be more likely to be acceptable, given the satisfaction of other criteria, than a gift offered after a brief therapeutic encounter. In this respect, both the quality and quantity of care that the psychiatrist had provided this patient might be a consideration indicating the appropriateness of the gift. Given Mr. Brown's social isolation (there was no one closer to him than the psychiatrist and no one so close as to be morally entitled to an inheritance), his financial means, and the many years of care that he had received from the psychiatrist, his gratitude seems understandable. It seems that Mr. Brown's motivation stemmed from a generous appreciation of the care he had received, and while the motivation behind gifts from some patients requires special scrutiny, this motivation seems straightforward.

All that said, other aspects of the case are potentially troubling. One would want to consider the relationship between the ultimate gift and the earlier request that the psychiatrist be identified as Mr. Brown's next of kin to make medical and financial decisions. As the psychiatrist recognized, becoming the patient's next of kin probably would have been an inappropriate boundary crossing, albeit a poignantly symbolic one in view of the patient's life story. The psychiatrist's refusal did not prevent the bequest in this case, perhaps because her elderly patient died so soon thereafter. Nonetheless, acceptance of the request would have been wrong—in part because it might have invited a slippery slope into a possible boundary violation.

Two other elements complicate this case—the size of the gift and the reaction of Mr. Brown's family. Because the family had previously disowned and perhaps neglected Mr. Brown, their claim to his estate seems unwarranted. Consequently, their resentment does not seem to be a relevant ethical consideration here. But it should remind us of another consideration that may need to be taken into account: appearances. Although there is no reason to think that the psychiatrist had exploited Mr. Brown, if it might have seemed to the family that she had, then perhaps she ought to have refused the bequest for the sake of avoiding the appearance of impropriety. The size of the gift may also be relevant: if it were relatively small by most worldly standards, then the argument from appearances would not be as compelling. Even if the bequest gave rise to no unethical appearances—let us say the family did not care or even know about it—accepting it may have served to erode the clinician's sense of herself as a professional. If her professional integrity was actually affected—an issue raised by her questioning of the bequest—then she should probably have declined the gift.

Case 4

Ms. Alan was an eighteen-year-old woman who attended a psychiatric partial hospital program for a period of two months for treatment of chronic psychiatric illness and difficulties in social and vocational functioning. She had been expelled from several schools and blamed her teachers for her problems, characterizing the teachers as incompetent and vindictive. She was similarly negative about members of her outpatient treatment team, whom she had recently fired. In the partial hospital program, her attendance and punctuality were spotty, and she tended to dominate groups by her self-referencing remarks. She regularly found fault with the staff and challenged attempts to set limits. She objected to program policies and procedures and would seek "special" modifications.

Under the leadership of an administrative psychiatrist, the partial hospital team made great efforts to forge an alliance with Ms. Alan and to contain the provocative challenges that she created. Over time, she was able to begin to understand that her difficulties had to do with the way she approached others. Fearful of being controlled, she instead sought to take control, often in ways that alienated others. At the conclusion of her partial hospital treatment, her psychiatric condition had improved. She was more attentive to her daily activities and the care of her apartment. She began a volunteer job, started to make friends, and agreed to see a new outpatient therapist and psychiatrist.

Ms. Alan's treatment in the partial hospital concluded with a family meeting. Her considerable progress was noted, and the family expressed appreciation for the dedication of the psychiatrist and the treatment team in overcoming difficulties. After the meeting, Ms. Alan's father offered the psychiatrist extremely desirable and hard-to-get theater tickets. The psychiatrist accepted and used the tickets, but later felt troubled. He wondered if the gift was simply an expression of appreciation from a grateful family or whether there were unspoken obligations assumed when he accepted the gift. How would he be expected to respond if Ms. Alan or her family sought services in the future? Would he be compromised in his clinical judgment or be expected to bend the rules beyond his level of comfort?

There is little need here to consider the consequences of accepting or declining this gift for the current treatment, which had concluded. The emotional impact on Ms. Alan of the psychiatrist's accepting or rejecting the gift is hard to judge, as Ms. Alan may not have even known that it was offered. If she did, she might have been impressed by the clinician's self-sacrificing behavior if he had refused the gift—or she might have been offended by his impoliteness if he had rebuffed such a friendly gesture. In neither situation would such considerations have been of clinical significance in the partial hospital program, as the treatment relationship there had ended.

Even if the treatment in the partial hospital were ongoing, it is important to note that exploration of the transference had not played a central role in this treatment relationship, which was primarily administrative and supportive. Furthermore, the gift was not offered by the patient but by a grateful parent. Therefore, it does not appear that a decision to accept or decline a gift would have had much direct bearing on an ongoing therapeutic process in the partial hospital. Instead, the most salient ethical issues in this case relate to a potential for future ethical conflicts, which would require thoughtful consideration if and when this patient returned to treatment. Would the clinician be more likely to treat her in the future or afford her special consideration because of anticipated gifts or favors? Might he be unable to confront or challenge her about difficult issues for fear that he would lose his special treatment from the family, or would he be able to approach a future treatment relationship with no regard to anticipated gifts or favors?

The psychiatrist in this case was appropriately concerned that the intention of the father's gift may have been bribery—a generous gratuity with future strings attached. Yet the giver's stated intention was gratitude. If the father did not acknowledge that an element of bribery was present, can the clinician be said to have acted unethically by accepting the gift and thereby accepting a bribe he did not know about? Of course, it would be an entirely different matter if the clinician knew that the gift was being used as a bribe and accepted it with an intention to act on it in the future (or to deceive the giver that he would). If he thought the gift was being offered as a bribe, the most ethical and tactful approach would be to have stated that he could accept such a gift only as an expression of gratitude, and that there could be no expectation of special consideration in the future as a result of it. The patient's father could then have withdrawn the gift or not, according to his predominant intentions.

The value of the gift relative to the resources of the family is important in determining the ethical propriety of acceptance, but we do not have the relevant information. The appropriateness of a gift in the context of a professional relationship depends partly on whether the donor can readily afford it. If so, the gift may be a nice and harmless gesture, but if not, it may be an act of fiscal self-injury and should not be accepted, however well intended. The value of the gift to the recipient may be more relevant here and seems to have contributed to the clinician's discomfort. The gift seemed extravagant to him and thus made him feel uncomfortable—but it is not clear that such a feeling in itself makes it unethical to accept such a gift. The clinician in such a situation might choose to consult with a colleague before accepting the gift, and if the clinician ultimately decides to accept it, he or she might then manage the ensuing discomfort about the extravagance of the gift in a variety of ways, perhaps by donating it to charity (though in the particular case before us, that particular option is perhaps not available).

Case 5

Paul, a sixteen-year-old youth from a wealthy family from the Midwest, was hospitalized for treatment of bipolar disorder. The family requested a consultation with a psychiatrist at the hospital who primarily performed clinical research. She agreed to do so and then remained in nearly daily communication with the family about the progress of their son during the lengthy and rocky hospitalization. Eventually this psychiatrist recommended a regimen of treatment that was successful in treating Paul, who began to function much better than he had done while under the care of previous clinicians. The family was eager for her to continue permanently as the treating psychiatrist for their son, but she explained that she had an extensive research commitment and could not take on a long-term patient. Nevertheless, she agreed to continue to see the son temporarily.

Paul continued to do well on an outpatient basis. Near the end of the first year of treatment, the psychiatrist unexpectedly received a gift of $15,000 from the family for her research fund. She gratefully acknowledged the gift and wrote to the family about possible projects that she planned to fund with the contribution. She continued to see Paul, being loath to pass his case on to another doctor in the wake of receiving such a generous gift, even though his medications were stabilized and he probably would have done equally well in the hands of another psychiatrist.

After another year elapsed, another gift of $15,000 arrived. The psychiatrist continued to see Paul, although she had no other private patients and refused to accept new patients, explaining that her research commitment precluded private practice. During the following year, she was approached by a hospital development officer who asked whether there were additional opportunities to seek donations from the family. The psychiatrist felt uncomfortable about the situation, but the development officer assured her that the family was very grateful to her and the hospital, and would easily be capable of making a contribution of several hundred thousand dollars. The development officer offered to help the psychiatrist, if she wished, in soliciting these funds.

The main ethical questions raised by this case are as follows: Is it proper for a psychiatrist to accept a substantial financial sum as a gift if it directly or indirectly benefits the psychiatrist in some way? Should a psychiatrist accept (and continue to accept) gifts that may be intended to influence her clinical decisions? Is it ethical for a psychiatrist to approach a benefactor for additional gifts for the institution with which she is affiliated?

With respect to the first question, one could argue plausibly that it is never appropriate for an individual psychiatrist to accept a gift of $15,000, because such a large amount of money is so likely to create a conflict of interest. But there is an important countervailing consideration in this case: the psychiatrist accepted the gift not for her own personal use, but to enhance her research efforts, which could have beneficial consequences for a large number of people in the future. At the same time, the psychiatrist clearly benefited from the donation, as it increased her funding and enhanced her career opportunities. Thoughtful deliberation and discussion with colleagues about how best to balance the relative risks and benefits of accepting a large gift are ethically warranted in a challenging situation of this kind.

The psychiatrist should have carefully considered whether such a gift was having an undue influence on the treatment itself: given the psychiatrist's decision to curtail her clinical work in order to focus on research activities, it appears that her treatment of Paul would not have continued were it not for the initial and subsequent gifts. Whatever the motivation of Paul's family—whether it was simple gratitude or inducement to continue treatment—the gift likely resulted in a different course of treatment than would have occurred otherwise. In particular, the psychiatrist may well have continued to work with Paul because she hoped for more gifts in the future or felt that it would be ungracious to terminate with him after receiving such generous gifts. Under such circumstances, a psychiatrist ought to reflect carefully on his or her motives and would be well advised to seek the advice of a trusted colleague or an ethics consultant.

The third question raised by the case of Paul concerns institutional ethics and the practice of soliciting contributions from individuals (and their families) who have mental illnesses and, consequently, a potential interest in funding psychiatric research. On one hand, asking for gifts from such individuals appears both reasonable and unproblematic because, in addition to having the ability to make substantial contributions for psychiatric research, they understand the importance of such research as a result of their direct experience of the devastating impact of mental illness. But soliciting from such individuals must be conducted with sensitivity and thoughtfulness because of several potential pitfalls. The patient or family may feel coerced to give the institution a gift for fear that they will not receive top-notch clinical care if they do not. They may feel pressured into making a decision to donate large sums of money under significant duress as they deal with the anguish of caring for a family member with mental illness. They may feel that their confidentiality has been compromised if a development officer approaches them for a gift before they have consented to such a solicitation. The psychiatrist who treated Paul was understandably uncomfortable and right to raise ethical questions about this issue. Respectful treatment of the patient and family in such cases depends on ethical behavior of both the clinician and the development office staff.

Discussion

These five cases and commentaries illustrate some of the complexity of ethical judgments about gift giving and some of the ways that these complexities multiply and interact within psychiatric practice. Factors such as the intention of the gift, its relative monetary or other value for the patient, and the effect—and even perceived effect—on the treatment of rejecting or accepting a gift are important when a gift is proffered in any medical setting. But in psychiatric practice, where emotional dimensions of the therapeutic relationship are so charged, such considerations may become magnified, carrying more weight and affecting the ethical dimensions more deeply.

Not only these considerations but others—as our vignettes illustrate—arise within the nuanced and context-sensitive arena of psychiatric practice. Paramount here, from a psychodynamic standpoint, are the gift's meanings to the patient, its conscious and unconscious connotations. There is the question of who gave the gift (perhaps the family rather than the patient) and what its ostensible purpose may be. There are considerations related to the gesture's part in the transference relationship and to the nature of the relationship more generally. Also, aspects of the patient's disorder and personality are critical, as is the type of therapy undertaken. For example, a gift from patient to psychiatrist may warrant more scrutiny in the context of a transference-based psychodynamic psychotherapy than in a medical-model psychopharmacologic treatment. In addition, these vignettes show that there are factors concerning the patient's perception of the treatment received, as well as cultural expectations and norms governing gratitude, gift giving, and interpersonal transactions. Finally, the patient's and family's social and economic life situation may be important elements altering the ethical imperatives involved.

While seeking to maximize therapeutic effect and to safeguard the best interests of the patient, the practitioner may be required to balance and weigh all the considerations enumerated above and also others. The composite cases offered here are only a tiny subset of the many possible cases we might have selected to illustrate the permutations and combinations of ethical considerations that arise for a psychiatrist offered a gift by a patient. They demonstrate the complexity and variation of gift-giving scenarios in psychiatry and the multitude of factors influencing sound ethical practice in this arena. If a conclusion may be drawn from our diverse observations, it is that the context-sensitivity of these boundary questions defies any easy or simple rule making. The pragmatic model we have outlined suggests that these challenges need to be handled on a case-by-case basis by paying careful attention to the patient's best interest and the practical result for the patient of accepting or declining the gift. While some gifts raise serious ethical problems that militate against accepting them, it is important to recognize that sometimes, even in psychiatry, a gift may just be a gift.

References

1. Gabbard, G. O. (1999). Boundary violations. In S. Bloch, P. Chodoff, & S. A. Green (Eds.), *Psychiatric ethics* (3rd ed., pp. 141–160). Oxford: Oxford University Press.

2. Gutheil, T. G., & Gabbard, G. O. (1998). Misuses and misunderstandings of boundary theory in clinical and regulatory settings. *American Journal of Psychiatry*, *155*, 409–414.

3. Radden, J. (2001). Boundary violation ethics: Some conceptual clarifications. *Journal of the American Academy of Psychiatry and the Law*, *29*, 319–326.

4. Hundert, E. M., & Appelbaum, P. S. (1995). Boundaries in psychotherapy: Model guidelines. *Psychiatry*, *58*, 345–356.

5. Martinez, R. (2000). A model for boundary dilemmas: Ethical decisionmaking in the patient-professional relationship. *Ethical Human Sciences and Services*, *2*, 43–61.

6. Glass, L. L. (2003). The gray areas of boundary crossings and violations. *American Journal of Psychotherapy*, *57*, 429–444.

7. Lyckholm, L. J. (1998). Should physicians accept gifts from patients? *Journal of the American Medical Association*, *280*, 1944–1946.

8. Weijer, C. (2001). Point-counterpoint: Should physicians accept gifts from their patients? No: gifts debase the true value of care. *Western Journal of Medicine*, *175*, 77.

9. Andereck, W. (2001). Point-counterpoint: Should physicians accept gifts from their patients? Yes: if they are given out of beneficence or appreciation. *Western Journal of Medicine*, *175*, 76.

10. Boisaubin, G. (2001). Controversies in professionalism: Accepting gifts from patients. *Texas Medicine*, *97*, 9–11.

11. Weiss G. G. (2002). Patients bearing gifts. *Medical Economics*, 79:58, 61.

12. Akhtar, S. (1983). On accepting gifts from patients. *American Journal of Psychiatry, 140*, 1105.

13. Hundert, E. M. (1998). Looking a gift horse in the mouth: The ethics of gift-giving in psychiatry. *Harvard Review of Psychiatry, 6*, 114–117.

14. Talan, K. H. (1989). Gifts in psychoanalysis: Theoretical and technical issues. *Psychoanalytic Study of the Child, 44*, 149–163.

15. Polster, D. S. (2001). Gifts. In Ethics Committee of the American Psychiatric Association (Eds.), *Ethics primer of the American Psychiatric Association* (pp. 45–50). Washington, DC: American Psychiatric Association.

16. Roberts, L. W. (2006). Ethical philanthropy in academic psychiatry. *American Journal of Psychiatry, 163*, 772–778.

17. Brendel, D. H. (2006). *Healing psychiatry: Bridging the science/humanism divide*. Cambridge, MA: MIT Press.

18. Fins, J. J., Miller, F. G., & Bacchetta, M. D. (1998). Clinical pragmatism: Bridging theory and practice. *Kennedy Institute of Ethics Journal, 8*, 37–42.

19. McGee, G. (Ed.). (2003). *Pragmatic bioethics* (2nd ed.). Cambridge, MA: MIT Press.

20. Miller, F. G., Fins, J. J., & Bacchetta, M. D. (1996). Clinical pragmatism: John Dewey and clinical ethics. *Journal of Contemporary Health Law and Policy, 13*, 27–51.

22

How Certain Boundaries and Ethics Diminish Therapeutic Effectiveness

Arnold A. Lazarus

Civilized interactions depend heavily on recognizing and respecting boundaries. To violate a boundary, whether of an entire nation or one individual, is to usurp someone's legitimate territory and invade his or her privacy by disregarding tacit or explicit limits. In quality relationships, people honor one another's rights and sensibilities and are careful not to intrude into the other's psychological space. It is therefore not surprising that the literature on psychotherapy continues to dwell on this important issue from many different perspectives.

Ethical considerations are closely related to matters of personal and interpersonal boundaries. The recently revised ethical principles of psychologists (*American Psychologist,* 1992, Vol. 47, no. 12) spells out numerous specific boundaries that all professional psychologists are required to respect. Many of the ethical principles and proscriptions emphasize the avoidance of harassment, exploitation, harm, and discrimination and underscore the significance of respect, integrity, confidentiality, and informed consent. Nevertheless, when taken too far, these well-intentioned guidelines can backfire. Furthermore, some psychotherapists have constructed artificial boundaries and tend to embrace prohibitions that often undermine their clinical effectiveness.

During my internship in the 1950s, I was severely reprimanded by one of my supervisors for allegedly stepping out of role (one type of boundary) and thereby potentially undermining my clinical effectiveness. (In many quarters, clearly demarcated client-therapist roles have been very strongly emphasized in recent years.) It had come to my supervisor's attention that at the end of a session, I had asked a client to do me the favor of dropping me off at a service station on his way home. My car was being repaired, and I had ascertained that the client would be heading home after the session and that I would not be taking him out of his way. My supervisor contended that therapy had to be a one-way street and that clients should not be called upon to provide anything other than the agreed-upon fees for service. Given my transgression, my supervisor claimed that I had jeopardized the client-therapist relationship. Interestingly, I recall that my rapport with the client in question was enhanced rather than damaged by our informal chat on the way to the service station.

The extent to which some clinicians espouse what I regard as dehumanizing boundaries is exemplified by the following incident. During a recent couples therapy session, the husband mentioned that he had undergone a biopsy for a suspected malignancy and would have the result later that week. Our next appointment was two weeks away, so I called their home after a few days to ask about the laboratory findings. The husband answered the telephone, reported that all was well, and expressed gratitude at my interest and concern. The wife, a licensed clinical psychologist, had a different reaction. She told a mutual colleague (the person who had referred the couple to me) that she was rather dismayed and put out at what I had done, referring to it as the violation of a professional boundary. A simple act of human decency and concern had been transformed into a clinical assault.

A different boundary issue was raised in the columns of a state journal. A therapist was treating an adolescent and wanted to arrange a meeting with the boy's mother. A busy professional, the mother's schedule was such that the most convenient time was during a lunch break, and she suggested they meet to discuss the matter at a local restaurant. The position taken by various correspondents was that this would not only transgress various boundaries but constitute a dual relationship. I wondered whether meeting in the park, or at the mother's place of work, in a hotel lobby, or in a car would be similarly discounted. Or could the venue indeed be a restaurant if no food but only coffee were ordered?[1]

During more than three decades of clinical practice, I have emphasized the need for flexibility and have stressed the clinical significance of individual differences. Dryden (1991), in an interview with me that he aptly subtitled "It Depends," clearly accentuated my contention that blanket rules for one and all will often bypass important individual nuances that have to be addressed. With some clients, anything other than a formal and clearly delimited doctor-patient relationship is inadvisable and is likely to prove counterproductive. With others, an open give-and-take, a sense of camaraderie, and a willingness to step outside the bounds of a sanctioned healer will enhance treatment outcomes. Thus I have partied and socialized with some clients, played tennis with others, taken long walks with some, graciously accepted small gifts, and given presents (usually books) to a fair number. At times, I have learned more at different sides of a tennis net or across a dining room table than might ever have come to light in my consulting room. (Regrettably, from the viewpoint of present-day risk management, in the face of allegations of sexual impropriety, it has been pointed out that such boundary crossings, no matter how innocent, will ipso facto be construed as evidence of sexual misconduct by judges, juries, ethics committees, and state licensing boards.)

Out of the many clients whom I have treated, the number with whom I have stepped outside the formal confines of the consulting room is not in the hundreds, but give or take a few dozen. And when I have done so, my motives were not based on capriciousness but arose from reasoned judgments that the treatment objectives would be enhanced. Nevertheless, it is usually inadvisable to disregard strict boundary limits in the presence of severe psychopathology involving passive-aggressive, histrionic, or manipulative behaviors; borderline personality features; or manifestations of suspiciousness and undue hostility.

Some years back, I was treating a "difficult" patient who was combative and contentious. He arrived early for his appointment one morning while I was still having breakfast. An intuitive whim led me to invite him to pull up a chair and have some toast and tea.[2] This was a turning point. The act of "breaking bread" resulted in a cooperative liaison in place of his former hostility. Let me not be misunderstood. I am not advocating or arguing for a transparent, pliant, casual, or informal therapeutic relationship with everyone. Rather, I am asserting that those therapists who always go by the book and apply predetermined and fixed rules of conduct (specific dos and don'ts) across the board will offend or at the very least fail to help people who might otherwise have benefited from their ministrations.

For example, a psychiatric resident was treating a young woman who often asked him personal questions. "How old are you?" "Where did you go to school?" "Do you enjoy the ballet?" "Are you married?" In keeping with his supervisor's counsel, he studiously sidestepped all of these questions and asked about their intent. But the therapy was going nowhere, and he joined one of my supervision groups. "I think the patient is about to drop out of therapy," he said. This matter was discussed at length, whereupon I advised him to apologize to his patient, to explain that he meant no disrespect but was merely following his previous supervisor's advice. I recommended that he answer each of her questions, even showing her the photo of his young son that he carried in his wallet. At the next supervisory meeting, he reported having carried out his assignment and stated that their therapeutic alliance seemed to have been greatly enhanced; for the first time ever, real gains had accrued. The patient continued making progress.

There is something demeaning and hostile about having one's questions dismissed and answered by another question:

Client: Have you seen the latest Tom Cruise movie?
Therapist: Why is this important?
Client: Is your car the blue Chevy with the white interior?
Therapist: Why do you want to know?

It is even more demeaning when therapists simply dismiss straightforward queries:

Client: Did you play hockey in high school?
Therapist: We are here to discuss you, not me.

Unless there are valid reasons for not being forthright, or unless the question goes beyond the bounds of propriety, why not answer it candidly and then inquire as to its significance? "Yes, I was quite an avid hockey player in high school. Why do you ask?"

An example of what strikes me as an excessive boundary issue was related by one of my students. He was seeing a client who had written a short poem that she wished to share with him. According to my student, his supervisor was concerned that he may have taken the poem and read it, rather than having asked the client to read it to him. The supervisor had allegedly stated, "It's best not to touch or handle clients' personal possessions." This type of rigid professionalism is most unfortunate and seems likely to breed alienation and distance and is likely to rupture the therapeutic relationship rather than foster it.

My thesis is that it doesn't hurt to temper rules and regulations with a touch of common sense. Thus a colleague referred a couple to me. After two sessions, it seemed that their individual agendas took priority over their dyadic transactions, and I suggested to my colleague that she might want to work with the wife while I treated the husband. A few weeks later, I asked my colleague if she felt, as I did, that the marriage was probably bankrupt. "I can't discuss this with you because I have not obtained [the wife's] permission to do so," she replied. Ethically, my colleague was certainly toeing the line, but to my way of thinking, she exercised poor clinical judgment. My question was not an idle, voyeuristic attempt to pry into her client's privacy. It was geared toward a potentially helpful collegial exchange of information. Besides, having seen the wife myself, I was not a casual outsider, but someone who was concerned about and involved with the dyadic system.

By contrast, I was approached by a colleague who was treating one of my former clients and wanted specific information about him. Strictly speaking, I should first have obtained a written release from the client. Instead of wasting time, I simply told my colleague about traps and barriers that the client had erected that had undermined the therapy. I was able to alert her to various pitfalls that the client was likely to dig and into which she (like I) would probably fall unless she exercised due caution. She subsequently informed me that my caveats were of enormous clinical value in forestalling a self-sabotaging client from destroying his life. My motives behind this collegial interchange were obviously entirely in the client's best interests.

I have crossed many boundaries to good effect. I have even treated relatives and friends in addition to colleagues and acquaintances, and some of my closest friends are former clients. Nevertheless, my plea for flexibility and my defense of unorthodoxy are not completely heretical. I remain totally opposed to any form of disparagement, exploitation, abuse, or harassment, and I am against any form of sexual contact with clients. But outside of these confines, I feel that most other limits and proscriptions are negotiable. But the litigious climate in which we live has made me more cautious in recent years. I would not take certain risks that I gave no thought to in the 1960s. For example, I accepted two clients into my home (at different times). One lived with my family for several weeks, the other for several days. Both were men from out of state who had relocated and were looking for a place to live. Similarly, I would have thought nothing of offering a client our spare bedroom on a snowy night or furnishing a couple of aspirins if someone asked for them. But like most of my colleagues, I have attended seminars on how to avoid malpractice suits that have made my blood run cold. It is difficult to come away from those lectures without viewing every client as a potential adversary or litigant. Fortunately, the effects tended to wear off after a few days, and I regained my spontaneity. But the ominous undertones remain firmly implanted and are reinforced by passages in books that explain how innocent psychologists can protect themselves against unwarranted lawsuits (Keith-Spiegel & Koocher, 1985). Consequently, being more guarded has rendered me a less humane practitioner today than I used to be in the 1960s and 1970s.

It is interesting that Freud gave some patients gifts, loaned them books, sent them postcards, offered a meal to the Rat Man, and even provided financial support in a few cases. Perhaps Freud's most striking boundary violation was the analysis of his own daughter, Anna. According to Gutheil and Gabbard (1993), "these behaviors are no longer acceptable practice regardless of their place in the history of our field" (p. 189).

While reading a book on psychodrama by Kellermann (1992), I was particularly impressed with his account of a client who had participated in psychodrama groups for many years. When asked what she had found most helpful, the client stated,

> The most important thing for me was that I established a close relationship with Zerka,[3] a kind of friendship which extended beyond the ordinary patient-therapist relation. She took me to restaurants and on trips and treated me like my own mother had never done. That friendship had such a great impact on me that I can feel its effects to this very day! (p. 133)

It is, of course, safer and easier to go by the book, to adhere to an inflexible set of rules, than to think for oneself. But practitioners who hide behind rigid boundaries, whose sense of ethics is uncompromising, will, in my opinion, fail to really help many of the clients who are unfortunate enough to consult them. The truly great therapists I have met were not frightened conformists but courageous and enterprising helpers, willing to take calculated risks. If I am to summarize my position in one sentence, I would say that one of the worst professional or ethical violations is that of permitting current risk-management principles to take precedence over humane interventions. By all means drive defensively, but try to practice psychotherapy responsibly—with compassion, benevolence, sensitivity, and caring.

Notes

1. It has been argued that meetings outside the office, followed by sessions during lunch, often lead to dinner dates, movies, and other social events, finally culminating in sexual intercourse (see Gabbard, 1989; Simon, 1989).

2. Except for a period of five years, when I worked out of a professional office, my private practice has been conducted out of my home. This, for many, is in and of itself a transgression of a significant boundary.

3. Psychodrama was founded by J. L. Moreno (1889–1974). His wife, Zerka, son, Jonathan, and many enthusiasts have carried on and extended the overall tradition.

References

Dryden, W. (1991). *A dialogue with Arnold Lazarus: "It depends."* Philadelphia: Open University Press.

Gabbard, G. O. (Ed.). (1989). *Sexual exploitation in professional relationships.* Washington, DC: American Psychiatric Press.

Gutheil, T. G., & Gabbard, G. O. (1993). The concept of boundaries in clinical practice: Theoretical and risk-management dimensions. *American Journal of Psychiatry, 150,* 188–196.

Keith-Spiegel, P., & Koocher, G. P. (1985). *Ethics in psychology: Professional standards and cases.* New York: Random House.

Kellermann, P. F. (1992). *Focus on psychodrama.* Philadelphia: Jessica Kingsley.

Simon, R. I. (1989). Sexual exploitation of patients: How it begins before it happens. *Psychiatric Annals, 19,* 104–122.

23

Boundary Issues in Social Work: Managing Dual Relationships

Frederic G. Reamer

Particularly since the early 1980s, social workers have developed an increasingly mature grasp of ethical issues. During the past two decades, social work's literature has expanded markedly with respect to identifying ethical conflicts and dilemmas in practice, developing conceptual frameworks and protocols for ethical decision making when professional duties conflict, and formulating risk management strategies to prevent ethics-related negligence and ethical misconduct (Berliner, 1989; Besharov, 1985; Levy, 1993; Linzer, 1999; Loewenberg & Dolgoff, 1996; Reamer, 1982, 1990, 1994, 1995a, 1998b, 1999; Rhodes, 1986).

As the social work literature clearly demonstrates, ethical issues related to professional boundaries are among the most problematic and challenging (Congress, 1996; Jayaratne, Croxton, & Mattison, 1997; Kagle & Giebelhausen, 1994; Strom-Gottfried, 1999). Briefly, boundary issues involve circumstances in which social workers encounter actual or potential conflicts between their professional duties and their social, sexual, religious, or business relationships. As explored more fully later, not all boundary issues are necessarily problematic or unethical, but many are. The primary purpose of this discussion is to identify—in the form of a typology—the range of boundary issues in social work, develop criteria to help social workers distinguish between problematic and nonproblematic boundary issues, and present guidelines to help practitioners manage boundary issues and risks that arise in practice.

Boundary Issues in Social Work

Social workers—be they clinicians, community organizers, policymakers, supervisors, researchers, administrators, or educators—often encounter circumstances that pose actual or potential boundary issues. Boundary issues occur when social workers face possible conflicts of interest in the form of what have become known as dual or multiple relationships. Dual or multiple relationships occur when professionals engage with clients or colleagues in more than one relationship, whether social, sexual, religious, or business (St. Germaine, 1993, 1996). According to Kagle and Giebelhausen (1994),

a professional enters into a dual relationship whenever he or she assumes a second role with a client, becoming social worker and friend, employer, teacher, business associate, family member, or sex partner. A practitioner can engage in a dual relationship whether the second relationship begins before, during, or after the social worker relationship. (p. 213)

Dual relationships occur primarily between social workers and their current or former clients and between social workers and their colleagues (including supervisees and students).

The social work literature contains few in-depth discussions of boundary issues (Jayaratne et al., 1997; Kagle & Giebelhausen, 1994; Strom-Gottfried, 1999). Most discussions have focused on dual relationships that are exploitive in nature, such as social workers' sexual involvement with clients. Certainly these are important and compelling issues. However, many boundary and dual-relationship issues in social work are subtler than these egregious forms of ethical misconduct. A recent empirical survey of a statewide sample of clinical social workers uncovered substantial disagreement concerning the appropriateness of behaviors such as developing friendships with clients, participating in social activities with clients, serving on community boards with clients, providing clients with one's home telephone number, accepting goods and services from clients instead of money, and discussing one's religious beliefs with clients (Jayaratne et al., 1997; see also Borys & Pope, 1989; Brownlee, 1996; Gutheil & Gabbard, 1993; Pope, Tabachnick, & Keith-Spiegel, 1988; Smith, 1999; Smith & Fitzpatrick, 1995; Strom- Gottfried, 1999). As Corey and Herlihy (1997) noted:

The pendulum of controversy over dual relationships, which has produced extreme reactions on both sides, has slowed and now swings in a narrower arc. It is clear that not all dual relationships can be avoided, and it is equally clear that some types of dual relationships (such as sexual intimacies with clients) should always be avoided. In the middle range, it would be fruitful for professionals to continue to work to clarify the distinctions between dual relationships that we should try to avoid and those into which we might enter, with appropriate precautions. (p. 190)

To achieve a more fine-tuned understanding of boundary issues, social workers must broaden their analysis and examine dual relationships through several conceptual lenses. First, social workers should distinguish between boundary violations and boundary crossings (Gutheil & Gabbard, 1993; Smith & Fitzpatrick, 1995). A boundary violation occurs when a social worker engages in a dual relationship with a client or colleague that is exploitive, manipulative, deceptive, or coercive. Examples include social workers who become sexually involved with current clients, recruit and collude with clients to bill insurance companies fraudulently, or influence terminally ill clients to include social workers in clients' wills. Boundary violations are inherently unethical.

One key feature of boundary violations is a conflict of interest that harms clients or colleagues (Epstein, 1994; Kitchener, 1988; Kutchins, 1991; Pope, 1988, 1991). Conflicts of interest occur when professionals find themselves in "a situation in which regard for one duty leads to disregard of another or might reasonably be expected to do so" (Gifis, 1991, p. 88). Thus, a clinical social worker providing services to a client with whom he or she would like to develop a sexual relationship faces a potential conflict of interest; the social worker's personal interests clash with professional duty. Similarly, a community organizer who invests money in a client's business is embedded in a conflict of interest; the social worker's financial interests may clash with the social worker's professional duty to the client (e.g., if the social worker's relationship with the client becomes strained because they disagree about some aspect of their shared business).

The concept of conflict of interest is addressed explicitly in the NASW *Code of Ethics* (2000):

Social workers should be alert to and avoid conflicts of interest that interfere with the exercise of professional discretion and impartial judgment. Social workers should inform clients when a real or potential conflict of interest arises and take reasonable steps to resolve the issue in a manner that makes the clients' interests primary and protects clients' interests to the greatest extent possible. In some cases, protecting clients' interests may require termination of the professional relationship with proper referral of the client. (Standard 1.06a)

The *Code* goes on to say that "social workers should not engage in dual or multiple relationships with clients or former clients in which there is a risk of exploitation or potential harm to the client" (Standard 1.06c).

Some conflicts of interest involve what lawyers call undue influence. Undue influence occurs when a social worker inappropriately pressures or exercises authority over a susceptible client in a manner that benefits the social worker and may not be in the client's best interest. In legal terminology, undue influence involves:

[the] exertion of improper influence and submission to the domination of the influencing party. . . . In such a case, the influencing party is said to have an unfair advantage over the other based, among other things, on real or apparent authority, knowledge of necessity or distress, or a fiduciary or confidential relationship. (Gifis, 1991, p. 508)

The NASW *Code of Ethics* also addresses the concept of undue influence: "Social workers should not take unfair advantage of any professional relationship or exploit others to further their personal, religious, political, or business interests" (Standard 1.06b).

In contrast, a boundary crossing occurs when a social worker is involved in a dual relationship with a client or colleague in a manner that is not intentionally exploitive, manipulative, deceptive, or coercive. Boundary crossings are not inherently unethical. In principle, the consequences of boundary crossings may be harmful, salutary, or neutral (Gutheil & Gabbard, 1993). Boundary crossings are harmful when the dual relationship has negative consequences for the social worker's client or colleague and, possibly, for the social worker as well. For example, a clinical social worker who discloses to a client personal, intimate details about his or her own life, ostensibly to be helpful to the client, ultimately may confuse the client and compromise the client's mental health because of complicated transference issues produced by the social worker's self-disclosure. A social work educator who accepts a student's dinner invitation may inadvertently harm the student by confusing the student about the nature of the social work educator's relationship. A social work administrator whose family vacations with an employee and his or her family may have difficulty managing future personnel problems involving that employee.

Alternatively, some boundary crossings may be helpful to clients and colleagues. Some social workers argue that, handled judiciously, a clinical social worker's modest self-disclosure or decision to accept an invitation to attend a client's graduation ceremony may prove, in some special circumstances, to be therapeutically useful to a client (Anderson & Mandell, 1989; Chapman, 1997; Reamer, 1997, 1998a). A social worker at a community mental health center who worships, coincidentally, at the same church a client attends may help the client "normalize" the professional-client relationship. A social work educator who hires a student to serve as a research assistant may boost the student's self-confidence in a way that greatly enriches the student's educational experience.

Yet other boundary crossings produce mixed results. A social worker's self-disclosure about personal challenges may be both helpful and harmful to the same client—helpful in that the client feels more "connected" to the social worker and harmful in that the self-disclosure undermines the client's confidence in the social worker. The social work administrator of a residential substance abuse treatment program who hires a former client may initially elevate the former client's self-confidence and create boundary problems when the former client subsequently wants to resume the status of an active client following a relapse.

In light of the impressive range of boundary issues in the profession, it is important for social workers to have access to a conceptual framework to help them identify and manage the dual relationships they encounter. What follows is a typology of boundary issues in social work, based on several data sources: insurance industry statistics summarizing malpractice and negligence claims, empirical surveys of social workers and other professionals about boundary issues, legal literature and court opinions in litigation involving boundaries, and my experiences as chair of a statewide ethics adjudication committee and expert witness in a large number of legal cases involving boundary issues (Reamer, 2001a).

Boundary issues in social work can be placed into five conceptual categories revolving around five central themes pertaining to social workers: (1) intimate relationships, (2) pursuit of personal benefit, (3) emotional and dependency needs, (4) altruistic gestures, and (5) responses to unanticipated circumstances (see table 23.1).

Table 23.1
Central themes in dual relationships

Intimate relationships	Sexual relationships Physical contact Services to former lover Intimate gestures
Personal benefit	Monetary gain Goods and services Useful information
Emotional and dependency needs	Extending relationships with clients Promoting client dependence Confusing personal and professional lives Reversing roles with clients
Altruistic gestures	Performing favors Providing nonprofessional services Giving gifts Being extraordinarily available
Unanticipated circumstances	Social and community events Joint affiliations and memberships Mutual acquaintances and friends

Intimacy

Many dual relationships in social work involve some form of intimacy. Typically these relationships entail a sexual relationship or physical contact, although they may also entail other intimate gestures, such as gift giving, friendship, and affectionate communication.

Sexual Relationships

A significant portion of intimate dual relationships entered into by social workers involves sexual contact (Akamatsu, 1988; American Psychological Association, 1989; Bouhoutsos, 1985; Bouhoutsos, Kolroyd, Lerman, Foster, & Greenberg, 1983; Coleman & Schaefer, 1986; Feldman-Summers & Jones, 1984; Gabbard, 1989; Gechtman, 1989; Pope, 1990; Pope & Bouhoutsos, 1986; Reamer, 1984, 1992, 1994; Sell, Gottlieb, & Schoenfeld, 1986). During a recent twenty-year period, nearly one in five lawsuits (18.5 percent) against social workers insured through the malpractice insurance program sponsored by the NASW Insurance Trust alleged some form of sexual impropriety, and more than two-fifths (41.3 percent) of insurance payments were the result of claims concerning sexual misconduct (Reamer, 1995b). According to research evidence gathered by Brodsky (1986), the prototypical therapist sued for sexual misconduct is male, middle aged, involved in unsatisfactory relationships in his own life, provides counseling to a mostly female caseload, becomes sexually involved with multiple clients who are many years younger, discloses his personal problems to the clients with whom he is sexually involved, is lonely, and is isolated professionally. Of course, there are many documented cases involving female practitioners as well, albeit a much smaller number proportionately.

Sexual misconduct in the helping professions generally is a significant problem. National data suggest that between 8.0 percent and 12.0 percent of male counselors or psychotherapists and between 1.7 percent and 3.0 percent of female counselors or psychotherapists admit having had sexual relationships with current or former clients (Olarte, 1997). Insurance industry data suggest that inappropriate dual relationships in the form of sexual misconduct constitute the most frequent reason for lawsuits filed against mental health professionals (Reamer, 1994).

Although social workers generally agree that sexual relationships with current clients are inappropriate (NASW, 2000, Standard 1.09a), there is less clarity about social workers' sexual relationships with former clients. The *Code of Ethics* states clearly that in general, sexual relationships with former clients are unethical: "Social workers should not engage in sexual activities or sexual contact with former clients because of the potential for harm to the client" (Standard 1.09c). However, in this same standard, the *Code* also implies that exceptions may be warranted under extraordinary circumstances, for example, when the social worker is involved in a nonclinical relationship with the client:

If social workers engage in conduct contrary to this prohibition or claim that an exception to this prohibition is warranted because of extraordinary circumstances, it is social workers—not their clients—who assume the full burden of demonstrating that the former client has not been exploited, coerced, or manipulated, intentionally or unintentionally. (Standard 1.09c)

Current ethical standards also prohibit social workers from engaging in sexual activities or sexual contact with clients' relatives, or other individuals with whom clients maintain a close personal relationship, when there is a risk of exploitation or potential harm to the clients. As the code asserts:

Sexual activity or sexual contact with clients' relatives or other individuals with whom clients maintain a personal relationship has the potential to be harmful to the client and may make it difficult for the social worker and client to maintain appropriate professional boundaries. Social workers—not their clients, their clients' relatives, or other individuals with whom the client maintains a personal relationship—assume the full burden for setting clear, appropriate, and culturally sensitive boundaries. (Standard 1.09b)

NASW's *Code of Ethics* (NASW, 2000) also contains standards that explicitly prohibit sexual relationships between social work supervisors or educators and supervisees, students, trainees, and other colleagues over whom they exercise professional authority (Standard 2.07a). In addition, the *Code* stipulates that social workers should avoid engaging in sexual relationships with professional colleagues when there is a potential for conflicts of interest (Standard 2.07b).

The profession's ethical standards are less clear with respect to non-clinical relationships that do not involve possible exploitation of authority. Social workers need to examine the unique circumstances surrounding intimate relationships between, for example, community organizers and community residents, or between social work researchers (program evaluators) and their clients (agency administrators), to determine whether they constitute a boundary violation that may lead to significant harm.

Physical Contact

Not all physical contact between social workers and clients is sexual in nature. Physical contact may be nonsexual and appropriate in a number of circumstances, for example, a brief hug at the termination of long-term treatment or placing one's arm around a distraught client in a residential program who just received bad family news. Such brief, limited physical contact is not likely to be harmful; many clients would find such physical contact comforting and "therapeutic." Moreover, physical contact may be culturally appropriate and encouraged in some ethnic or social communities (Stake & Oliver, 1991). As Smith and Fitzpatrick (1995) observed:

There are also cultural factors to be considered. For example, in Montreal where the dominant culture is French-Canadian, kissing on both cheeks is a widely practiced greeting among friends and even casual acquaintances. When it occurs between a therapist and client (as it sometimes does on special occasions), it does not carry the erotically charged meaning it might elsewhere in North America. (pp. 502–503)

In contrast are situations involving physical touch that have more potential for psychological harm. In clinical relationships, physical touch may exacerbate a client's transference in destructive ways and may suggest that the social worker is interested in more than a professional relationship. For example, a clinical social worker provided counseling to a twenty-eight-year-old woman who had been sexually abused as a child. As an adult, the client sought counseling to help her understand the impact of the early victimization, especially pertaining to her intimate relationships. As part of the therapy, the social worker would occasionally dim the office lights, turn on soft music, and sit on the floor while cradling and talking with the client. In nonclinical relationships, too, physical touch may cause psychological harm. An example involved a social work administrator in a psychiatric hospital who was fired after evidence demonstrated that he sexually harassed two social workers on his staff in the form of inappropriate physical contact in the workplace.

For the first time in the history of the social work profession, the current NASW *Code of Ethics* (NASW, 2000) includes a standard pertaining specifically to the concept of physical touch:

Social workers should not engage in physical contact with clients when there is a possibility of psychological harm to the client as a result of the contact (such as cradling or caressing clients). Social workers who engage in appropriate physical contact with clients are responsible for setting clear, appropriate, and culturally sensitive boundaries that govern such physical contact. (Standard 1.10)

Counseling a Former Lover

Providing clinical services to someone with whom the social worker was once intimately, romantically, or sexually involved also constitutes a dual relationship. The relationship history is likely to make it difficult for the social worker and client to interact with each other solely as professional and client; inevitably the dynamics of the prior relationship will influence the professional-client relationship—how the parties view and respond to each other possibly in ways that are detrimental to the client's best interests. The *Code of Ethics* comments on this phenomenon:

Social workers should not provide clinical services to individuals with whom they have had a prior sexual relationship. Providing clinical services to a former sexual partner has the potential to be harmful to the individual and is likely to make it difficult for the social worker and individual to maintain appropriate professional boundaries. (Standard 1.09d)

Intimate Gestures

Boundary issues can also emerge when social workers and clients or colleagues engage in other intimate gestures, such as gift giving and expressions of friendship (including sending affectionate notes, for example, on the social worker's personal stationery). It is not unusual for clients to give social workers a modest gift. Certainly, in many instances, a client's gift represents nothing more than an appreciative gesture. In some instances, however, a client's gift may carry great meaning. For example, the gift may reflect the client's fantasies about a friendship or more intimate relationship with the social worker. Thus, it behooves social workers to consider carefully the meaning of clients' gifts and establish prudent guidelines governing the acceptance of gifts. Similarly, gifts from a social work supervisor to a supervisee might be interpreted as evidence of favoritism, which may damage other employees' morale and pose a conflict for the supervisor when she must conduct personnel evaluations.

In many social services settings—such as family services agencies, community mental health centers, hospitals, rehabilitation facilities, schools, and public human services departments—staff are not permitted to accept gifts because of a potential conflict of interest or appearance of impropriety or are permitted to accept gifts only of modest value. Some agencies permit staff to accept gifts only with the understanding—which is conveyed to clients—that the gifts represent a contribution to the agency, not to the individual social worker.

There is consensus among social workers that friendships with current clients constitute an inappropriate dual relationship. There is less clarity, however, about friendships between social workers and former clients. Although social workers generally understand the risk involved in befriending a former client—due to the possibility of confused boundaries—some social workers argue that friendships with former clients are not inherently unethical and reflect a more egalitarian, non-hierarchical approach to practice. These social workers typically claim that emotionally mature social workers and former clients are quite capable of entering into new kinds of relationships following termination of the professional-client relationship and that such new relationships often are, in fact, evidence of the former client's substantial therapeutic progress.

Social workers involved in nonclinical relationships—such as social work researchers or community organizers—may argue that strict prohibition of relationships with former clients should not automatically apply to them. Again, social workers may need to examine critically the unique circumstances involved to determine the nature and extent of conflicts of interest and potential harm.

Personal Benefit

Beyond these various manifestations of intimacy, social workers can become involved in dual relationships that produce other forms of personal benefit. The personal benefit to the social worker may take the form of monetary gain, goods, services, or useful information.

Monetary Gain

In some situations social workers stand to benefit financially because of a dual relationship (Bonosky, 1995). In one case, the former client of a social worker in private practice decided to change careers and become a social worker. After graduating from social work school, the former client contacted the social worker for supervision (such supervision was required for a state license). The social worker was tempted to provide the client with supervision for a fee, in part because the social worker enjoyed their relationship and in part because of the financial benefit. The social worker also recognized that the shift in relationship from social worker–client to collegial would introduce a number of boundary issues. In another case, a client in a substance abuse program named the social worker in his will. Following the client's death and probate of the will, the client's family accused the social worker of undue influence (the family alleged that the social worker encouraged the client to bequeath a portion of the client's estate to the social worker and that the client was not mentally competent).

Goods and Services

On occasion social workers receive goods or services—rather than money—as payment for their professional services. In one case, a clinical social worker's client lost his insurance coverage, yet still needed counseling services. The client, a house painter, offered to paint the social worker's home in exchange for clinical services. The social worker decided not to enter into the barter arrangement; after consulting with colleagues, the social worker realized that the client's interests could be undermined should some problem emerge with the paint job that would require some remedy or negotiation (e.g., if the paint job proved to be inferior in some way). In another case, a social worker who worked as a geriatric consultant received several paintings from a client—an artist— as payment for services rendered. This social worker reasoned that accepting "goods" of this sort was not likely to undermine the professional-client relationship, whereas accepting a service might.

In 1996 NASW included, for the first time, a specific standard on barter. The NASW Code of Ethics Revision Committee struggled to decide whether to prohibit or merely discourage all forms of barter (Reamer, 1998a). On the one hand, bartering entails potential conflicts of interest; on the other hand, bartering is an accepted practice in some communities (Schank & Skovholt, 1997; Woody, 1998). Ultimately the committee decided to discourage barter because of the risks involved, at the same time recognizing that barter is not inherently unethical. Further, the *Code* establishes strict standards for the use of barter by social workers:

Social workers should avoid accepting goods or services from clients as payment for professional services. Bartering arrangements, particularly involving services, create the potential for conflicts of interest, exploitation, and inappropriate boundaries in social workers' relationships with clients. Social workers should explore and may participate in bartering only *in very limited circumstances* when it can be demonstrated that such arrangements are an accepted practice among professionals in the local community, considered to be essential for the provision of services, negotiated without coercion, and entered into at the client's initiative and with the client's informed consent. Social workers who accept goods or services from clients as payment for professional services assume the full burden of demonstrating that this arrangement will not be detrimental to the client or the professional relationship. [italics added] (Standard 1.13b)

Useful Information

Social workers occasionally have an opportunity to benefit from clients' unique knowledge. A social worker with a complex health problem may be tempted to consult a client who is a physician and who happens to specialize in the area relevant to the social worker's illness. A social worker who is interested in adopting a child and whose client is an obstetrics/gynecology nurse may be tempted to talk to her client about adoption opportunities through the client's hospital. A social work administrator who is an active stock market investor may be tempted to consult one of the agency's clients who happens to be a stockbroker. A social worker with automobile problems may be tempted to consult a client who happens to be an automobile mechanic. In these situations there is clearly the potential for an inappropriate dual relationship, where a social worker engages with the client in a self-serving manner and where a social worker's judgment and services may be shaped and influenced by his or her access to a client's specialized knowledge. Conversely, relatively brief, casual, and nonexploitive conversations with clients concerning topics on which clients are expert may empower clients, facilitate therapeutic progress and the delivery of both clinical and nonclinical services, and challenge traditionally hierarchical relationships between social workers and clients.

Emotional and Dependency Needs

A number of boundary issues arise out of social workers' efforts to address their own emotional needs. Many of these issues are subtle in nature, and some are more glaring and egregious. Among the more egregious are the following examples:

The administrator of a state child welfare agency that serves abused and neglected children was having difficulty coping with his failing marriage. He was feeling isolated and depressed. The administrator was arrested on the basis of evidence that he developed a sexual relationship with a sixteen-year-old boy who was in the department's custody and used illegal drugs with the boy.

* * *

A social worker in a private psychiatric hospital provided counseling to a resident who was diagnosed with paranoid schizophrenia. The social worker, who was religiously observant, began to read biblical passages to the client in the context of counseling sessions. The client was not religiously observant and complained to other hospital staff about the social worker's conduct.

* * *

A clinical social worker in private practice provided counseling to a forty-two-year-old woman who had been sexually abused as a child. During the course of their relationship, the social worker invited the client home for several candlelight dinners, went on a camping trip with the client, gave the client several expensive gifts, and wrote the client several very affectionately worded notes on personal stationery.

* * *

A social worker in a public child welfare agency was responsible for licensing foster homes. The social worker, who was recently divorced, became very friendly with a couple who had applied to be foster parents and also became very involved in the foster parents' church. The social worker, who approved the couple's application and was responsible for monitoring the foster home placement in the couples' home, moved with her son into a mobile home on the foster parents' large farm.

* * *

A social work supervisor who was socially isolated in his personal life spent an inordinate amount of time supervising one staff member with whom he felt a special bond.

In contrast, some boundary issues are subtler. Examples include social workers whose clients invite them to attend important life cycle events (such as clients' weddings or graduations or key religious ceremonies), social workers who conduct home visits and whose clients invite them to sit-down meals being served at the time of the visits, and social workers who themselves are in recovery and encounter clients or supervisees at Alcoholics Anonymous (AA) or Narcotics Anonymous (NA) meetings. In these situations, social workers sometimes disagree about the most appropriate way to handle boundary issues (Doyle, 1997). For example, some social workers are adamantly opposed to attending clients' life cycle events because of potential boundary problems (e.g., the possibility that a client might interpret the gesture as an indication of the social worker's interest in a social relationship or friendship); others, however, believe that attending such events can be ethically appropriate and, in fact, therapeutically helpful as long as the clinical dynamics are handled skillfully. Some social workers believe that practitioners in recovery should never attend or participate in AA or NA meetings where clients or colleagues are present because of the difficulty clients and colleagues may have reconciling social workers' professional roles and personal lives. Others, however, argue that recovering social workers have a right to meet their own needs and can serve as compelling role models to clients and colleagues in recovery.

Altruistic Gestures

Some boundary issues and dual relationships arise out of social workers' genuine efforts to be helpful. Unlike social workers' involvement in sexual relationships or dual relationships that are intentionally self-serving, altruistic gestures are benevolently motivated. Although these dual relationships are not necessarily unethical, they do require careful management using the protocol discussed later.

A social worker in private practice was contacted by a long-standing friend who was in the midst of a marital crisis. The friend told the social worker that she and her husband "really trust" the social worker and want the social worker's professional help. The social worker agreed to see the couple professionally, but later realized that it was very hard for him to be objective.

* * *

A social worker in a family services agency provided casework services to a client who had a substance abuse problem. The client asked the social worker if she would like to purchase wrapping paper that the client's daughter was selling as a school fundraiser.

* * *

A social worker in a community mental health center provided counseling over a long period to a young man with a history of clinical depression. The client asked the social worker if he would "say a few words" during the ceremony at the client's upcoming wedding.

* * *

A school social worker in a small rural community provided counseling services to a ten-year-old boy who struggled with self-esteem issues. In his spare time, the social worker coached the community's only basketball team, which was unaffiliated with the school. The social worker believed that the boy would benefit from joining his basketball team (e.g., by developing social skills and new relationships).

Unanticipated Circumstances

The final category of boundary issues involves situations that social workers do not anticipate and over which they have little or no initial control. The challenge for social workers in these circumstances is to manage boundary issues in ways that minimize possible harm to clients and colleagues.

A social worker in private practice attended a family holiday gathering. The social worker's sister introduced him to her new boyfriend, who is the social worker's former client.

* * *

The client of a clinical social worker in a rural community was a grade school teacher. Because of an unexpected administrative decision, the client became the teacher in the classroom in which the social worker's child is a student.

* * *

A social work administrator in a community mental health center joined a local physical fitness club. During one of her visits, the social worker discovered that one of her clients is also an active member of the club.

Managing Dual Relationships

To manage boundary issues effectively, social workers must develop a clear understanding of what distinguishes ethical and unethical dual relationships. A dual relationship is unethical when it has several characteristics (Corey & Herlihy, 1997; Epstein, 1994; NASW, 2000; Reamer, 1998a, 2001b), such as that the relationship is likely to

- interfere with the social worker's exercise of professional discretion
- interfere with the social worker's exercise of impartial judgment
- exploit clients, colleagues, or third parties to further the social worker's personal interests
- harm clients, colleagues, or third parties

Social workers must be especially careful to consider how cultural and ethnic norms are relevant to boundary issues (see NASW, 2000, Standard 1.05; see also Lee & Kurilla, 1997; Pinderhughes, 1994). For example, a social worker who conducts home visits may be reluctant to accept a family member's invitation to join the family for a meal, but may agree to have crackers and a nonalcoholic beverage so as not to violate the family's deep-seated ethnic norms related to offering food to guests. Similar issues may arise related to social workers' attending family life cycle events. A pregnant community organizer may need to be very tactful when residents of a largely ethnic community invite the social worker to a neighborhood-sponsored shower held in her behalf. The social worker would need to think through the implications of attending the event and accepting gifts. As the NASW *Code of Ethics* (2000) states,

In instances when dual or multiple relationships are unavoidable, social workers should take steps to protect clients and are responsible for setting clear, appropriate, and *culturally sensitive boundaries*. [italics added] (Standard 1.06c)

To protect clients and minimize possible harm—and to minimize the possibility of ethics complaints and lawsuits that allege misconduct or professional negligence—social workers should establish clear risk management criteria and procedures. A sound risk management protocol to deal with boundary issues should contain six major elements:

1. Be alert to potential or actual conflicts of interest.

2. Inform clients and colleagues about potential or actual conflicts of interest; explore reasonable remedies.

3. Consult colleagues and supervisors, and relevant professional literature, regulations, policies, and ethical standards (codes of ethics) to identify pertinent boundary issues and constructive options.

4. Design a plan of action that addresses the boundary issues and protects the parties involved to the greatest extent possible.

5. Document all discussions, consultation, supervision, and other steps taken to address boundary issues.

6. Develop a strategy to monitor implementation of action plan.

First, social workers should always be vigilant in their efforts to be alert to potential or actual conflicts of interest in their relationships with clients and colleagues. Social workers should be cognizant of red flags that may signal a boundary problem. For example, clinical social workers should be wary of situations in which they find themselves attracted to a particular client, going out of their way to extend the client's counseling sessions (facilitated by scheduling the favored client at the end of the day), treating the client as someone "special," disclosing confidential information about other clients, acting impulsively in relation to the client, allowing the client to accumulate a large unpaid bill, and disclosing very personal details to the client (Simon, 1999). Similarly, nonclinical social workers (e.g., administrators, researchers, community organizers) should be alert to comparable warning signs, such as granting extraordinary special favors to clients or colleagues and granting unprecedented exceptions to clients or colleagues who have not fulfilled contractual agreements.

Second, social workers should inform clients and appropriate colleagues when they encounter boundary issues, including actual or potential conflicts of interest, and explore reasonable remedies. Third, social workers should consult colleagues and supervisors; relevant professional literature, regulations, and policies; and ethical standards (relevant codes of ethics) to identify pertinent boundary issues and constructive options. Special care should be taken in high-risk circumstances. For example, clinical social workers who attempt to make decisions about a possible friendship with a former client should consider prevailing ethical standards that take into consideration such factors as the amount of time that has passed since the termination of the professional-client relationship; the extent to which the former client is mentally competent and emotionally stable; the issues addressed in the professional-client relationship; the length of the professional-client relationship; the circumstances surrounding the termination of the professional-client relationship; the amount of influence the social worker has in the client's life; available, reasonable alternatives; and the extent to which there is foreseeable harm to the former client or others as a result of the new relationship (Ebert, 1997; Reamer, 1998a).

Fourth, social workers should design a plan of action that addresses the boundary issues and protects clients, colleagues, and third parties to the greatest extent possible. In some circumstances, protecting a client's interests may require termination of the professional relationship with proper referral of the client. It is particularly useful for social workers to imagine how a thoughtful panel of peers in the profession would perceive their course of action. Fifth, social workers should document all discussions, consultations, supervision, and other steps taken to address boundary issues (e.g., consultation with colleagues or supervisors about whether to accept a client's invitation to attend a life cycle event or terminate services to a client when conflict-of-interest issues arise). Finally, social workers should develop a strategy to monitor the implementation of their action plan, for example, by periodically assessing with relevant parties (clients, colleagues, supervisors, and lawyers) whether the strategy minimized or eliminated the boundary problems.

To promote practitioners' actual implementation of this protocol, social workers can sponsor staff training and continuing education workshops. In addition to presenting conceptual content related to boundary issues and dual relationships, such workshops can role-play realistic case scenarios to enhance social workers' ability to protect clients, colleagues, and third parties and to reduce risk.

There is no question that social workers have developed a richer, more nuanced understanding of boundary issues in the profession. To further enhance this understanding, social workers must examine dual relationships that are exploitive in nature and those that are more ambiguous. Practitioners' firm grasp of boundary issues involving their intimate relationships with clients and colleagues, responses to their own emotional and dependency needs, pursuits of personal benefits, altruistic gestures, and responses to unanticipated circumstances will increase their ability to protect clients, colleagues, and themselves. Most important, skillful management of boundary issues enhances social work's ethical integrity, one of the key hallmarks of a profession.

References

Akamatsu, T. J. (1988). Intimate relationships with former clients: National survey of attitudes and behavior among practitioners. *Professional Psychology, Research and Practice, 19,* 454–458.

American Psychological Association, Committee on Women in Psychology. (1989). If sex enters into the psychotherapy relationship. *Professional Psychology, Research and Practice, 20,* 112–115.

Anderson, S., & Mandell, D. (1989). The use of self disclosure by professional social workers. *Social Casework, 70,* 259–267.

Berliner, A. K. (1989). Misconduct in social work practice [Briefly Stated]. *Social Work, 34,* 69–72.

Besharov, D. J. (1985). *The vulnerable social worker.* Silver Spring, MD: National Association of Social Workers.

Bonosky, N. (1995). Boundary violations in social work supervision: Clinical, educational and legal implications. *Clinical Supervisor, 13,* 79–95.

Borys, D. S., & Pope, K. S. (1989). Dual relationships between therapists and clients: National study of psychologists, psychiatrists and social workers. *Professional Psychology, Research and Practice, 20,* 283–293.

Bouhoutsos, J. (1985). Therapist-client sexual involvement: A challenge for mental health professionals. *American Journal of Orthopsychiatry, 55,* 177–182.

Bouhoutsos, J., Kolroyd, J., Lerman, H., Foster, B. R., & Greenberg, M. (1983). Sexual intimacy between psychotherapists and patients. *Professional Psychology, Research and Practice, 14,* 185–196.

Brodsky, A. M. (1986). The distressed psychologist: Sexual intimacies and exploitation. In R. R. Kilburg, P. E. Nathan, & R. W. Thoreson (Eds.), *Professionals in distress: Issues, syndromes, and solutions in psychology* (pp. 153–171). Washington, DC: American Psychological Association.

Brownlee, K. (1996). The ethics of non-sexual dual relationships: A dilemma for the rural mental health professional. *Community Mental Health Journal, 32,* 497–503.

Chapman, C. (1997). Dual relationships in substance abuse treatment. *Alcoholism Treatment Quarterly, 15,* 73–79.

Coleman, E., & Schaefer, S. (1986). Boundaries of sex and intimacy between client and counselor. *Journal of Counseling and Development, 64,* 341–344.

Congress, E. P. (1996). Dual relationships in academia: Dilemmas for social work educators. *Journal of Social Work Education, 32,* 329–338.

Corey, G., & Herlihy, B. (1997). Dual/multiple relationships: Toward a consensus of thinking. In Hatherleigh Editorial Board (Ed.), *The Hatherleigh guide to ethics in therapy* (pp. 183–194). New York: Hatherleigh Press.

Doyle, K. (1997). Substance abuse counselors in recovery: Implications for the ethical issue of dual relationships. *Journal of Counseling and Development, 75,* 428–432.

Ebert, B. W. (1997). Dual-relationship prohibitions: A concept whose time never should have come. *Applied and Preventive Psychology, 6,* 137–156.

Epstein, R. (1994). *Keeping boundaries: Maintaining safety and integrity in the psychotherapeutic process.* Washington, DC: American Psychiatric Press.

Feldman-Summers, S., & Jones, G. (1984). Psychological impacts of sexual contact between therapists or other health care practitioners and their clients. *Journal of Consulting and Clinical Psychology, 52,* 1054–1061.

Gabbard, G. (Ed.). (1989). *Sexual exploitation in professional relationships.* Washington, DC: American Psychiatric Press.

Gechtman, L. (1989). Sexual contact between social workers and their clients. In G. Gabbard (Ed.), *Sexual exploitation in professional relationships* (pp. 27–38). Washington, DC: American Psychiatric Press.

Gifis, S. H. (Ed.). (1991). *Law dictionary* (3rd ed.). Happauge, NY: Barron.

Gutheil, T. G., & Gabbard, G. O. (1993). The concept of boundaries in clinical practice: Theoretical and risk-management dimensions. *American Journal of Psychiatry, 150,* 188–196.

Jayaratne, S., Croxton, T., & Mattison, D. (1997). Social work professional standards: An exploratory study. *Social Work, 42,* 187–199.

Kagle, J. D., & Giebelhausen, P. N. (1994). Dual relationships and professional boundaries. *Social Work, 39,* 213–220.

Kitchener, K. S. (1988). Dual role relationships: What makes them so problematic? *Journal of Counseling and Development, 67,* 217–221.

Kutchins, H. (1991). The fiduciary relationship: The legal basis for social workers' responsibilities to clients. *Social Work, 36,* 106–113.

Lee, C. C., & Kurilla, V. (1997). Ethics and multiculturalism: The challenge of diversity. In Hatherleigh Editorial Board (Ed.), *The Hatherleigh guide to ethics in therapy* (pp. 235–248). New York: Hatherleigh Press.

Levy, C. S. (1993). *Social work ethics on the line.* New York: Haworth Press.

Linzer, N. L. (1999). *Resolving ethical dilemmas in social work practice.* Boston: Allyn & Bacon.

Loewenberg, F., & Dolgoff, R. (1996). *Ethical decisions for social work practice* (5th ed.). Itasca, IL: F. E. Peacock.

National Association of Social Workers. (2000). *Code of ethics of the National Association of Social Workers.* Washington, DC: Author.

Olarte, S. W. (1997). Sexual boundary violations. In Hatherleigh Editorial Board (Ed.), *The Hatherleigh guide to ethics in therapy* (pp. 195–209). New York: Hatherleigh Press.

Pinderhughes, E. (1994). Diversity and populations at risk: Ethnic minorities and people of color. In F. G. Reamer (Ed.), *The foundations of social work knowledge* (pp. 264–308). New York: Columbia University Press.

Pope, K. S. (1988). Dual relationships: A source of ethical, legal and chemical problems. *In Practice, 8,* 17–25.

Pope, K. S. (1990). Abuse of psychotherapy: Psychotherapist- patient intimacy. *Psychotherapy and Psychosomatics, 53,* 191–198.

Pope, K. S. (1991). Dual relationships in psychotherapy. *Ethics and Behavior, 1,* 21–34.

Pope, K., & Bouhoutsos, J. (1986). *Sexual intimacy between therapists and patients.* New York: Praeger.

Pope, K., Tabachnick, B., & Keith-Spiegel, P. (1988). Good and bad practice in psychotherapy: National survey of beliefs of psychologists. *Professional Psychology, 19,* 547–552.

Reamer, F. G. (1982). Conflicts of professional duty in social work. *Social Casework, 63,* 579–585.

Reamer, F. G. (1984). Enforcing ethics in social work. *Health Matrix, 2,* 17–25.

Reamer, F. G. (1990). *Ethical dilemmas in social service* (2nd ed.). New York: Columbia University Press.

Reamer, F. G. (1992). The impaired social worker. *Social Work, 37,* 165–170.

Reamer, F. G. (1994). *Social work malpractice and liability.* New York: Columbia University Press.

Reamer, F. G. (1995a). Ethics and values. In R. L. Edwards (Ed.), *Encyclopedia of social work* (19th ed., Vol. 1, pp. 893–902). Washington, DC: NASW Press.

Reamer, F. G. (1995b). Malpractice claims against social workers: First facts. *Social Work, 40,* 595–601.

Reamer, F. G. (1997). Ethical standards in social work: The NASW Code of Ethics. In R. L. Edwards (Ed.-in-Chief), *Encyclopedia of social work* (19th ed., Suppl., pp. 113–123). Washington, DC: NASW Press.

Reamer, F. G. (1998a). *Ethical standards in social work: A critical review of the NASW Code of Ethics.* Washington, DC: NASW Press.

Reamer, F. G. (1998b). The evolution of social work ethics. *Social Work, 43,* 488–500.

Reamer, F. G. (1999). *Social work values and ethics* (2nd ed.). New York: Columbia University Press.

Reamer, F. G. (2001a). *Tangled relationships: Managing boundary issues in the human services.* New York: Columbia University Press.

Reamer, F. G. (2001b). *The social work ethics audit: A risk management tool.* Washington, DC: NASW Press.

Rhodes, M. L. (1986). *Ethical dilemmas in social work practice.* Boston: Routledge & Kegan Paul.

Schank, J. A., & Skovholt, T. M. (1997). Dual relationship dilemmas of rural and small-community psychologists. *Professional Psychology, Research and Practice, 28,* 44–49.

Sell, J., Gottlieb, M., & Schoenfeld, L. (1986). Ethical considerations of social/romantic relationships with present and former clients. *Professional Psychology, Research and Practice, 17,* 504–508.

Simon, R. I. (1999). Therapist-patient sex: From boundary violations to sexual misconduct. *Forensic Psychiatry, 22,* 31–47.

Smith, D., & Fitzpatrick, M. (1995). Patient-therapist boundary issues: An integrative review of theory and research. *Professional Psychology, Research and Practice, 26,* 499–506.

Smith, J. (1999). Holding the dance: A flexible approach to boundaries in general practice. In J. Lees (Ed.), *Clinical counseling in primary care* (pp. 43–60). New York: Routledge.

Stake, J. E., & Oliver, J. (1991). Sexual contact and touching between therapist and client: A survey of psychologists' attitudes and behavior. *Professional Psychology, Research and Practice, 22,* 297–307.

St. Germaine, J. (1993). Dual relationships: What's wrong with them? *American Counselor, 2,* 25–30.

St. Germaine, J. (1996). Dual relationships and certified alcohol and drug counselors: A national study of ethical beliefs and behaviors. *Alcoholism Treatment Quarterly, 14,* 29–44.

Strom-Gottfried, K. (1999). Professional boundaries: An analysis of violations by social workers. *Families in Society, 80,* 439–449.

Woody, R. H. (1998). Bartering for psychological services. *Professional Psychology, Research and Practice, 29,* 174–178.

24

Patient-Targeted Googling: The Ethics of Searching Online for Patient Information

Brian K. Clinton, Benjamin C. Silverman, and David H. Brendel

The Internet has changed the way that medicine and psychiatry are practiced, as patients and physicians now routinely search online for medical and personal information. In the literature, physicians have considered the pros and cons of online searches for information regarding diagnosis, treatment, and research.[1-7] Recently, others have considered the complexities of patients' searching online for information, both professional or personal, about physicians.[8-10] Little consideration has been given, however, to the converse situation—namely, to physicians' searching online for information about patients. We believe that this practice—which we call *patient-targeted Googling* (PTG)—is widespread and deserving of professional and ethical consideration. Throughout this article, we will use the words *Googling* or *to Google* to refer to the practice of online searching, whether or not that practice involves the Google search engine. In popular usage, *Googling* has become synonymous with "Internet searching."

Through informal surveys of several dozen of our colleagues over the past year, we have learned that most psychiatrists have engaged in PTG. We have (ourselves) searched for patient information, and we have witnessed groups of other physicians Google patients—for example, during formal clinical rounds. We have witnessed and heard reports of PTG across diverse practice settings, including emergency rooms, inpatient units, and long-term outpatient psychotherapy relationships. In the course of such searches, physicians obtain a broad range of personal information about patients: photographs, videos, news stories, criminal records, and details of substance use, intimate relationships, sexual activity, and finances.[11-13] Content may also include clinically important material such as suicide plans.[14] Social networking Web sites, such as MySpace and Facebook, have provided popular forums in which personal information can be both easily posted and searched online. Recent surveys report that approximately one-third of adult Internet users have profiles on social networking sites, with higher rates among younger adults (e.g., half of adults aged twenty-five to thirty-four and three-quarters of adults aged eighteen to twenty-four).[15]

Although we have noted PTG occurring among all types of physicians, the practice is especially complicated in a relationship between a patient and a psychiatrist (or other mental health clinician). In addition to taking into account medical information, such relationships focus on personal details and often deal with analysis of transference and countertransference as a key element of the treatment. PTG has the potential to either enhance or interfere with this process, depending on a particular patient's circumstances. For example, a patient who tends to attract exploitative relationships might enact this pattern by tempting the psychiatrist to engage in unnecessary PTG. By contrast, if a patient with rejection sensitivity and fear of abandonment asks a psychiatrist to explore a personal Internet site, a clinician's refusal might have a deleterious impact on the therapy relationship. Due to these unique characteristics, psychiatry has a long history of carefully framing treatment relationships and discussing boundary crossings and violations,[16] which highlights the special need to consider the impact of PTG in our discipline.

The lack of commentary on the practice of PTG may reflect the delayed emergence of the Internet as a source of detailed personal information, relative to its earlier evolution as a source of useful, but impersonal, information. Psychiatrists, particularly younger physicians and trainees, embrace the power of Internet searches in every aspect of their lives but may be naive to the impact of the Internet searches on their professional relationships. Consistent with the previously noted Internet usage trends, PTG is likely becoming commonplace as a new generation of physicians and trainees, who use Internet search technologies and social networking sites on a frequent and routine basis, move into professional practice.[17-19] The omnipresence of the Internet in our daily lives may lead psychiatrists to engage in PTG without considering the unique ethical questions and concerns posed by its practice.

Psychiatrists search online for patient information for a variety of reasons. PTG includes ethically problematic situations as well as those that are required clinically. As an example of the latter, we have experience working with an elderly patient with dementia who had been admitted to an inpatient psychiatric unit after having lost contact with his family. We were able to locate his family members and develop an optimal treatment plan for him only through PTG, after all other traditional measures for contacting his family members had failed (e.g., searches of hospital records and telephone books). In this case, we conducted PTG with a focused goal and without any obvious adverse consequences. Similarly, the psychiatric literature has commented briefly on the use of the Internet as a source of important collateral information. One case example reports that a resident searched online for collateral information, aiding in the safety assessment of a suicidal patient in an emergency room.[20]

Another article considers forensic evaluations of problematic Internet use and suggests that PTG can be a useful tool for forensic psychiatrists.[21] Based on these examples, the outcome of PTG appears to be beneficial, but these select cases do not demonstrate the diverse ethical challenges of PTG in psychiatric contexts. Among the ethically problematic motivations are curiosity, voyeurism, and habit. Some searches by psychiatrists may start with a clear empathic goal, such as gaining an appreciation of a patient's online persona in order to enhance treatment, but may grow more troublesome due to unexpected findings. PTG may occur with or without a patient's consent and with or without the patient in the room. Unexpected findings, such as the discovery of photographs of a patient engaged in substance use or sexual activity, may lead to unforeseen ethical dilemmas, including questions about whether to share knowledge of the online material with the patient or to document the findings in the patient's medical record.

Although Internet postings are considered to be in the public domain, the viewing of any information that a patient has not specifically shared in a treatment setting requires careful ethical consideration by clinicians. For example, discovering details about a patient's home (e.g., address, value of the home, or real estate taxes) or viewing photographs of the home (e.g., through satellite images on Google Maps) has become nearly effortless. Due to the ease and ubiquity of such searches, psychiatrists may engage in these examples of PTG without thorough ethical consideration. Such searches could be analogous, however—prior to PTG—to driving by a patient's home or otherwise infringing on a patient's privacy in a way that most psychiatrists would view as a boundary violation. The accessibility, anonymity, and universality of the Internet have made it easier, and perhaps more tempting, for psychiatrists to engage in such ethically questionable activity.

The practice of PTG has received little consideration in the psychiatric literature, with a notable absence of discussion of the more ethically challenging types of cases we have described. No formal or professional guidelines have dealt with PTG—likely due, in part, to its recent emergence, but possibly also due to potential feelings of shame and guilt associated with admitting to the practice of PTG. As Internet searching continues to grow and becomes an almost reflexive behavior, psychiatrists will benefit from an ethical framework for considering PTG in clinical practice and also, in turn, for training residents and students, the populations most likely to engage in the practice.

Before searching online for patients, psychiatrists should consider the intention of the search, its potential value or risk to the patient, and the anticipated effect of gaining previously unknown information. The psychiatrist is obligated to act in a way that will respect the patient's best interests and that adheres to professional ethics. However, the results and potential dangers of PTG are not always intuitive or consciously available prior to searches. Abstract moral principles such as beneficence provide insufficient guidance to clinicians in particular PTG scenarios. By avoiding PTG altogether (as some clinicians might choose to do), psychiatrists can avoid the associated risk of exploiting their patients, but this approach ignores the current reality of clinical practice and the further intertwining of the Internet and clinical practice that is likely in the future. It also violates other important principles of clinical ethics, such as flexibility in the service of a particular patient's best interests at a particular moment. For example, if a patient's asking a therapist to look at his online profile represents a significant therapeutic step toward the patient's understanding his view of himself and his interactions with friends, would the clinician want to avoid this search on the general principle that PTG may exploit some patients in other situations? Considerations of PTG need to be examined on a case-by-case basis, supporting the need for a consistent framework for evaluating the ethics of searching online for patients.

In this article, we propose a pragmatic model for considering PTG that focuses on practical results of searches and that aims to minimize the risk of exploiting patients. This framework of clinical pragmatism has been applied to other ethical issues in psychiatric practice, such as accepting gifts from patients,[22] and provides an approach to clinical ethics that specifies several core values that ought to be balanced in patient care.[23-25] In the case of PTG, a core value of clinical pragmatism is that the psychiatrist should focus ethical deliberations on the specific results of that decision for the patient in question, not only on general moral principles. The psychiatrist must consider how PTG would affect the treatment relationship and the progress toward treatment goals—a thought process that may involve discussions with the patient, the patient's family, and a clinician's community of supervisors, colleagues, and consultants. In the following sections, we present a pragmatic model for PTG and describe three cases of PTG, highlighting important ethical dilemmas in multiple practice settings. Each case is discussed from the standpoint of the pragmatic model and as an example of how this model can help guide psychiatrists in their decision making about PTG.

Pragmatic Framework

Before searching online for patients, a psychiatrist should engage in a conscious and complex decision-making process on a case-by-case basis. We propose the following pragmatic model for considering PTG, focusing on the practical results of searches and aiming to minimize the risk of exploiting patients. Our model avoids ideological assumptions about PTG. On one hand, we believe PTG can be an acceptable and ethically sound clinical tool (and even clinically required in some cases, as described above). On the other hand, we do not advocate unbridled PTG simply because online information about patients is legally available in the public domain. Instead, our pragmatic framework focuses on the practical questions of whether PTG serves a particular patient's best interests and might promote the therapeutic process. The pragmatic model does not specify whether a psychiatrist should or should not engage in PTG in any particular situation, but it urges the clinician, at the very least, to address the following six questions whenever he or she considers searching online for a patient.

1. Why Do I Want to Conduct This Search?
If the answer to this question about conducting a search involves nothing other than curiosity, voyeurism, prurient interest, or exploitation, then the psychiatrist should not go forward with the search. In addition, the psychiatrist in these circumstances should consider obtaining consultation or supervision regarding his or her potentially problematic thoughts and feelings about the patient. If the answer is that the search may ultimately promote the patient's best interests, then the psychiatrist should move on to question 2. In all cases, the psychiatrist should be thoughtful about whether he or she is deceiving himself or herself into believing that the online search is primarily in the service of the patient's best interests rather than primarily in the service of personal curiosity or voyeurism.

2. Would My Search Advance or Compromise the Treatment?

The psychiatrist must try to predict what information obtained online about a patient might promote the patient's best interests and guide important treatment decisions. For example, learning about a patient's suicidal thoughts or plans on a blog might lead to a critical, potentially lifesaving clinical intervention.[26] Conversely, the psychiatrist ought to consider whether any information obtained online might compromise the treatment relationship. For example, if the psychiatrist discovered that the patient held political beliefs contrary to his or her own, might the psychiatrist withdraw from the patient and thereby compromise the therapeutic alliance? The psychiatrist must also try to predict the validity of information obtained online. What if the psychiatrist reads about a patient on another individual's blog, a context in which false information can be easily posted? Alternatively, if the psychiatrist reads about someone with the patient's name on a reliable newspaper Web site, how can he or she be sure that it is the patient and not simply someone else with the same name? Another important consideration is that patients may intentionally represent themselves online in ways that are playful or dissonant with their real-world behaviors.[27] Would obtaining the information online, rather than by interviewing, affect the treatment relationship in a unique way? If the psychiatrist believes that PTG might advance the treatment and not seriously harm it in any obvious or identifiable way, then he or she can move forward to question 3. Before doing so, however, the psychiatrist should assess whether another approach or strategy might achieve the desired benefits without creating the risks inherent in PTG. For example, talking with a patient's family members as a source of collateral information in a safety assessment might pose less risk than engaging in PTG.

3. Should I Obtain Informed Consent from the Patient Prior to Searching?

While there is no established norm for obtaining consent before engaging in PTG, the clinician should reflect on its possible role in preserving the patient's privacy and enhancing the patient-doctor relationship. The process of informed consent for PTG would include discussion of all possible risks, including breaches of patient privacy and the potential for harm to the psychotherapeutic relationship, along with an acknowledgment of possible unpredictable and unknown consequences. The consent process itself might also contribute to treatment progress by enabling a discussion of the factors (e.g., countertransference or patient behaviors) that led the psychiatrist to consider PTG. If the clinician is certain that the patient would feel hurt or violated if he or she learned that the psychiatrist searched online without consent, then the psychiatrist should seriously consider seeking formal consent prior to searching.

If the clinician is uncertain about the patient's feelings about PTG, then he or she should carefully consider the risk benefit ratio of engaging in PTG without prior informed consent. If there is a high likelihood of clinical benefit from the search and a low likelihood that the patient will feel angry or wronged if he or she later found out about it, then the search may be justifiable even in the absence of prior consent (but, as discussed below in question 4, the psychiatrist will have to decide whether to share the results of the search with the patient post hoc). Finally, if a prospective search presents a low likelihood of clinical benefit and a high likelihood of offending or otherwise upsetting the patient, then the clinician ought to seriously consider forgoing the search.

4. Should I Share the Results of the Search with the Patient?

After the online search has occurred, the psychiatrist needs to think carefully about how to use the information obtained and whether to share or discuss that information with the patient. This task may be easier if the patient consented to the search before it was conducted, as the patient in that scenario would already know that such a search might occur. If the psychiatrist conducted the search without prior consent, he or she has to consider benefits and burdens of sharing the information post hoc. In this scenario, the complexities of the particular patient-doctor relationship will determine whether and how the psychiatrist should share information about the occurrence of the search and the data that it revealed. In circumstances where the psychiatrist feels that the patient should know about the search but worries that the patient may feel upset, violated, or otherwise harmed if told about it (or about the information that the psychiatrist obtained online), the clinician might need to consider consulting with a clinical peer, an ethicist, a risk-management specialist, or other expert, as the particular situation dictates. If the psychiatrist chooses not to reveal to the patient either the occurrence of the search or the information thereby obtained, the psychiatrist must carefully consider the effects of this hidden knowledge on countertransference and on the psychotherapeutic relationship—and again might benefit from a consultation.

5. Should I Document the Findings of the Search in the Medical Record?

There is no clear medico-legal guidance about how psychiatrists should document PTG findings in the medical record. In general, psychiatrists should aim to document all relevant clinical data in the record accurately, but in a way that is sensitive to the fact that the patient may read the record at some point. PTG presents several complexities with regard to documentation. If the psychiatrist performs an online search without the patient's consent and in the course of that search discovers compromising information about the patient, it may not be clear if this information should be entered in the record. For example, if the psychiatrist performs an unauthorized search and discovers online that the patient smokes cigarettes, abuses illegal substances, or engages in other risky behaviors, entering that information in the record could lead to insurance or employment discrimination against the patient in the future. In the case of electronic medical records, the information would also be readily available to other current and future treaters. Such occurrences might seriously violate the patient's privacy and confidentiality rights. The clinician who obtains sensitive information via PTG may therefore need to consult with an attorney in order to make a sound decision about whether to enter the findings in the medical record.

6.   How Do I Monitor My Motivations and the Ongoing Risk-Benefit Profile of Searching?

To ensure ethical and patient-centered treatment, psychiatrists should reflect continually on their own needs, desires, drives, and emotions. When they consider learning about their patients via PTG, they must strive to acknowledge honestly to themselves the full range of their motivations, which may include straightforward curiosity and voyeuristic interest. As a psychiatrist assesses the possible risks and benefits of PTG with regard to an individual patient, he or she should avoid self-deception about the complex motivations that may underlie the consideration of an online search. This self-assessment should occur on a regular basis for any given patient, as the psychiatrist's thoughts and feelings about the patient may evolve over time. The psychiatrist should seek help—whether through personal psychotherapy, clinical supervision, ethical or legal consultation, or otherwise—whenever he or she faces an especially challenging situation that involves PTG or consideration thereof.

Case Vignettes

We now present three cases that demonstrate ethical dilemmas arising in the context of PTG and reflect on each case from the standpoint of the pragmatic model. The cases describe a wide spectrum of clinical scenarios in which PTG may occur. The cases are disguised and contain a composite of patients with whom we have worked directly, scenarios shared by colleagues, and plausible examples generated for demonstration. The cases have been chosen to contain typical clinical scenarios spanning treatment settings in which psychiatrists commonly work and train. Following each case, we consider the applicability of the pragmatic approach.

Case 1

Jennifer is a sixteen-year-old girl who was brought in to the psychiatric emergency department by her mother for missing school and staying out past midnight on a daily basis. Jennifer has a history of self-harm in the form of superficially cutting her upper arms. She has been seeing an outpatient therapist for dialectical behavior therapy since her first cutting episode, two years earlier. She had not cut herself in nine months, has never been psychiatrically hospitalized, and has been a B– to C– student in high school. She would like to attend college to study psychology. She lives with her mother, stepfather, and sister and usually has a close relationship with her immediate family.

Recently, Jennifer has missed seven days of school over the past month and has been receiving failing grades. Her mother reported she has been "out of control" since starting a new relationship with a thirty-five-year-old man and has not been returning home at night or following her mother's directions. Her mother brought Jennifer into the emergency department after they had an argument and the mother felt she could not control her daughter's behavior.

In the emergency department, Jennifer described being in a consensual relationship with her new boyfriend and felt her mother was "blowing it out of proportion." She said, "I am just having some fun. Anyway, he loves me. My mom doesn't understand." She wanted to return home and promised to start listening to her mother and to return to school. The psychiatry resident in the emergency department called Jennifer's outpatient therapist in order to gain collateral information as part of a safety assessment. Her therapist felt Jennifer was safe to return home, though incidentally brought up that Jennifer reported her boyfriend had been taking provocative pictures of her and posting them on his Web site. The therapist had not seen the alleged pictures and indicated Jennifer told her about them as a "secret" from Jennifer's mother.

To complete a more comprehensive safety assessment prior to discharging Jennifer home with her mother, the psychiatry resident decided it would be important to know more about the online pictures. He considered that the photos might be exploiting the underage patient in a way that would be illegal or that the Web page might identify the patient's school or contact information in a way that put the patient at risk. In the emergency department, he searched for the alleged pictures on the Internet but was unable to find the boyfriend's Web site. The psychiatrist next contacted the on-call social worker, who evaluated Jennifer and filed a case with Child Protective Services on the basis of the allegations concerning the photos. The social worker noted that even if the pictures had been found on the Internet, the emergency department team would not have been able to verify the identities, ages, or existence of other photographs to a sufficient degree to eliminate concerns for the patient's safety. Regardless of what the psychiatrist had found on the Internet, a case would have been filed with Child Protective Services.

Discussion   In this case, a psychiatry resident engaged in PTG in the context of a safety assessment in the psychiatric emergency department. The psychiatry resident unsuccessfully attempted to search for alleged photographs of the patient and ended up filing a case with Child Protective Services. The resident's primary motivation in the case was to protect the child patient. The intervention of filing a case with Child Protective Services, however, could have been accomplished without an Internet search. Other methods of protecting the child patient, such as inpatient hospitalization, could have been considered rather than attempting to rely on an assessment of online information.

Would other motives have influenced the psychiatrist to venture down the path of PTG rather than exploring other possibilities? One motive, conscious or unconscious, could have been the resident's personal desire to view provocative pictures of his patient—a possibility that raises a number of concerns about patient exploitation and boundary violations.

Although the psychiatry resident's PTG in this case yielded no results, he did not fully consider the potential range or consequences of the information—which could and should have been thought about before undertaking the online search. For example, how would he identify the individuals in any alleged photographs? In a case with forensic implications, how would he document any Internet findings (or the absence of findings)? How would viewing possibly lewd photographs of his patient alter his care for her and their relationship? Would the psychiatrist tell the patient about the search? And if she perceived the search as violating a "secret" shared with her therapist, would that prevent her from reengaging in psychiatric or psychological care in the future? If the psychiatrist had attempted to obtain informed consent in advance of the search, might that have led to an empathic connection and allowed the patient to reveal more about her current life circumstances? Without consent, would she feel harassed by the psychiatrist of the opposite sex and file a complaint against him?

In this case, the primary motivation to protect a child patient would initially seem to justify the practice of PTG, but it is clear that the psychiatrist did not consider all of his possible motivations and did not consider all of the implications of his actions before the search. In the end, PTG had no benefit or impact on the treatment plan, and other avenues were available to protect this patient, possibly without exposing her or the resident to the risks of PTG. In the fast-paced emergency department, the resident relied on a now standard practice in his life—that is, searching for needed information online, in the face of a clinical question. Going straight to PTG without first consulting with a supervisor or other senior psychiatrist, and without considering other alternatives, may have placed this patient and psychiatrist at unnecessary risk.

Case 2

Thomas is a twenty-two-year-old college student who was referred for an outpatient consultation for treatment of generalized anxiety disorder and panic attacks. He was referred by his primary care physician, who had been treating him with a selective serotonin reuptake inhibitor but felt the patient would benefit from psychotherapy as well, given his voiced difficulties in his relationships with his parents and girlfriend.

Thomas entered weekly psychodynamic therapy with a psychiatrist and, after two months, began to speak openly and insightfully about his feelings of anger toward his parents over their lack of emotional support. He began to feel less anxious and never missed a weekly appointment. Thomas communicated the positive results to his therapist: "This is really working. I really look forward to our sessions each week." After three months, however, Thomas noted that he would have difficulty affording the full fee for his therapy sessions as a result of his impending tuition payments for the upcoming semester. The psychiatrist worked out a sliding-scale reduced fee with Thomas based on his means and continued weekly therapy. Over the next several months, Thomas began deferring payments and accrued a large bill. His psychiatrist discussed this topic in multiple sessions, but Thomas quickly brushed off the issue: "I am sorry. School has just been so busy. I have the money. I'll put a check in the mail this week. This is very important to me, and I want to keep seeing you."

In reviewing Thomas's bill, his psychiatrist noted that Thomas's street address was in a wealthy neighborhood. The psychiatrist searched for this street address with Google Maps, which enabled him to see photographs of the house and to verify the address as a large mansion. Additional Internet searches provided the psychiatrist with the last appraised and sale values of the house, both being several million dollars. The psychiatrist had feelings of anger that Thomas may have been misrepresenting his financial means to obtain a reduced fee. On Thomas's next visit, the psychiatrist confronted him about his unpaid bills: "It's surprising that you live in such an affluent neighborhood and yet you find yourself unable to pay even the reduced fee we agreed to. Your house looks quite large online." Thomas explained that he was renting a room in the basement of the mansion for a small fee, in addition to performing chores around the house, such as landscaping work. He felt offended by the psychiatrist's Internet search and did not come back for future therapy sessions. He did send a check in the mail the following week to cover all of his outstanding balance.

Discussion   In this case, a psychiatrist was able to learn about his patient's living environment (e.g., photographs and costs) in a matter of minutes, a process that, prior to the Internet, would have taken hours to days of library research or have even required driving through a patient's neighborhood. Although most psychiatrists would not make the effort to drive to a patient's house and would likely find such behavior to be in violation of the patient's privacy, the ease of an online search may be more tempting.

The psychiatrist's goal for PTG in this case was to determine the veracity of Thomas's need for a reduced fee. At a deeper level, the psychiatrists' motivations likely ranged from selfish greed and a desire for justice to a voyeuristic curiosity to see the patient's home and a clinical desire to see how this information might provide an example of how the patient perceives himself in the world. In advance of the search, the psychiatrist did not fully consider alternatives to the search, the question of whether to secure consent, or the impact that the information obtained would have on the treatment relationship. The information proved to be accurate (house location, photographs, cost) but was misconstrued (e.g., in thinking Thomas or his family had the financial resources to own such as a house). The psychiatrist felt compelled to confront the patient with concrete information, in the hope of obtaining a higher fee. The unintended consequence was to end what had been a beneficial therapy relationship. The PTG also led the psychiatrist away from a more traditional therapy, which may have considered Thomas's late payments in the context of a transferential relationship and as a form of resistance to therapy. Maybe Thomas wanted his psychiatrist to end their relationship and thus played a role in enacting the PTG. If so, PTG served one of the psychiatrist's motives (wanting to get paid appropriately), but in a way that was likely countertherapeutic for the patient.

The psychiatrist was ultimately left with the task of documenting the PTG in a termination note in Thomas's medical record. If the psychiatrist had fully considered his or her motives prior to engaging in PTG, he or she might have delayed the Internet search in favor of addressing the perceived resistance directly in therapy or, at the very least, asking Thomas to consent to the PTG in advance of the search (a conversation that likely would have provided the psychiatrist with the desired information and may have avoided PTG and its associated risks altogether). Alternatively, after engaging in PTG, the psychiatrist could have avoided sharing the search or obtained data with Thomas (e.g., confronting him as in the vignette) and continued more traditional psychotherapeutic techniques of addressing the missed payments and Thomas's financial situation in therapy. In that circumstance, the psychiatrist would need to carefully monitor countertransferential feelings and would likely benefit from consultation.

Case 3

Angela is a twenty-five-year-old business school student, who presented to the clinic with a request for a psychotherapist. During her intake with Dr. P, a second-year female psychiatry resident, Angela reported a history of mildly depressed mood beginning during her college years. Angela stated, "A year ago, I found out my last real boyfriend was cheating on me using the Internet. Since then, I always do my research, but I don't trust men now." Dr. P eagerly began weekly psychotherapy with Angela, enjoying their similar age and experience. Across the next six months, Dr. P found it fascinating to explore Angela's romantic relationships, which sparked nostalgic memories in Dr. P.

Dr. P was supervised weekly by Dr. H, a senior faculty member. Dr. H recommended increasing the frequency of visits to further explore transferential issues with the patient. Dr. P welcomed the prospect of a more intimate connection. However, Dr. P then began talking less in therapy, taking more notes, and limiting her comments to what she felt Dr. H would approve. Dr. P began to feel more distant from Angela. After two months of closely supervised, biweekly therapy sessions, Dr. P was unable to meet with Dr. H for four weeks due to his travel plans.

While Dr. H was away, Angela revealed to Dr. P that she had begun to meet men through her MySpace page, but had been embarrassed to mention it for several months. She said to Dr. P, "It never works out. Maybe you should write my profile." Dr. P. replied cautiously, "I wonder what you think I would write." Between sessions, Dr. P. found herself curious about Angela's online persona, wondering if it might attract incompatible romantic partners. Dr. P searched online for the patient's MySpace page and found the description "Single: Nice body and brains to go with it . . . looking for a man who loves the finer things in life." Dr. P read the replies of men at the bottom of the Web page and found herself curious enough to view their personal pages. Dr. P did not disclose her Internet search to Angela, but during the next therapy session, Dr. P felt a new zest in the psychotherapy and felt her own comments to be more incisive. In the following weeks Dr. P continued to check the MySpace page for updates between sessions. She also viewed satellite pictures of the patient's apartment on Google Maps, and she searched for information about the patient's college and high school. Each session brought new detail that could be explored online. Dr. P continued to feel a renewed connection and empathy with Angela. After several weeks away, Dr. H returned from vacation. As Dr. P considered supervision with Dr. H, she felt ashamed of her intense curiosity about Angela. Should she have told Dr. H about her Internet searching? Did he know much about the Internet? Might he suggest disclosing the search to Angela?

Discussion   In this case, a psychiatrist in training entered into an intensive psychotherapy with a patient and is supervised closely on the case. Dr. P began the therapy eagerly with a sense of camaraderie but, feeling frustrated by a lack of progress, began a more intensive treatment schedule to explore transferential issues within the case. To her surprise, a change in therapy style contributed to a feeling of distance from the patient—which, in turn, fueled curiosity when she was given an opportunity to learn more on the Internet. In this case, PTG occurred during an extended absence from her supervisor and after the patient mentioned her previously undisclosed online dating activity that was relevant to the material discussed in therapy.

This therapist was motivated to perform an Internet search by a wish to gain insight into the case and perhaps also a by desire to feel closer to this patient with whom she identified. Despite her retrospective shame about PTG, the therapist's experience was that it advanced the treatment by intensifying the therapy. In this case, however, PTG cannot be justified in terms of clinical necessity. The therapist did not pause to consider the necessity, risks, or alternatives to the search. For example, in advance of viewing the MySpace page, the therapist might have discussed it with the patient, thereby providing an opportunity to obtain informed consent and to comment on transference. Another option was to determine whether the patient would agree to view the profile together during a therapy session.

Disclosing the results of the Internet search to the patient post hoc may harm the therapy relationship due to feelings of privacy violation. Furthermore, documenting this Internet search in the medical record could have several consequences for both the patient and the therapist. Documentation of PTG can have unanticipated results. For example, in a large hospital or clinic setting, patients are sometimes able to obtain their medical records without the therapist's consent or knowledge, in which case the discovery of a documented but undisclosed Internet search may anger the patient. As in the case example, the perceived risks related to disclosure of PTG to a patient can reduce the willingness of mental health practitioners to discuss or document PTG.

The awkwardness of PTG entered this therapist's mind only when she realized she might end up divulging the incident in supervision. In that respect, the case highlights that the supervision available to trainees may prove an invaluable means of gaining understanding of PTG. In particular, the supervisor can be helpful in deciding how to use the Internet information, whether to tell the patient, how it facilitates or obscures the trainee's understanding of the case, and how the data might be used therapeutically. Supervision is also vital in this case because the therapist developed a pattern of repeatedly searching online, in part to strengthen a sense of connection with the patient. It would be important to clarify the role of PTG in this treatment and in the trainee's development. Why was the experience of secretively experiencing the patient online so resonant for this therapist? While PTG may have helped the trainee to understand the patient and to overcome her sense of stagnation in the therapy, the trainee should have sought supervision before engaging in PTG to ensure that doing so was in service of the patient.

The trainee's ambivalence in telling her supervisor also points to a reality: supervisors differ with regard to their experience with the Internet, their views of current social expectations of personal privacy on the Internet, and their ideas about the possible countertherapeutic impact of surreptitious attempts to gain information about patients. This trainee felt ashamed about sharing the Internet search in supervision—despite her belief that no harm was done. In part, the shame results from not knowing what to expect from her supervisor concerning an issue that had not been discussed in training. Also, the trainee may have been reluctant to discuss the Internet search in supervision because she did not want to relinquish the emotional rewards of this new habit. In our own experience, supervisors range from those who have unabashedly recommended searching for patients on the Internet, at one extreme, to those who condemn the practice in any therapy relationship, at the other. This polarity of supervisory views highlights the lack of professional dialogue or guidelines about this phenomenon.

Discussion

In the three cases presented, we have proposed and applied a pragmatic model for considering the practice of searching online for patient information. This practice, which we call patient-targeted Googling, is now occurring on a regular basis and continues to grow as younger physicians enter the profession. Nevertheless, despite the obvious need for teaching and, more broadly, for further discussion and analysis, there continues to be no formal teaching about it. Our pragmatic approach to PTG is an effort to provide guidance to clinicians and trainees and to develop a model for professional ethics in this area. The goals of the pragmatic model are to respect the patient's best interests and to minimize the risk of exploiting patients. Within this model, important factors include the intention of the Internet search, the potential impact of the search on the treatment, and the clinician's motivations for the search, along with questions about informed consent, disclosure, and documentation.

Our pragmatic model avoids reliance on specific abstract moral principles and does not specify whether a psychiatrist should or should not engage in PTG in any particular situation. Instead, it draws two major conclusions: (1) the questions raised by PTG need to be handled on a case-by-case basis by paying careful attention to the patient's best interests and the practical results of Internet searches, and (2) clinicians must consider the issues surrounding PTG *before* engaging in the practice with respect to any particular patient. We hope that the pragmatic model will empower psychiatrists to think in a structured way about issues such as the balances between patient privacy and clinical necessity, and between exploitation or voyeurism and beneficence, *before* engaging in PTG. Our vignettes repeatedly point the psychiatrist to deliberate and to consult (e.g., with a supervisor, colleague, or ethicist) *before* engaging in PTG.

Many psychiatrists, psychiatry residents, and clinicians from other fields of medicine are actively involved in PTG. Younger clinicians, particularly residents graduating from college since the founding of social networking Web sites in the early 2000s, are accustomed both to looking up information on the Internet and to interacting with others on social networking sites. The need to develop formal training in this area is readily apparent, and we hope that our pragmatic model will help to move that process along.

We envision future work in this area to include formal surveys of psychiatrists (both trainees and senior clinicians) to investigate their use of the Internet in clinical practice. The goal would be to gain an empiric understanding of this phenomenon, the motivations behind its practice, and its perceived impact on patients. Aside from studies of boundary violations (not involving PTG), we have few data to indicate how patients might react to the suspicion or discovery that a provider has engaged in PTG. Further research could include prospective trials with patients—for example, in which participants engaged in specific Internet-based communications with clinicians, as through social networking sites, in order to examine the effects of PTG on psychotherapeutic relationships.

On a wider scale, the practice of PTG requires us to think carefully about patient privacy. Patients have long sought help from psychiatrists (and other physicians), with the hope and expectation of compassion, competence, and confidentiality. With the continuing growth of the Internet as a public domain for information, the concepts of privacy and confidentiality evolve. Patients may currently experience a *perceived* privacy because they assume that their psychiatrists would not search online for them (e.g., much as they would assume that their psychiatrists would not eavesdrop on their conversations in restaurants) and also because they tend to think of online information as impermanent.[28] This sense of perceived privacy may also be reinforced by patients' perception that their online information is functionally invisible because it is buried in a vast sea of online material. Any privacy of that kind has been compromised, however, by the ever-growing precision of Internet search engines such as Google and by the easy searchability of social networking sites such as MySpace and Facebook. And even the publication of articles such as this one—on the clinical use of the Internet—will ultimately alter patients' perceptions of online privacy in relation to psychiatry. On the other side of the equation, clinicians may be assuming that their Internet searches are anonymous, but there have been notable occasions on which search records have been unexpectedly released in the past.[29] An awareness of PTG and its potential consequences may thus prompt both clinicians and patients to use the Internet more carefully and, more generally, may lead to a more careful and cautious assessment of the role of the Internet in psychotherapeutic relationships, especially regarding the use of online searches as a means of gathering information about patients.

References

1. Styra, R. (2004). The Internet's impact on the practice of psychiatry. *Canadian Journal of Psychiatry, 49*, 5–11.

2. Tang, H., & Ng, J. H. (2006). Googling for a diagnosis—use of Google as a diagnostic aid: Internet based study. *BMJ (Clinical Research Ed.), 333,* 1143–1145.

3. Lowes, R. (2007). Can Google make you a better doctor? *Medical Economics, 84,* 24–25.

4. Sim, M. G., Khong, E., & Jiwa, M. (2008). Does general practice Google? *Australian Family Physician, 37,* 471–474.

5. Mathy, R. M., Kerr, D. L., & Haydin, B. M. (2003). Methodological rigor and ethical considerations in Internet-mediated research. *Psychotherapy (Chicago, Ill.), 40,* 77–85.

6. Pittenger, D. J. (2003). Internet research: An opportunity to revisit classic ethical problems in behavioral research. *Ethics and Behavior, 13,* 45–60.

7. Moreno, M. A., Fost, N. C., & Christakis, D. A. (2008). Research ethics in the MySpace era. *Pediatrics, 121,* 157–161.

8. Gorrindo, T., & Groves, J. E. (2008). Web searching for information about physicians. *Journal of the American Medical Association, 300,* 213–215.

9. Sinnott, J. T., & Joseph, J. P. (2008). Web searches about physicians. *Journal of the American Medical Association, 300,* 2249–2250.

10. Gorrindo, T., & Groves, J. E. (2008). Web searches about physicians—reply. *Journal of the American Medical Association, 300,* 2250.

11. Moreno, M. A., Parks, M., & Richardson, L. P. (2007). What are adolescents showing the world about their health risk behaviors on MySpace? *MedGenMed: Medscape General Medicine, 9,* 9.

12. Hinduja, S., & Patchin, J. W. (2008). Personal information of adolescents on the Internet: A quantitative content analysis of MySpace. *Journal of Adolescence, 31,* 125–146.

13. Williams, A. L., & Merten, M. J. (2008). A review of online social networking profiles by adolescents: Implications for future research and intervention. *Adolescence, 43,* 253–274.

14. Baume, P., Cantor, C. H., & Rolfe, A. (1997). Cybersuicide: The role of interactive suicide notes on the Internet. *Crisis, 18*, 73–79.

15. Lenhart, A. *Adults and social network websites.* 2009. At http://www.pewinternet.org/Reports/2009/Adults-and-Social-Network-Websites.aspx.

16. Gutheil, T. G., & Brodsky, A. (2008). *Preventing boundary violations in clinical practice.* New York: Guilford Press.

17. Thompson, L. A., Dawson, K., Ferdig, R., et al. (2008). The intersection of online social networking with medical professionalism. *Journal of General Internal Medicine, 23*, 954–957.

18. Gorrindo, T., Gorrindo, P. C., & Groves, J. E. (2008). Intersection of online social networking with medical professionalism: Can medicine police the Facebook boom? *Journal of General Internal Medicine, 23*, 2155; author reply 2156.

19. Guseh, J. S., Brendel, R. W., & Brendel, D. H. (2009). Medical professionalism in the age of online social networking. *Journal of Medical Ethics, 35*, 584–586.

20. Neimark, G., Hurford, M. O., & DiGiacomo, J. (2006). The Internet as collateral informant. *American Journal of Psychiatry, 163*, 1842.

21. Recupero, P. R. (2008). Forensic evaluation of problematic Internet use. *Journal of the American Academy of Psychiatry and the Law, 36*, 505–514.

22. Brendel, D. H., Chu, J., Radden, J., et al. (2007). The price of a gift: An approach to receiving gifts from patients in psychiatric practice. *Harvard Review of Psychiatry, 15*, 43–51.

23. Brendel, D. H. (2006). *Healing psychiatry: Bridging the science/humanism divide.* Cambridge, MA: MIT Press.

24. Fins, J. J., Miller, F. G., & Bacchetta, M. D. (1998). Clinical pragmatism: Bridging theory and practice. *Kennedy Institute of Ethics Journal, 8*, 37–42.

25. McGee, G. (Ed.). (2003). *Pragmatic bioethics* (2nd ed.). Cambridge, MA: MIT Press.

26. Tan, L. (2008). Psychotherapy 2.0: MySpace blogging as self-therapy. *American Journal of Psychotherapy, 62*, 143–163.

27. Gibbs, P. L. (2007). Reality in cyberspace: Analysands' use of the Internet and ordinary everyday psychosis. *Psychoanalytic Review, 94*, 11–38.

28. Huang, M. P., & Alessi, N. E. (1996). The Internet and the future of psychiatry. *American Journal of Psychiatry, 153*, 861–869.

29. Barbaro, M., & Zeller, T. (2006). A face is exposed for AOL searcher no. 4417749. *New York Times*, August 9.

25

Professional Boundaries in the Era of the Internet

Glen O. Gabbard, Kristin A. Kassaw, and Gonzalo Perez-Garcia

In a previous communication (1), we identified the emerging clinical and ethical problems in the era of electronic communication. We now turn to the novel ethical and clinical dilemmas involved in defining professional boundaries in light of the expanded dimensions of the Internet. Over the past decade, the capacity to search for information quickly and accurately has grown through search engines such as Google, Yahoo, and Bing. Also, individuals have greater ability to share personal information through blogs and social networking sites such as Facebook and MySpace. The availability of personal and professional details to be had with a click or two redefines anonymity and privacy for everyone, but our interest in this communication is how it affects psychiatrists and other mental health professionals. At present, there are no firm guidelines for psychiatrists regarding how to manage information on the Internet. Also, many psychiatrists are unaware of the measures that may be taken to protect their privacy. In the following, we describe the clinical and ethical issues, educate readers about preventive strategies, and outline some potential recommendations.

Literature Review

Four years passed between the launch of the social networking site Facebook in February 2004 (2) and its first mention in the medical literature in February 2008 (3), when researchers studied the dangers of social networking sites for sexual solicitation of underage youth. In another 2008 study, at the University of Florida (4), researchers found that 64.3 percent of medical students and 12.8 percent of residents had Facebook accounts. A random subset of ten profiles found seven with photographs involving alcohol and three with unprofessional content such as drunkenness, overt sexuality, foul language, and patient-privacy violations. In a recent article (5), medical school deans were surveyed on professionalism issues involving medical student use of the Internet. Of the seventy-eight deans surveyed, 60 percent reported incidents of students posting unprofessional content online, and 13 percent reported students violating patient confidentiality online within the previous year. Deans also gave examples of medical students who requested inappropriate friendships with patients on Facebook, posted online content suggesting intoxication or illicit substance use, and used disparaging language about a course, professor, or classmate online. Only 19 percent reported having a committee or task force responsible for addressing student-posted online content. In another recent article (6), a medical intern discussed his conflict in allowing a former patient to add him as a friend on Facebook, as well as his relief when he found that the main reason for the patient's reaching out was to seek advice on applying to medical school.

In addition to social networking sites, blogs are popular in the health care community. In 2008, researchers examined 271 blogs with health content written by a doctor or nurse (7). Over half had identifiable authors, and 22 percent displayed a photo of the author. Of all the blogs studied, 18 percent described patients in a negative light, including insulting comments, and 30 percent featured negative comments about the health professions. Another study (8) found 331 English-language medical blogs that had updated content during the previous month. Bloggers with available contact information were surveyed, and 80 responded. The majority had been blogging for over two years, and 75 percent wrote under their real names. They were also active writers outside the Internet, with 54 percent having published a scientific paper, 44 percent having published a book or book chapter, and 41 percent having published a newspaper article.

In this communication, we will confine our discussion to professional boundaries as they apply in a mental health setting, because these boundaries are generally more stringent than in other medical settings. We will also attempt to delineate which issues are more properly classified as clinical or professionalism dilemmas.

Social Networking Sites, Blogs, and Search Engines

Social networking sites, such as Facebook and MySpace, have been widely adopted as a means of communication. In early 2009, Facebook had over 150 million users, with those over the age of thirty representing the fastest- growing demographic (9). Because of its wide popularity, we will use Facebook to illustrate concerns about social networking sites in general.

A number of aspects of Facebook may compromise the privacy of patients as well as the privacy of psychiatrists. First, a patient may send a "friend request" to a psychiatrist. A friend request, if accepted, allows each party full access to the other's Facebook profiles, including updates, photos, interest groups, and other content. Most users see Facebook as a forum for self-expression through posts, affiliations, and photos. These items are, of course, more personally revealing than what is generally disclosed in a treatment relationship. Also, Facebook users may post photos and tag or label another Facebook user by name without the knowledge or consent of the individual in the picture. Facebook users may discover that they are tagged in a professionally unbecoming photograph long after numerous others have seen it.

Another concern with Facebook is the potential for breaching patient privacy in a nonclinical setting. A status post about a challenging patient may contain enough recognizable information to compromise confidentiality. Although disguised information about a patient is often used in case reports, the intent there is educational. Posting information about patients as a status update is generally self-serving in its intent. It is possible to use privacy settings to control who has access to a Facebook page. However, as many as 80 percent of Facebook users do not actively manage their privacy settings, meaning that the content of their profile is available to any users of Facebook, whether they are an accepted friend or not (10). In the Florida study noted earlier (4), only 37.5 percent of medical students and residents used their privacy settings. Anyone, including patients, colleagues, and program directors, for example, may access a profile. Currently, there are no means to know who has access to and who has viewed a profile. Finally, even with most privacy settings activated, many individuals leave their profile picture accessible for searches. One ill-chosen photograph can have unforeseen consequences. Moreover, Facebook users commonly list their sexual orientation, marital status, religion, age, hometown, and political affiliation in their profiles, most of which is information not typically shared with patients.

Related to social networking sites are online dating sites (match.com, eHarmony, jdate, and others). A user creates a profile, usually with a photograph, to attract potential romantic partners. Unlike social networking sites, where real names must be used, an online dating site user may create a name. A user's profile, complete with photo and personal information, will appear along with others meeting the same search criteria. Users may be contacted through the site, but direct contact information such as an e-mail address or phone number is not revealed. Users may choose to ignore or respond to messages sent through the site. A patient who uses online dating sites may recognize a psychiatrist using the service and may learn significant amounts of sensitive information that the psychiatrist has unintentionally revealed.

Blogs

Although one can never be absolutely certain who has viewed a social networking or online dating profile, this problem is more pervasive in blogs. The term *weblog* was coined in 1997 by Jorn Barger, editor of the Web site Robot Wisdom, and this word was eventually shorted to *blog* (11). Key differences between social networking and blogging make blogging more problematic for psychiatrists. The first is accessibility. Although limiting a Facebook profile so that it is only seen by those whom one knows and trusts is relatively common and simple, such limiting happens less often and can be more complex in a blog, because bloggers tend to enjoy sharing ideas and Web links with others. In a 2008 survey of medical bloggers (8), 99 percent noted that they received attention from their blog from other bloggers. Also, 74 percent noted that their motivation for blogging was "to share practical knowledge and skills," and 56 percent professed a desire "to influence the way other people think."

Furthermore, whereas a Facebook user is more likely to journal quick thoughts or statements on a profile, a blogger is more prone to write many paragraphs, or even many different entries over time, focusing on a single topic. This output creates more opportunities for a psychiatrist-blogger to post potentially problematic entries, such as breaking patient confidentiality or writing about unprofessional activities in which he or she might engage.

A blog also leaves a more permanent footprint on the Internet. Currently, there is no way to quickly search through someone's Facebook profile to see what he or she has written in the past. Readers have to scroll to the bottom of a profile and click on "older posts" ad nauseum until they find something written some time ago. The more active the user is, the more times one needs to click on "older posts." By contrast, most blogs are searchable by date or keywords so that a blog entry written a year ago can be quickly accessed. Furthermore, another Web site can post a link back to a psychiatrist's blog or easily copy and paste a psychiatrist's blog entry, referencing the psychiatrist as the original author. In a situation such as this, even if the psychiatrist later decides to delete a blog entry, he or she cannot control what another blogger has posted on a different Web site. One must particularly be aware that the antipsychiatry movement is also active in the blogosphere.

Search Engines

Much of the redefinition of privacy has been with the full cooperation of the people who choose to blog or to post on social networking sites. The ubiquity of search engines has created a related but different problem in the realm of privacy. Even those who do not wish to indulge in self-disclosures on a social networking site or blog find that all kinds of details about their private lives are available to those who wish to search for it.

Psychoanalysts and psychotherapists have long emphasized the asymmetry of disclosure in the doctor-patient relationship and operated with the assumption that little knowledge of their personal lives would be shared with the patient. However, prospective patients now routinely "Google" psychiatrists before agreeing to see them, and patients can find out a great deal of information about a psychiatrist's family through search engines. As part of their research or due diligence in deciding whether to see a particular psychiatrist, patients can also access various sites that rate doctors. On these sites are many statements by disgruntled patients. Some of these comments, of course, accurately portray deficiencies in the psychiatrist, but other statements may reflect rage at not being prescribed a controlled substance or negative transferences that really say very little about the psychiatrist's actual competence.

There was a time when clinicians would go to meetings or other out-of-town events without informing their patients of their destination; rather, they would simply say that they would be away for a week, without going into detail. Search engines have also radically changed this form of anonymity. Patients can now find out details about where their psychotherapists may be speaking or staying and what they might be doing.

There is an extraordinary availability of public documents through search engines. What a psychiatrist paid for his or her home can be learned by accessing property tax documents. If an unmarried therapist is living with someone, this information is also accessible. The extent of political contributions that a therapist made can be discovered in seconds. Patients who wish to trace the genealogy of their therapist can find out a great deal about family histories. The psychiatrist practicing psycho-therapy today is likely to feel violated, invaded, and exposed. If a psy-chotherapist brings up the patient's intrusiveness as a therapeutic issue, however, the patient may well respond, "This is public information avail-able to anyone. I am not invading your privacy." This retort may stymie the therapist and lead to a variation of a therapeutic impasse in the treatment.

The differences between search engines and social networking or blog-ging are significant. The doctor has no choice regarding participation. Also, search engines are really without bounds as compared with the limits of blogging or social networking sites. Everything about a clinician is fair game. One of the major difficulties with search engines is that there may be misinformation on such things as Web sites that rate doctors, the doctor's private life, or data about family members. Many people may have the same name, and patients or prospective patients can read highly negative (or positive) information about someone they presume to be their psychiatrist when in fact they are reading about somebody else.

Search engines have truly altered the conceptual framework of privacy, anonymity, and self-disclosure in the clinical setting. Psychiatrists can no longer assume that they are a "blank screen" to patients, but must now assume that patients know a good deal about them and must rethink the stance that their private life is beyond reach of the patient.

Implications

The professional-boundary questions that have risen in the expanded world of cyberspace generally fall into three areas: ethical concerns, professionalism issues, and clinical dilemmas. Only the first category involves true boundary problems as they are generally defined.

Ethical Concerns

Beauchamp (12) has outlined four clusters of moral principles that are the underpinnings of biomedical ethics codes: respect for autonomy (an acknowledgment that patients are free to make decisions), nonmalefi-cence (the fundamental principle of avoiding the potential for harm), beneficence (a consideration of the equation of weighing benefits versus risks), and justice (fairness in how burdens and benefits are distributed). Some of the situations described in the previous section are clearly viola-tions of ethics. For example, breaches of confidentiality by writing about patients on a blog or social networking system have the potential to harm patients or patients' families. Even if a name is not mentioned but identifying features have been provided, some readers may be able to detect the identity of the patient. Although several guidelines suggest ways to protect patient confidentiality in writing scientific papers (13), the off-the-cuff venting that occurs on blogs and social network sites generally does not take these factors into account because the content is not designed for publication in a journal.

Another concern involves dual relationships. If a patient is a Facebook friend of a doctor, or vice versa, an expectation follows from that designation that may compromise the boundaries of the doctor-patient relationship. Such relationships may also jeopardize the ethics principle of nonmaleficence in that the capacity to make good use of a psychiatrist in the patient role may be more difficult if one is also a friend. Inherent in the caution against dual relationships is the idea that psychiatrists optimize the treatment setting by making it clear to the patient that the psychiatrist will never be anything other than a treater, even after termination. Patients then know that there are no consequences in any outside relationship if they reveal something shameful or painful to their psychiatrist (14). One can find definitions of a "Facebook friend" online that restrict it to relationships that only occur in cyberspace at the present time, even if they started with a real-life connection. However, this difference breaks down when the "friend" is a patient, because there are therapeutic contacts that do not take place in cyberspace. Moreover, patients may have no idea about this definition and take it to mean that they are friends with their psychiatrist in the literal sense of the word.

Another ethical principle, respect for autonomy, may come to the fore in situations where patients "Google" their psychiatrists. Psychiatrists who are accustomed to traditional anonymity and privacy and feel violated may issue an edict that patients should not intrude into the psychiatrist's private life and must avoid accessing information available on the Internet. The ethical principle of respect for autonomy makes it clear that psychiatrists should not place constraints on patients' freedom to pursue public information. The term *boundary violation* is not applicable to the patient who investigates the doctor online through public information. Patients have no ethics code and therefore are not violating professional boundaries when they seek out information about their doctor. Clearly, this ethical principle is at times overridden by concerns about danger to self or others. However, operating a search engine does not fall into that category. Psychiatrists who feel that their personal space is being intruded by the patient must deal with this matter as a counter-transference issue for supervision, consultation, or personal treatment while exploring with patients the meanings of their curiosity. In other words, psychiatrists must resolve their reaction within themselves. They cannot block certain aspects of their lives from their patients, and they must learn to adapt to the new world that cyberspace has created.

Professionalism Issues

Some of the phenomena associated with blogs and social networking sites fall into the area of professionalism. Both medical educators and psychiatric educators have vastly increased their emphasis on professionalism as part of training to the point where it is now considered one of the core competencies in training physicians and psychiatrists (15). Physician-educators have variously defined professionalism. One useful definition is from the American Board of Internal Medicine (16), which suggests that professionalism "requires the physician to serve the interests of the patient above his or her self-interest. Professionalism aspires to altruism, accountability, excellence, duty, honor, integrity, and respect for others." Some prefer to think of professionalism as simply a matter of how one behaves with patients, colleagues, and others in public places when no one is watching. With the expansion of the Internet, all physicians and physicians-in-training must remember that they are viewed by others as in that professional role to some extent whenever they are in public, even if they are not at work. The emphasis on professionalism education now raises the standards for the behavior of graduate psychiatrists and educators who are role models for trainees, whether residents or medical students. Photos of a psychiatrist or psychiatric resident that suggest intoxication or illicit substance use, for example, may appear on social networking sites or blogs. Although the activity may have occurred off duty, the effect on those who see such photos may be devastating nevertheless. Similarly, making negative comments about colleagues on a blog or a social networking site becomes equivalent to publicly denouncing a colleague. Even if one is talking about patients generically, one can appear unprofessional if a comment disparages patients. Although no ethics code is being violated in such instances, standards of professionalism certainly are.

Clinical Dilemmas

Answering the standard questions from Facebook's initial page can reveal a good deal of information about a doctor, as can providing the information required by online dating sites. These are bits of personal data that one does not generally convey to patients in treatment, but patients may come across this information online. Even though it is not a matter of ethics or a boundary violation to make this demographic information available, doing so can certainly create a clinical dilemma for the treating clinician to explore. Patients may have reactions that are useful to examine in the psychotherapeutic context. Excessive self-disclosure is generally regarded as a potential boundary violation in the treatment relationship (14,17), but disclosure of this information on a social networking site is not intended to be in a treatment context. Hence, psychiatrists cannot be held accountable for unethical behavior by virtue of listing this information on a site that has privacy detection built in. Even if the psychiatrist has failed to use the privacy option, the information is not conveyed within the doctor-patient relationship.

Another phenomenon that commonly occurs is often referred to as "extratherapeutic contacts." A psychiatrist may bump into a patient at a restaurant or concert and must navigate this rather awkward situation with respect for the patient's privacy. This situation is not an ethical matter (unless a confidentiality breach occurs) because it was not planned but, rather, accidental. Planning a meeting with the patient outside the office, such as for lunch or a walk in the park, does violate the usual boundaries of the doctor-patient relationship and is cause for concern. In an analogous manner, extratherapeutic contacts that are inadvertent, such as on an online dating service or social networking site, are difficult but not unethical. Because of the complicated nature of those contacts, psychiatrists may wish to use a consultant who has clinical experience to help them negotiate the optimal management of such situations. When a patient encounters erroneous information about a doctor, either because someone else has the same name as the psychiatrist or simply because of errors in reporting the facts, this too is a dilemma for the doctor to work out clinically. If a distortion of the physician's prescribing practices appears on a Web site that rates doctors, the physician can explore the patient's reaction and clarify what the actual prescribing practices are.

One other situation that arises in discussions of the new world of boundaries involves whether it is ethical for a psychiatrist to look up a patient on the Internet. Some (18) have suggested that seeking this information might violate doctor-patient boundaries. However, just as the information about the doctor is public, so is information on the Internet about patients. It is customary when evaluating patients to often get collateral sources of data from other individuals who know the patient,

Table 25.1
Recommended guidelines for maintaining professional boundaries online

---

1. Psychiatrists and other mental health professionals who use social networking sites should activate all available privacy settings (5,19,20).

2. Web searches should be conducted periodically to monitor false information or photographs of concern (20). If these items are discovered, the Web site administrator can be contacted to remove problematic information.

3. The following items should not be included in blogs or networking sites: (a) Patient information and other confidential material. (b) Disparaging comments about colleagues or groups of patients. (c) Any comment on lawsuits, clinical cases, or administrative actions in which one is involved, because they can potentially compromise one's defense (22). (d) Photographs that may be perceived as unprofessional (e.g., sexually suggestive poses or drinking or drug use).

4. Although looking up information about a patient on the Internet is not unethical because it is public, psychiatrists who choose to do so must be prepared for clinical complications that require careful and thoughtful management. Some patients may experience the psychiatrist's interest in this information as a boundary violation or a compromise of trust (23).

5. One should avoid becoming "Facebook friends" or entering into other dual relationships on the Internet with patients (19,21). One strategy is to have separate profiles for separate roles, that is, personal versus professional (R. Hsiung, personal communication, December 14, 2009).

6. One must not assume that anything posted anonymously on the Internet will remain anonymous, because posts can be traced to their sources (22). Psychiatrists or psychiatric residents who wish to post their availability on online dating sites are free to do so but must be fully prepared for the possibility that patients will see them and have intense reactions.

7. Training institutions should educate their trainees about professionalism and boundary issues as part of their professionalism curriculum and assist them in their mastery of technology.

8. All training institutions should develop policies for handling breaches of ethics or professionalism through Internet activity.

9. Psychotherapy training should include consideration of the clinical dilemmas presented by social networking sites, blogging, and search engines, as well as potential boundary issues.

---

usually with the permission of the patient. The treating psychiatrist may want to ask permission of the patient but can certainly access public information without a release if it is thought to be essential or helpful for the treatment.

Recommendations

Useful recommendations for physicians and medical students are now appearing in the literature (5,19,20). Recently, there has been an online movement to establish a code of ethics among healthcare bloggers. The Healthcare Blogger Code of Ethics (21) focuses on five qualities to which medical bloggers should adhere: clearly representing their perspective, respecting confidentiality, announcing commercial disclosures, providing reliable information, and being courteous to others. Medical bloggers can submit their blogs for approval and, after a review process, be accepted as a blog that adheres to this ethical code.

Although this approach bears promise, psychiatry has a special set of requirements for professional boundaries. As yet, no detailed and systematic recommendations for psychiatrists and psychiatric residents have appeared. In table 25.1, we outline some preliminary recommendations with the hope that they will lead to further discussion and debate and, ultimately, policy statements for the profession. Free speech and freedom to associate with whomever one wishes are protected by the Constitution, but ethics codes have always been more restrictive than constitutional regulation. The recommendations we propose are in keeping with the wish to prevent harm or the potential for harm in treatment and interprofessional relationships. These principles should become a component of psychiatric resident education and be operationalized with other training policies. They can be equally useful to psychiatrists in practice in both institutional and noninstitutional settings.

References

1. Kassaw, K., & Gabbard, G. O. (2002). The ethics of e-mail communication in psychiatry. *Psychiatric Clinics of North America, 25*, 665–674.

2. Facebook: Facebook Factsheet. Available at http://www.facebook.com/press/info.php?factsheet.

3. Ybarra, M. L., & Mitchell, K. J. (2008). How risky are social networking sites? A comparison of places online where youth solicitation and harassment occurs. *Pediatrics, 121*(2), e350–e357.

4. Thompson, L. A., Dawson, K., Ferdig, R., et al. (2008). The intersection of online social networking with medical professionalism. *Journal of General Internal Medicine, 23*, 954–957.

5. Chretien, K. C., Greysen, S. R., Chretien, J. P., et al. (2009). Online posting of unprofessional content by medical students. *Journal of the American Medical Association, 302*, 1309–1315.

6. Jain, S. H. (2009). Practicing medicine in the age of Facebook. *New England Journal of Medicine, 361*, 649–651.

7. Lagu, T., Kaufman, E. J., Asch, D. A., et al. (2008). Content of weblogs written by health professionals. *Journal of General Internal Medicine, 23*, 1642–1646.

8. Kovic, I., Lulic, I., & Brumini, G. (2008). Examining the medical blogosphere: An online survey of medical bloggers. *Journal of Medical Internet Research, 10*(3), e28.

9. Grossman, L. (2009). Why Facebook is for old fogies. *Time Magazine, 173*, 94.

10. Stone, B. (2009). Is Facebook growing up too fast? Sunday Business, *New York Times,* March 29, 1.

11. McCullagh, D., & Broache, A. (2007). Blogs turn 10—who's the father? *CNET News.* March 20. Available at http://news.cnet.com/2100-1025_3 -6168681.html.

12. Beauchamp, T. L. (2009). The philosophical basis of psychiatric ethics. In S. Bloch & S. A. Green (Eds.), *Psychiatric Ethics* (pp. 25–48). New York: Oxford University Press.

13. Gabbard, G. O. (2000). Disguise or consent: Problems and recommendations concerning the publication and presentation of clinical material. *International Journal of Psycho-Analysis, 81*(Pt. 6), 1071–1086.

14. Gutheil, T. G., & Gabbard, G. O. (1993). The concept of boundaries in clinical practice: Theoretical and risk-management dimensions. *American Journal of Psychiatry, 150*, 188–196.

15. Gabbard G. O. (In press). *Professionalism in Psychiatry.* Arlington, VA: American Psychiatric Publishing.

16. American Board of Internal Medicine (ABIM) Foundation. (2002). American Board of Internal Medicine ACP-ASIM, Foundation American College of Physicians—American Society of Internal Medicine, European Federation of Internal Medicine: Medical Professionalism in the New Millennium: the Physician Charter. *Annals of Internal Medicine, 136*, 243–246.

17. Gutheil, T. G., & Gabbard, G. O. (1998). Misuses and misunderstandings of boundary theory in clinical and regulatory settings. *American Journal of Psychiatry, 155*, 409–414.

18. Huremovic, D., & Rao, N. (2009). Beyond doctor-patient relationship in cyberspace: Pitfalls, transgressions and guidelines (when therapists and patients Google each other). Paper presented at the APA Annual Meeting, San Francisco.

19. Guseh, J. S., II, Brendel, R. W., & Brendel, D. H. (2009). Medical professionalism in the age of online social networking. *Journal of Medical Ethics, 35*, 584–586.

20. Gorrindo, T., & Groves, J. E. (2008). Web searching for information about physicians. *Journal of the American Medical Association, 300,* 213–215.

21. Healthcare Blogger Code of Ethics. *The Code.* Available at http://medblogger code.com/the-code/.

22. PRMS. (2009). Risk management tips for physician bloggers. *Psychiatric News, 44*(18), 31.

23. White, H. (2009). Locating clinical boundaries in the World Wide Web. *American Journal of Psychiatry, 166,* 620–621.

Contributors

Paul S. Appelbaum, MD   Elizabeth K. Dollard Professor of Psychiatry, Medicine and Law; director, Division of Law, Ethics, and Psychiatry, Department of Psychiatry, Columbia University, New York, New York

James A. Beshai, PhD   Psychologist, Veterans Administration Medical Center, Lebanon, Pennsylvania

Michelle Black, MSc, LLB   Associate, Stewart McKelvey, Halifax, Nova Scotia, Canada

J. Alexander Bodkin, MD   Chair, McLean Hospital Ethics Committee; associate psychiatrist, McLean Hospital, Belmont, Massachusetts; assistant professor, Department of Psychiatry, Harvard Medical School, Boston, Massachusetts

David H. Brendel, MD, PhD   Medical director of psychiatric services, Walden Behavioral Care, Waltham, Massachusetts; private practice, Belmont, Massachusetts

Kim Bullock, MD   Clinical associate professor, Behavior Medicine Clinic, Stanford University School of Medicine, Stanford, California

Rebecca Campbell, PhD   Professor of community psychology and program evaluation, Department of Psychology, Michigan State University, East Lansing

Arthur L. Caplan, PhD   Director, Division of Medical Ethics, Department of Population Health, New York University Langone Medical Center, New York, New York

James A. Chu, MD   Consultant in psychiatry, McLean Hospital, Belmont, Massachusetts; associate clinical professor of psychiatry, Harvard Medical School, Boston, Massachusetts

Brian K. Clinton, MD, PhD   Assistant clinical professor of psychiatry, Columbia University Medical Center, New York, New York

William J. Curran, JD, LLM, SMHyg   Taught law at the University of Santa Clara and the University of North Carolina and was professor of legal medicine at the Harvard Schools of Medicine and Public Health. He died in 1996.

Jocelyn Downie, MA, MLitt, LLB, LLM, SJD   Canada Research Chair in Health Law and Policy, professor in the faculties of law and medicine, Dalhousie University, Halifax, Nova Scotia, Canada

Glen O. Gabbard, MD   Professor of psychiatry, State University of New York, Upstate Medical University, Syracuse, New York; clinical professor of psychiatry,

Baylor College of Medicine, Houston, Texas; training and supervising analyst, Center for Psychoanalytic Studies in Houston, Texas; private practice, The Gabbard Center, Houston, Texas

Margery Gans, EdD   Psychologist, Arlington, Massachusetts

William B. Gunn Jr., PhD   Assistant professor of community and family medicine, Department of Community and Family Medicine, Dartmouth Medical School, Hanover, New Hampshire

Toksoz B. Karasu, MD   Professor and Dorothy and Marty Silverman Chair in Psychiatry, Department of Psychiatry and Behavioral Sciences, Albert Einstein College of Medicine, New York, New York

Kristin A. Kassaw, MD   Associate professor and associate director, Baylor Psychiatric Clinic, and director of undergraduate medical education, Baylor College of Medicine, Houston, Texas

Arnold A. Lazarus, PhD, ABPP   Distinguished Professor Emeritus, Rutgers University; president, The Lazarus Institute, Skillman, New Jersey

Howard Leeper, MEd   Served as a member of the Ethics Committee, McLean Hospital, Belmont, Massachusetts

Ralph B. Little, MD   Served at the Institute of the Pennsylvania Hospital, Philadelphia, Pennsylvania

Jonathan M. Lukens, PhD   Assistant professor of social work, Salem State University, Salem, Massachusetts

A. Thomas McLellan, PhD   Chief executive officer, Treatment Research Institute, Philadelphia, Pennsylvania

Charles P. O'Brien, MD, PhD   Kenneth Appel Professor, Department of Psychiatry, University of Pennsylvania, Philadelphia

Gonzalo Perez-Garcia, MD   Clinical assistant professor, Department of Psychiatry, University of Texas Southwestern Medical Center, Dallas, Texas

Harrison G. Pope Jr., MD   Professor of Psychiatry, Harvard Medical School, Boston, Massachusetts; director, Biological Psychiatry Laboratory, McLean Hospital, Belmont, Massachusetts

Claire L. Pouncey, MD, PhD   Psychiatrist in private practice, Philadelphia, Pennsylvania

Jennifer Radden, PhD   Professor of philosophy emerita, University of Massachusetts Boston; consultant on medical ethics, McLean Hospital, Belmont, Massachusetts

Frederic Reamer, PhD   Professor, Graduate Program of the School of Social Work, Rhode Island College, Providence

Craig Reinarman, PhD   Professor of sociology and legal studies, University of California, Santa Cruz

John A. Rich, MD, MPH   Professor and chair of health management and policy, Drexel University School of Public Health, Philadelphia, Pennsylvania

Hila Rimon-Greenspan, MA   Served as research coordinator for the Scattergood Program for Applied Ethics of Behavioral Healthcare at the University of Pennsylvania, Philadelphia. She is currently a researcher at Bizchut, the Israeli Human Rights Center for People with Disabilities.

Laura Weiss Roberts, MD, MA   Chairman and Katharine Dexter McCormick and Stanley McCormick Memorial Professor, Department of Psychiatry and Behavioral Sciences, Stanford University School of Medicine, Stanford, California

Charles E. Rosenberg, PhD   Professor of the history of science and Ernest E. Monrad Professor in the Social Sciences, Department of the History of Science, Harvard University, Cambridge, Massachusetts

John Z. Sadler, MD   Daniel W. Foster MD Professor of Medical Ethics, professor of psychiatry and clinical sciences, Distinguished Teaching Professor, Department of Psychiatry, University of Texas Southwestern Medical Center, Dallas, Texas

Jacqueline Samson, PhD   Assistant professor of psychology, Department of Psychiatry, McLean Hospital, Belmont, Massachusetts

Benjamin C. Silverman, MD   Psychiatrist-in-charge, McLean Center at Fernside, Princeton, Massachusetts; instructor in psychiatry, Harvard Medical School, Boston, Massachusetts

Dominic A. Sisti, PhD   Assistant professor, Department of Medical Ethics and Health Policy; director, The Scattergood Program for Applied Ethics of Behavioral Healthcare, Perelman School of Medicine, University of Pennsylvania, Philadelphia

David A. Stone, PhD   Associate vice president for research and associate professor, Public Health, Northern Illinois University, DeKalb, Illinois

Edward A. Strecker, MD   Served as chief medical officer of the Institute of Pennsylvania Hospital, professor and head of nervous and mental diseases at Jefferson Medical College, and professor and head of the Department of Psychiatry at the University of Pennsylvania. He was president of the American Psychiatric Association in 1943.

Thomas S. Szasz, MD   Professor of psychiatry emeritus, State University of New York Health Science Center, Syracuse, New York; adjunct scholar, Cato Institute, Washington, D.C.; author and lecturer. He died in 2012.

George Szmukler, MD, FRCPsych, FKC   Professor of psychiatry and society, Institute of Psychiatry, King's College, London, United Kingdom

Gail Tsimprea, PhD   Associate in psychiatry, Harvard Medical School; chief quality and risk management officer, McLean Hospital, Belmont, Massachusetts

Richard J. Tushup, PhD   Adjunct instructor of psychology, Lebanon Valley College, Annville, Pennsylvania; staff psychologist, VA Medical Center, Lebanon, Pennsylvania

Robert Henley Woody, PhD, ScD, JD   Professor of psychology, University of Nebraska at Omaha

Permissions and Credits

"'Personality Disorder' and Capacity to Make Treatment Decisions" was reproduced from the *Journal of Medical Ethics*, Szmukler G., Vol. 35, pgs. 647–650, Copyright 2009, with permission from BMJ Publishing Group Ltd.

"Sanctity of Human Life in War: Ethics and Post-traumatic Stress Disorder" was reproduced with permission of authors and publisher from: Beshai, J., & Tuhup, R. J. *Psychological Reports*, 2006, 98, 217–225. © Psychological Reports 2006.

"The Experience of Violent Injury for Young African American Men: The Meaning of Being a 'Sucker'" was republished with kind permission from Springer Science+Business Media: *Journal of General Internal Medicine*, 11, 1996, 77–82, Rich, J. A., Stone, D. A.

"The Psychological Impact of Rape Victims' Experiences with the Legal, Medical, and Mental Health Systems." Copyright © 2008 by the American Psychological Association. Reproduced with permission. The official citation that should be used in referencing this material is: Campbell R. The psychological impact of rape victims. *Am Psychol*. 2008 Nov; 63(8):702–17. The use of this information does not imply endorsement by the publisher.

"Addiction as Accomplishment: The Discursive Construction of Disease." Reinarman, C., *Addiction Research & Theory*, 2005; 13(4):307–320, copyright ©2005, Informa Healthcare. Reproduced with permission of Informa Healthcare.

"The Ethics of Addiction" was reprinted from Szasz T. S., *American Journal of Psychiatry*, Nov 1971; 128 (5); 541–546. Reprinted with permission from the *American Journal of Psychiatry* (Copyright ©1971). American Psychiatric Association.

"Myths about the Treatment of Addiction" was reprinted from *The Lancet*, Vol. 347, No. 8996, O'Brien, C. P., & McLellan, A. T., pgs. 237–240, Copyright (1996), with permission from Elsevier.

"Ethical Considerations in Caring for People Living with Addictions," Roberts L. W., & Bullock K., *FOCUS* 2011;9: 66–69. Reprinted with permission from *Focus* (Copyright ©2011). American Psychiatric Association.

"Confidentiality and the Prediction of Dangerousness in Psychiatry" was republished from the *New England Journal of Medicine*, Vol. 293, pgs. 285–286, William J. Curran, 1975, with permission from the *New England Journal of Medicine*. Copyright (1975), Massachusetts Medical Society.

"Madness versus Badness: The Ethical Tension between the Recovery Movement and Forensic Psychiatry" is reprinted with kind permission from Springer Science+Business Media: *Theoretical Medicine and Bioethics*, Vol. 31, 2010, pgs. 93–105, Pouncey, C. L., & Lukens, J. M.

"Ethical Considerations of Multiple Roles in Forensic Services" was reprinted by permission of the publisher (Taylor & Francis Ltd, http://www.tandf.co.uk/journals). Woody, R. H. (January 1, 2009). *Ethics and Behavior, 19,* 1, 79–87.

"Watch Your Language: A Review of the Use of Stigmatizing Language by Canadian Judges" originally appeared in Black, M., and Downie, J., 2010, *Journal of Ethics in Mental Health* 5(1):1–8. Reprinted with permission from the authors and from the *Journal of Ethics in Mental Health*.

"Boundary Violation Ethics: Some Conceptual Clarifications" was reprinted with permission from the American Academy of Psychiatry and the Law from Radden, J. (January 1, 2001). *The Journal of the American Academy of Psychiatry and the Law, 29,* 3, 319–26.

"The Price of a Gift: An Approach to Receiving Gifts from Patients in Psychiatric Practice" originally appeared in Brendel, D. H., Chu, J., Radden, J., Leeper, H., Pope, H. G., Samson, J., Tsimprea, G., Bodkin, J. A., *Harvard Review of Psychiatry,* 2007; 15 (2): 43–51, copyright © 2007, Informa Healthcare. Reproduced with permission of Informa Healthcare.

"How Certain Boundaries and Ethics Diminish Therapeutic Effectiveness" first appeared in Lazarus, A. A, 1994, *Ethics & Behavior* 4(3):255–261. Reprinted by permission of the publisher (Taylor & Francis Group, http://www.informaworld.com).

"Boundary Issues in Social Work: Managing Dual Relationships" was republished with permission of The National Association of Social Workers, from *Social Work,* Reamer, F. G., Vol. 48, No. 1, 2003; permission conveyed through Copyright Clearance Center, Inc.

"Patient-Targeted Googling: The Ethics of Searching Online for Patient Information" originally appeared in Clinton, B. K., Silverman, B. C., & Brendel, D.H., *Harvard Review of Psychiatry,* 2010; 18(2):103–112, copyright ©2010, Informa Healthcare. Reproduced with permission of Informa Healthcare.

"Professional Boundaries in the Era of the Internet" is from Gabbard, G. O., Kassaw, K. A., & Perez-Garcia, G. (May 1, 2011). *Academic Psychiatry, 35,* 3, 168–174. Reprinted with permission from *Academic Psychiatry* (Copyright ©2011). American Psychiatric Association.

Index

Basic Bioethics

Arthur Caplan, editor

Books Acquired under the Editorship of Glenn McGee and Arthur Caplan

Karen F. Greif and Jon F. Merz, *Current Controversies in the Biological Sciences: Case Studies of Policy Challenges from New Technologies*

Deborah Blizzard, *Looking Within: A Sociocultural Examination of Fetoscopy*

Ronald Cole-Turner, ed., *Design and Destiny: Jewish and Christian Perspectives on Human Germline Modification*

Holly Fernandez Lynch, *Conflicts of Conscience in Health Care: An Institutional Compromise*

Mark A. Bedau and Emily C. Parke, eds., *The Ethics of Protocells: Moral and Social Implications of Creating Life in the Laboratory*

Jonathan D. Moreno and Sam Berger, eds., *Progress in Bioethics: Science, Policy, and Politics*

Eric Racine, *Pragmatic Neuroethics: Improving Understanding and Treatment of the Mind-Brain*

Martha J. Farah, ed., *Neuroethics: An Introduction with Readings*

Jeremy R. Garrett, ed., *The Ethics of Animal Research: Exploring the Controversy*

Books Acquired under the Editorship of Arthur Caplan

Sheila Jasanoff, ed., *Reframing Rights: Bioconstitutionalism in the Genetic Age*

Christine Overall, *Why Have Children? The Ethical Debate*

Yechiel Michael Barilan, *Human Dignity, Human Rights, and Responsibility: The New Language of Global Bioethics and Bio-Law*

Tom Koch, *Thieves of Virtue: When Bioethics Stole Medicine*

Timothy F. Murphy, *Ethics, Sexual Orientation, and Choices about Children*

Daniel Callahan, *In Search of the Good: A Life in Bioethics*

Robert Blank, *Intervention in the Brain: Politics, Policy, and Ethics*

Gregory E. Kaebnick and Thomas H. Murray, eds., *Synthetic Biology and Morality: Artificial Life and the Bounds of Nature*

Dominic A. Sisti, Arthur L. Caplan, and Hila Rimon-Greenspan, eds., *Applied Ethics in Mental Health Care: An Interdisciplinary Reader*